Medical and Public Health Building (later MacNider Hall). The only building on the medical campus when Dr. W. Reece Berryhill became Dean of the UNC School of Medicine in 1941. *(NCC)*

Bettering the Health of the People

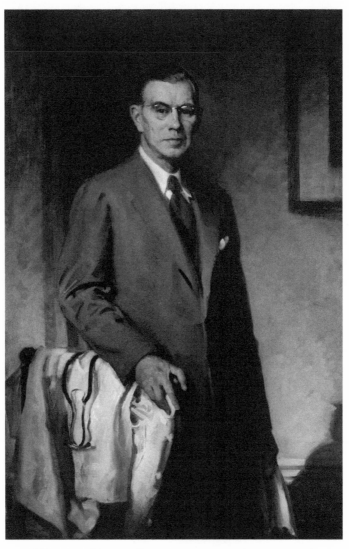

WALTER REECE BERRYHILL, MD (1900–1979)

The University of a State, when it truly fulfills its duty, should be its chief strength and glory, a light for the people, the fountain-head of their higher life, the source of their uplifting and upbuilding, the bulwark of their liberties . . . It moulds the leaders of the people . . . Great movements for the bettering of the condition of the people . . . spring from it.

University Day address by President Francis P. Venable at the University of North Carolina, Chapel Hill, October 12, 1900. Reprinted in the *Charlotte Daily Observer* on October 14, 1900, the day of the birth of Walter Reece Berryhill near Charlotte.

Bettering the Health of the People

W. Reece Berryhill,
the UNC School of Medicine,
and the
North Carolina Good Health Movement

WILLIAM W. MCLENDON
FLOYD W. DENNY, JR.
WILLIAM B. BLYTHE

For Kristen M. Swanson, RN, PhD

with admiration for your nursing and academic accomplishments, and with gratitude for your inspiring leadership as Dean of the UNC school of Nursing.

William W. McLendon
28 September 2013

The University of North Carolina at Chapel Hill Library
in association with
The Medical Foundation of North Carolina, Inc.
Chapel Hill

William W. McLendon, MD, is professor emeritus
of pathology and laboratory medicine at the
University of North Carolina at Chapel Hill (UNC).
The late *Floyd W. Denny, Jr., MD,* was professor
and chair emeritus of pediatrics at UNC.
The late *William B. Blythe, MD,* was professor
emeritus of medicine at UNC.

First printing.

Library of Congress Cataloging-in-Publication Data

McLendon, William W.
   Bettering the health of the people : W. Reece Berryhill, the UNC School
of Medicine, and the North Carolina good health movement /
William W. McLendon, Floyd W. Denny Jr., William B. Blythe.
      p. ; cm.
   Includes bibliographical references and index.
   ISBN 978-0-8078-3195-3 (alk. paper)
1. Berryhill, W. Reece (Walter Reece), 1900–1979. 2. Physicians—North Carolina—
Biography. 3. Medical teaching personnel—North Carolina—Biography. 4. University
of North Carolina at Chapel Hill. School of Medicine—History. I. Denny, Floyd W.,
1923– II. Blythe, William B., (William Brevard), 1928– III. University of North Carolina at Chapel Hill. Library. IV. Medical Foundation of North Carolina. V. Title.
[DNLM: 1. Berryhill, W. Reece (Walter Reece), 1900–1979. 2. Berryhill, Norma. 3. University of North Carolina at Chapel Hill. School of Medicine. 4. Faculty, Medical—North
Carolina—Biography. 5. Physicians—North Carolina—Biography. 6. Faculty, Medical
—history—North Carolina. 7. History, 20th Century—North Carolina—Biography.
8. Hospitals, University—history—North Carolina. 9. Public Health—history—North
Carolina. 10. Schools, Medical—history—North Carolina.   WZ 100 B5347M 2007]
   R154.B558M35 2007
   610.92—dc22
   [B]   2007041467

Design and production by BW&A Books, Inc., Durham, North Carolina

Distributed by
The University of North Carolina Press
Chapel Hill, North Carolina 27515-2288
1-800-848-6224
www.uncpress.unc.edu

Photo Credits

Frontispiece: the portrait of Walter Reece Berryhill is by Baker Studio, New York City;

Text: Unless otherwise noted, the photos are from the authors; the Berryhill family;
or the North Carolina Collection (NCC) of the Wilson Library, UNC, Chapel Hill.
Archival collections in the NCC include the photos from Medical Illustrations,
School of Medicine, UNC (Med. Illustrations) and the UNC Photo Lab.

Contents

Preface

$\mathcal{T}$*he suggestion* for a biography of Walter Reece Berryhill came from Floyd W. Denny, Jr., the second chair of the UNC Department of Pediatrics, after he and his colleagues had completed a history of the Department of Pediatrics. He then recruited William B. Blythe and William W. McLendon, both retired professors at the UNC School of Medicine, to participate in the project. At the time of Bill Blythe's sudden death in 2000 and then of Floyd Denny's demise in 2001, a number of interviews had been done and most of the material had been gathered. The outline for the book had been completed and three of the chapters were in early draft form. Although the undersigned completed the writing and the preparation for publication, Floyd Denny and Bill Blythe are truly coauthors, for this work would not exist without their inspiration, their insights, and their many contributions. Their passing was not only a deep personal loss, but was a major loss to the School of Medicine, the university, and the people of the state, all of whom they had served so well.

If this biography were written by someone who did not know the Berry- hills and had had no previous contacts with the university and its School of Medicine—whether a professional historian or a graduate student doing a doctoral dissertation—it would be an entirely different work. This volume is rather a labor of love, because the three authors knew the Berryhills for decades and lived through much of the history portrayed. One of the authors (Denny), who was born and raised in South Carolina, was recruited by Dean Berryhill from the Western Reserve School of Medicine in 1960 as a department chair and worked closely with him in developing his department. He knew the dean for almost two decades and Norma for four. He frequently observed, "Every brick and stone in this medical center is a monument to the dedicated efforts of Dr. Berryhill." The other two authors, born and raised in North Carolina, were undergraduates, medical students, and resident physicians at UNC in the 1940s and 1950s while Berryhill was dean of the School of Medicine. They both later became faculty members at the UNC School of Medicine. The father of one (Blythe), like Berry- hill, was born in Mecklenburg County and was a member of the remarkable UNC undergraduate class of 1921. He and the Berryhills were lifelong friends. The father of the other coauthor (McLendon) was raised in rural Anson County not too far from Berryhill's childhood home, was a graduate of the UNC Law School, and was Berryhill's ally in the 1940s and 1950s during the political and funding battles for the expansion of the School of Medicine and the location of the teaching hospital in Chapel Hill.

The authors thus cannot claim complete objectivity, but we have attempted to present a balanced and informed view with regard to controversial issues, such as Dean Berryhill's conflicts within the Division of Health Affairs in the 1950s and 1960s as well his initial difficulty in accepting the racial integration of the School of Medicine. We hope the reader will find that any lack of absolute objectivity is compensated for by the authors' experiences and insights.

In 1979 Berryhill, Blythe, and Manning published a short history of the first 100 years of medical education at Chapel Hill. Brief histories of the North Carolina Good Health Movement and longer histories of various components of the UNC School of Medicine also have been written, but none are easily accessible to the general public. Furthermore, the passage of a half century since the founding of the expanded school and teaching hospital in Chapel Hill in 1952 now provides a useful perspective on many of the critical decisions that were made in the 1940s and 1950s.

We believe that biography is a good medium for portraying a complex history such as North Carolina's movement to promote good health for its citizens. The historian Barbara Tuchman reminds us, "As a prism of history, biography attracts and holds the reader's interest in the larger subject. People are interested in other people, in the fortunes of the individual." She elaborates, "Biography is useful because it encompasses the universal in the particular. It is a focus that allows both the writer to narrow his field to manageable dimensions and the reader to more easily comprehend the subject." Thus a biography can be the story of both an individual's life and also the story of the times in which that life was lived. Accordingly we have attempted to use this biography as a means to personalize the impact on our subject—and on the institutions with which he was associated—of the Civil War, World War I, the influenza pandemic of 1918, the Great Depression, World War II, and the explosive postwar growth of biomedical research and of patient care facilities and services. We also hope to demonstrate that, as Kenneth M. Ludmerer wrote in *Time to Heal* (1999), "the future is not predetermined" by such monumental events, and "that individuals can make a difference."

Biographer Leon Edel states, "The secret of biography resides in finding the link between talent and achievement. A biography seems irrelevant if it doesn't discover the overlap between what the individual did and the life that made this possible." He warns, "Without discovering that, you have shapeless happenings and gossip." We have attempted to avoid this trap by framing the questions we wish to address about Berryhill's life and times in the prologue and then providing our assessments in the epilogue.

The "great man" approach to writing history as the story of superhuman leaders is now appropriately discredited. We have attempted to show that Reece Berryhill was the kind of man Ludmerer described in *Time to Heal:* an "ordinary flawed [person] who was not seen as particularly heroic by [his] contemporaries." He was a very human individual with doubts and frustrations as well as occasional flashes of anger and even paranoia. His greatness was not in being superhuman, but in tenaciously pursing for many years a larger vision for bringing better health to the people of his state. His unselfish service, his integrity, and his propensity to give credit to others characterized his life. Finally, this is not the story of a "great man," but rather the account of an extraordinary partnership of a man and a woman, Reece and Norma Berryhill.

Several appendices are included to provide both the general reader and the historian of medical education with some documentation of the evolution of medical education in North Carolina for the past 150 years and of its relationship to national trends in medical education. They provide chronologies of medical education in North Carolina and the nation; excerpts from the reports by Flexner (1910), Poe (1944–1945), and Sanger (1946) that profoundly affected North Carolina medical education; and Berryhill's 1950 presentation arguing for the location of medical schools on the parent university campus. The development of medical and health sciences education on the UNC campus at Chapel Hill during the second half of the twentieth century is documented with organizational charts and maps.

In acknowledging those who generously contributed to this endeavor I run the risk of overlooking some, but I ask their forgiveness.

Traditionally the author's spouse is mentioned last. I am reversing that by first thanking my bride of fifty-five years, Anne, for her patience through what must have seemed to her to be an endless pursuit. Without her unselfish support during many challenges, this work would never have seen the light of day.

Next I thank the Berryhill family, beginning with the remarkable and unique Norma, who passed away at 103 years of age after a life full of love for her family and of service to others. I am grateful for the interviews she gave to George Johnson, Jr., and for the insights she provided into her life and into the challenges she and Reece Berryhill faced. The Berryhills' daughters, Catherine Berryhill Williams and the late Jane Berryhill Neblett, generously provided information, documents, and photographs. They were supportive and provided feedback without ever attempting to censor the result.

As an amateur historian I am grateful to Professor (and later chair) Lloyd S. Kramer of the UNC Department of History for allowing me to fully participate in his History 200 course in the fall of 1998. This course on historical methods and historiography covered the approaches to, and resources for, writing history. It is required for all graduate students in the department and provided me with unique insights and resources that would otherwise have escaped me.

As a retired professor in the UNC Department of Pathology and Laboratory

Medicine, I am indebted to J. Charles Jennette, chair, and Nancy Nye, department administrator, for providing a shared emeritus professor office where reference materials could be housed and writing done.

Many persons have reviewed and provided feedback to the authors concerning the various chapters in this manuscript, and I am most appreciative to each of them. Those who undertook the laborious task of reviewing the entire manuscript—Stuart Bondurant, John Sanders, and Kate Torrey—provided invaluable constructive criticism and encouraged its completion and publication. Reviewers Charles Kaplan and Tom Karnes, both of whom are newcomers to the state, provided objective constructive feedback as well as valuable insights from their careers as professors of English and history, respectively.

I am especially indebted to Glenn Pickard, Jr., one of the early members in the 1960s of the UNC Medical School's Division of Research and Education in Community Medical Care. He was actively involved in the writing and revision of the community medicine chapter, and it would have been a much more difficult task without his knowledge, time, and effort. I am also grateful to Bryant Galusha, the first director of the Charlotte Area Health Education Center (AHEC), and to William J. Cromartie, former associate dean of the School of Medicine, for their critical reviews of several drafts of this chapter and for their enthusiastic encouragement that it be published. Tom Bacon, director of the North Carolina AHEC Program, provided support for the circulation of a prepublication version of the community medicine chapter to the AHEC directors and faculty throughout the state. This resulted in helpful feedback in several areas as well as encouragement to publish it.

Many others in the School of Medicine, the other health sciences schools, the hospitals, and the university were most helpful in reviewing specific sections or chapters and in responding to the author's queries for specific information or feedback. Marie Mitchell in the dean's office of the School of Medicine was most helpful in coordinating many of these requests.

Those who shared their anecdotes and observations on the Berryhills are acknowledged in the text or the notes. Their contributions have been essential in adding life to what otherwise might simply be a recounting of historical events or facts. We trust these accounts will bring both of them to life for those who did not know them and will be an accurate reflection of their lives for those who did.

Many contributed in making available essential source materials for this project, and to all I am most grateful: The directors and staff of the Southern Historical Collection (SHC) in the UNC Wilson Library; Janice Holder in the University Archives of the SHC; Robert Anthony, director of the North Carolina Collection (NCC) in Wilson Library, and his staff, especially Alice Cotten; and Diane M. McKenzie in the UNC Health Sciences Library. Eleanor Morris of Chapel Hill provided an essential resource in the form of a scrapbook of mid-1940s clippings from many North Carolina newspapers about the expansion of the School of Medicine and the Good Health Movement. This was compiled by her father, the late J. Marion "Spike" Saunders, who was the longtime secretary of the UNC General Alumni Association. After publication of this work, the scrapbook will be donated to the NCC.

Several secondary publications were valuable resources for the writing of this work. Berryhill, Blythe and Manning's centennial history of medical education at Chapel Hill provided a framework for the discussion of the three failed attempts to establish a state-supported MD-granting medical school in the first half of the twentieth century. Furthermore, this work provided insights into Berryhill's thinking about people and events, for as he noted in the Introduction, "the account of the years 1941–1964 is in a measure, and perhaps inevitably so, autobiographical—as was that of the period 1905–1933 for Dr. Manning."

William S. Powell's many publications on North Carolina and UNC history and William D. Snider's bicentennial history of UNC at Chapel Hill, *Light on the Hill,* provided historical context for many of the events in Berryhill's life. Kenneth M. Ludmerer, a physician and medical historian on the faculty at Washington University, St. Louis, Missouri, provided a broader historical perspective through his insightful histories of American medical education in the twentieth century.

Photographs and illustrative materials were found and copies provided by Jerry Cotten and Stephen J. Fletcher, successive directors of the Photographic Archives of the NCC; Douglas M. Mokaren, director of medical illustrations in the School of Medicine; Andrew Berner of the North Carolina AHEC Program; and Janet F. Lovell of the Medical Alumni Office. James D. Hundley of Wilmington, NC, a graduate of the medical class of 1967, generously donated the colorized architectural schematic of the original North Carolina Memorial Hospital that now hangs in the concourse of the UNC Hospitals and that graces the dust jacket of this volume.

The funding of this publication was made possible by a generous donation from the Medical Foundation of North Carolina, Inc., along with publication grants by William Roper, dean of the School of Medicine; James R. Harper, associate dean for alumni affairs; and Sarah Michalak, University Librarian. The successive presidents of the Medical Foundation, James L. Copeland and David B. Anderson, and their staffs have been generous with their time and effort in support of this publication and of a previous volume, *The Norma Berryhill Lectures, 1985–1999.*

We are grateful to the UNC Library for publishing this volume and to Richard V. Szary, director of Wilson Library and associate university librarian for Special Collections, for his expertise and support. We are indebted to the University of North Carolina Press and its director, Kate Torrey, for distribution and order fulfillment of this work.

The publication of this work has been a pleasure due to the enthusiastic and professional work of Chris Crochetière and Barbara Williams of BW&A Books,

Inc., Durham, North Carolina, who provided the design and managed all aspects of the production and printing. Barbara Norton of Norton Editorial, Durham, went far beyond the usual copyediting tasks to provide useful suggestions for improving readability and clarifying the presentation. The author is most grateful for her valuable assistance.

While grateful for all of the assistance provided by many others, the authors are solely responsible for the final work.

William W. McLendon

Bettering the Health of the People

PROLOGUE

Leaders of one era are frequently glorified by subsequent generations, but most of history's leaders have been ordinary flawed people who were not seen as particularly heroic by their contemporaries. True leaders are generally notable for their convictions, not for their charisma. They ask how their organization or institution can make a difference, they champion and exemplify worthy values and purposes, and they articulate a mission or cause beyond just making money.

—Kenneth M. Ludmerer, *Time to Heal*, 1999

Reece's reason for being was his interest in the State of North Carolina, the University, and the Medical School.

—Norma Berryhill

Although he has been the moving force behind creation of the four-year school, Dr. Berryhill for the most part has gone unnoticed in the eyes of the North Carolina public. Paradoxically, he is undoubtedly one of the greatest—yet least known—men in the Old North State today. By nature a retiring man, the 49-year-old dean never speaks of his accomplishments. In fact, even many of his close friends—who call him Reece—do not realize the effort and devotion he has put into bringing to the University and to Chapel Hill a complete medical school.

—"Tar Heel of the Week," *Raleigh News and Observer*, February 1950

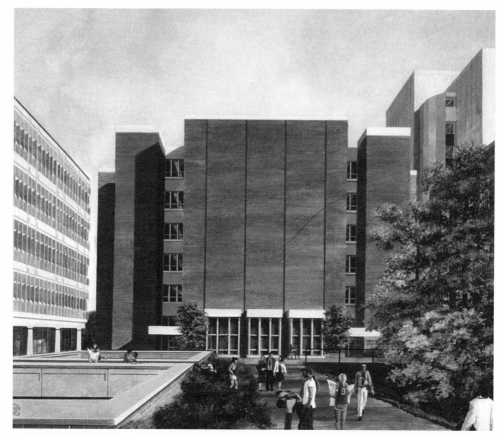

Architectural rendering of Berryhill Hall. *(Med. Illustrations, NCC)*

The Dean of North Carolina Medicine

Thursday, March 22, 1973, was a chilly but beautiful day in Chapel Hill as a crowd of several hundred gathered outside around a speaker's platform on the medical campus of the University of North Carolina (UNC) to dedicate the Basic Medical Sciences Building as Berryhill Hall in honor of W. Reece Berryhill, MD, who was dean of the medical school from 1941 to 1964.[1]

The almost windowless eight-story red-brick building had been the site of great activity since opening in January 1971.[2] It served as the teaching center for the instruction of first- and second-year medical and dental students as well as for students in nursing, public health, and allied health science, for a total of several thousand students per semester. It housed a television studio, the latest audiovisual equipment and scientific apparatus, two large auditoriums, smaller lecture rooms, and multiple teaching laboratories, including those for gross anatomy. Five multidisciplinary laboratories on each of two floors contained individual desks for each of the first- and second-year medical students. These laboratories provided a welcome relief for students who previously had had to carry heavy microscopes and books between classes and who had been forced to search for a quiet place to study at nights or on weekends. A snack bar named in honor of William Osler, MD, the first professor of medicine at the pioneering Johns Hopkins Medical School and the foremost physician in the English-speaking world in the early twentieth century, provided a break in the routine and a place for informal discussions among students and between students and faculty.

Former North Carolina governor Luther Hodges and other state and university officials were among the many friends and colleagues of the Berryhills in the audience. They were joined by a number of loyal medical school alumni who were in Chapel Hill for clinical rounds in the hospital and continuing medical education sessions on timely medical topics.[3]

The honoree, W. Reece Berryhill (AB, UNC, 1921; Cert. Med.,[4] UNC, 1925; MD, Harvard, 1927), had been the architect of the conversion of a respected two-year basic sciences medical school to a nationally renowned academic medical center with a teaching hospital, a full MD-granting curriculum in medicine,

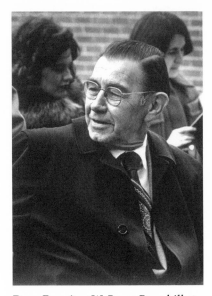

Dean Emeritus W. Reece Berryhill at the dedication ceremony for Berryhill Hall, 1973. *(Med. Illustrations, NCC)*

postgraduate education in all the major primary and specialty care areas, and an active biomedical research program. The medical school he had helped develop and nurture was one of only a few in the nation that were co-located on the parent university campus with a teaching hospital and schools of dentistry, nursing, pharmacy, and public health.[5]

Dr. and Mrs. Berryhill sat on the front row in the audience. Their two daughters, Jane and Catherine, and other family and friends sat nearby. Although Berryhill had been described in his college annual as "Reece, who could pass a pleasant and jovial smile [and] whose laugh was free,"[6] his years of medical training and practice had resulted in the scholarly and serious demeanor typical of the physicians of his day. He was tall, slim, and dignified, with thinning dark hair and metal-rimmed glasses. A careful observer and a good listener, he was a man of few words, and when he spoke it was with authority. He had a prodigious knowledge of the names and faces of state political and medical leaders, of faculty colleagues, and of alumni and students. His only vice, to anyone's knowledge, was his habit of having a lighted cigarette in his hand or mouth at most times. This habit contributed to his death a few years later, but only after he had lived a full and productive seventy-nine years.

At Berryhill's side was his wife of more than forty-two years, Norma Connell Berryhill. She was a native of Warren County, in the northeastern part of North Carolina. They had met when she was a student at Peace College in Raleigh and he was an undergraduate at UNC. They were married nine years later, in 1930, when Berryhill was a chief resident in medicine at Western Reserve University in Cleveland, and in 1933 they returned to their beloved Chapel Hill to stay. Norma Berryhill was a gracious and caring Southern lady with great dignity, but she never hesitated to speak her mind whenever the occasion warranted. A former student and later dean of the medical school stated, "She played her role as first lady [of the medical school] with grace, effectiveness and skill," adding, "She and Dr. Berryhill were quite a team. I wouldn't doubt they talked over everything. Her influence was substantial."[7]

The dedication program began with remarks by William C. Friday, president of the University of North Carolina system; Ferebee Taylor, chancellor of the University of North Carolina at Chapel Hill; and Christopher C. Fordham, III, MD, dean of the medical school at Chapel Hill.[8]

The dedicatory address was made by Erle E. Peacock, MD, a native of Chapel Hill whose father had been a UNC professor and who himself was a 1947 graduate of the two-year medical school. He was an internationally recognized hand surgeon and was a professor and chair of surgery at the University of Arizona at Tucson. He focused his comments on an apparent dichotomy among medical educators: the basic science teacher is concerned with truth as discovered by the scientific method, while the usual clinical teacher is concerned with solving practical clinical problems.[9] He held hope that

> these schizophrenic-appearing traits of undergraduate medical education can possibly be corrected in this new building if it houses the same type of creativity that its namesake is known for throughout the academic world. It is suggested, therefore, that we look to the man, as have so many in the past, for a clue as to how this might be achieved. It is there—there have never been any secrets—first and foremost, there is a plan. This School, among other factors, literally is the result of a man obsessed with a plan for quality education of physicians in North Carolina. His life, as I have known him, has been the very antithesis of the old admonition, "If you aim for nothing, you will hit it every time."

Peacock confessed the difficulty in finding "exactly the right words to express what is in all of our hearts for the man, and his family, who made this wonderful moment in North Carolina medical education history possible." After asking Dr. Berryhill and his family for their "characteristic charity," he concluded:

> Dedication of this building this afternoon, in the larger sense, can be an invitation to a great university to rededicate its mission to the highest standards of quality medical education. Placing the name of Reece Berryhill upon this building provides our campus with a permanent reminder that the ferment of creativity can be instantly imparted. True greatness, dear and glorious physician, has made others believe in greatness.

As Reece Berryhill basked in the kind words and the lovely day, he undoubtedly thought back over the events and people that had brought them and the medical school to this special occasion.

Berryhill had come from the rural Steele Creek community in Mecklenburg County to the university campus at Chapel Hill in 1917 as a seventeen-year-old freshman in the class of 1921. He had become a leader in an illustrious class that elected him senior class president and voted him "best all 'round" member of his class. His undergraduate years were, as described by the class historian, "four years of such intensity and soul-stirring effort that they might have been spread over a half century of ordinary time."[10] America had been involved in the Great War (World War I). Some of Berryhill's classmates went off to France, while he and the remaining students were inducted into the Student Army Training Corps in the fall of 1918 and demobilized following the armistice on November 11, 1918. The worldwide influenza pandemic had struck the campus in October 1918, with more than 500 cases at the university. Complications of the flu precipitously took from their midst three students and a young university president, Edward Kidder Graham, who had imbued Berryhill and his fellow students with the vision that the university should be "in warm, sensitive touch with every problem in North Carolina life, small and great."[11] During their senior year, the new president, Harry Woodburn Chase, who would become known as "the architect of the modern university of North Carolina,"[12] had made their class realize their pivotal place in university history when he told them, "Your class is the connecting link between the old University and the new."[13]

When Berryhill was deciding, during his undergraduate years at UNC, to become a physician rather than a minister, he took note of the medical school building, Caldwell Hall. Located at the edge of the main campus across from the Coker Arboretum and named for the first president of the university, it was occupied in 1912 as the first building on the campus specifically designed for the medical curriculum. The medical school, which was founded as a one-year preclinical school in 1879 and adopted a two-year curriculum in 1896, had previously shared space in other academic buildings on the university campus. It would remain a two-year school until 1952, when the efforts of Berryhill and others resulted in opening of the four-year MD-granting school and teaching hospital at Chapel Hill.

Berryhill was still a youngster at Steele Creek during the first of what were to be four attempts during the first half of the twentieth century to establish an MD-granting school for the people of the state.[14] Such a school did exist from 1902 until 1910 in Raleigh as the Medical Department of the University of North Carolina. Medical students, after completing two years of basic medical sciences at Chapel Hill, could transfer to Raleigh, where the patients in Raleigh's hospitals and clinics were used for clinical instruction, and local practicing physicians were the professors. This unit of the university had seventy-six MD graduates, sixty-six of whom were to become practicing physicians in North Carolina.[15] UNC President Francis Venable had to discontinue the Raleigh Medical Department when the state could not provide the funds to meet the high standards mandated in the Carnegie Foundation's report on medical education in the United States and Canada, compiled by Abraham Flexner.[16] The 1910 Flexner Report thus contained no mention of the clinical school at Raleigh, but it was generally positive about the two-year basic science school at Chapel Hill, which was described as "an organic part of the university."[17] (See Appendix D.)

Not long after the demise of the UNC Medical Department in Raleigh, the North Carolina Medical College at Charlotte, an MD-granting proprietary school originally established at Davidson College in 1887, moved to Richmond and merged with the Medical College of Virginia.[18] The Leonard Medical School of Shaw University in Raleigh, an MD-granting, philanthropically supported medical school for African Americans established in 1882, also soon closed because of the lack of financial support to meet the modern standards of medical education.[19]

Thus, just a few years after the Flexner Report, North Carolina was left with no MD-granting medical schools. Young North Carolinians wanting to become physicians could attend the relatively inexpensive two-year schools at the university at Chapel Hill or the one established in 1902 at Wake Forest College, but they were faced with the considerable expense of going to out-of-state medical schools for their clinical years and the MD degree. Furthermore, both the medical students and the two-year schools themselves were faced with the uncertainty that places might not always be available for transfer to the MD-granting schools for the clinical years.

Berryhill was teaching in Charlotte in exchange for his free UNC undergraduate tuition when the second attempt to establish a state-supported, MD-granting medical school at Chapel Hill also failed. Planning was far enough along in late 1922 to allow the university to present a funding request for the school's expansion to the legislature when President William P. Few of Trinity College in Durham (soon to become Duke University) proposed a jointly operated MD-granting medical school using the existing two-year medical school at Chapel Hill, with the clinical years to be spent in Durham. Funding was to come from the Duke family and from state appropriations. The proposal for an academic medical center jointly operated by a Methodist-supported college and a state-supported university quickly ran into devastating opposition from those concerned with the separation of church and state. This opposition—plus competition from other cities for the university hospital, concerns about a "divided" medical school (with the basic science and clinical years not on the same campus), and President Chase's need for large state appropriations for other university buildings—led to the collapse of this attempt in early 1923. The Duke Endowment was established in 1924, Duke Hospital and the Duke School of Medicine opened in Durham in 1930, and the first MD degrees were awarded at Duke University in 1932 to eighteen students who had transferred to the new school from two-year schools.[20]

When the third attempt to establish a state-supported, MD-granting medical school also failed, Berryhill was a junior medical school faculty member at UNC, having returned to Chapel Hill in 1933 as university physician and faculty member of the medical school. While away from the state he had received the MD degree from Harvard, had trained in internal medicine in Boston, and had served as a junior faculty member at Western Reserve Medical School. The General Assembly in 1937 had called for a study to determine whether the state should establish an MD-granting medical school. The study commission, appointed by Governor Hoey, was preparing to make an affirmative recommendation to the 1939 General Assembly when it was made known that an anonymous donor was willing to help with the funding of such an endeavor if the expanded school were to be built in a designated city. Because of strong opposition among some committee members—especially Dean William de Berniere MacNider—to having a divided medical school, the motion to consider the informal offer was voted down, and the recommendation to the legislature for a four-year school and teaching hospital at Chapel Hill was not acted upon. In the meantime, the Bowman Gray family of Winston-Salem offered the money to the two-year medical school at Wake Forest College on the condition that it move to Winston-Salem and utilize the existing North Carolina Baptist Hospital for its clinical teaching. The school, renamed the Bowman Gray School of Medicine of Wake Forest College, moved to Winston-Salem in 1941 and awarded its first MD degrees in 1943. Wake Forest College moved from Wake Forest in Wake County to a new campus in Winston-Salem in 1956 and became Wake Forest University in 1967.[21]

Berryhill's acceptance of the appointment as dean of the medical school in 1941 began the fourth and finally successful effort to have a teaching hospital and a four-year MD-granting medical school at UNC for the people of North Carolina. After having served as acting dean during 1940–1941, he reluctantly accepted the deanship for a five-year term with an understanding from UNC's president, Frank Porter Graham, that the university was committed to a four-year medical school as soon after the war as was feasible.

Dean Berryhill wasted no time in beginning the push for the medical school expansion. In his first annual report to the president of the university in 1941, he had said, "In spite of the national emergency we should not lose sight of our ultimate goal of establishing a four year school . . . It is inevitable that we take this step if this school if to survive, and what is more important, if the State and University are to fulfill their obligations to the people of the State."[22]

Discussions by Berryhill and others in 1943 had led to the appointment by Graham of a committee of physicians to make recommendations to Governor J. Melville Broughton concerning a health-improvement program for the state. The governor presented their proposal to the university board of trustees on January 31, 1944, with the statement that "the ultimate purpose of this program should be that no person in North Carolina shall lack adequate hospital care or medical treatment by reason of poverty or low income."

The trustees unanimously approved the governor's proposal and authorized appointment of a group to study the needs and make a proposal for implementation to the General Assembly in 1945. Broughton appointed an ad hoc Hospital and Medical Care Commission composed of sixty leaders from all parts of North Carolina and led by Dr. Clarence Poe of Raleigh, the respected editor of the *Progressive Farmer*. The work of the commission was energized by the knowledge of "the shockingly high 57% rejection rate of North Carolina boys in the American armies," the worst rate of all forty-eight states during World War II.[23]

The seven subcommittees of the commission worked diligently for months on their reports. Berryhill, Dean Coy Carpenter of the Bowman Gray Medical School, and Dean Wilbur Davison of the Duke Medical School served on the subcommittee for the four-year medical school and expansion of hospital facilities, and Berryhill was drafted to write their report.

The commission approved a preliminary report on October 11, 1944, after presentations to Governor Broughton. To respond to this and other identified health needs in the state, the report called for "More Hospitals, More Doctors and More Insurance" for the people of North Carolina. As part of this statewide effort, the commission gave "its unqualified endorsement to the proposal that the present two-year medical school at the University of North Carolina be expanded into a standard four-year medical school with a central hospital of 600 beds." It was their opinion that "North Carolina students trained in North Carolina will likely remain in North Carolina to follow their chosen profession."

The commission's final report was made on February 10, 1945, to the new governor, R. Gregg Cherry, and to the General Assembly. The General Assembly accepted the report and established a permanent state-supported Medical Care Commission, which in July 1945 (a month before the end of World War II) assumed the leadership for coordinating the planning and implementation of the statewide plan for improved health care for North Carolinians.

One of the Medical Care Commission's first actions was to have a national committee of medical educators make recommendations about the need for and feasibility of expanding the medical school at Chapel Hill. This committee, led by William Sanger, PhD, president of the Medical College of Virginia, made a majority recommendation in 1946 supporting the expansion of the medical school at Chapel Hill with various stipulations. The Sanger Report called for the University of North Carolina to "develop a philosophy of medical education, research, and medical care which will make it a service facility for the whole State."[24]

In 1946 the North Carolina Good Health Association was established to publicize throughout the state the recommendation of the Medical Care Commission and to gather broad-based support for its implementation. In spite of the resulting publicity, Berryhill and other proponents had to struggle to establish political support for the location of the academic medical center and for the necessary state appropriations to begin planning and construction. The conventional wisdom at the time was that teaching hospitals should be located in major cities where there were large numbers of charity patients for teaching purposes, not in a community such as Chapel Hill, with a population of only a few thousand. The perceived economic advantages and prestige of a medical school hospital had led a total of eight North Carolina communities to express interest in the teaching hospital.[25] On the other side of the argument, a thoughtful observer during the earlier debate on this topic in the 1920s cited both the Mayo Clinic and Leonard Tuft's hotel in Pinehurst as examples of highly successful endeavors in small communities.[26] Berryhill, Frank Graham, and others argued convincingly that a state academic medical center should be located on the university campus so that it would benefit from the educational and scientific synergy with the parent university.[27] (See Appendix K.)

Berryhill would never forget the drama that ensued in the overflowing cham-

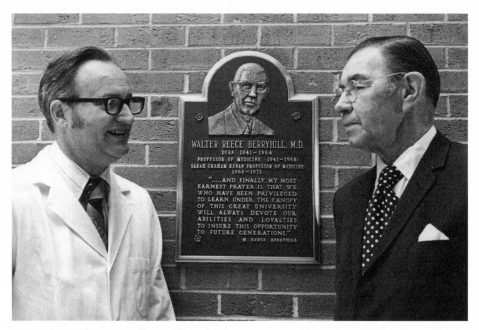

Dean Christopher C. Fordham, III, and Dean Emeritus W. Reece Berryhill with the plaque in the lobby of Berryhill Hall, 1973. *(Berryhill Family)*

ber of the state House of Representatives in Raleigh on February 13, 1947, when opponents and supporters debated the issues concerning the expanded medical school at Chapel Hill and the statewide Good Health Program. The arguments supporting the statewide program of hospital construction and the expansion of the UNC Medical School prevailed, and in March 1947 the General Assembly approved the initial state appropriations. These monies, coupled with federal matching funds under the Hill-Burton Act of 1946, resulted in an unprecedented growth of health care facilities in the state.

Berryhill must have remembered another ceremony in 1949, when the cornerstone for the teaching hospital was laid on the university campus. During the construction of the hospital and other buildings, Berryhill had been busy recruiting the first chairs of the clinical departments and giving them the resources to create their new departments. He recruited nationally for the chairs and took advantage of his many contacts from his years at Harvard and Western Reserve.

Berryhill's dream was fulfilled when the first patient was admitted to the new North Carolina Memorial Hospital in September 1952, at the same time the first class of third-year medical students began their clinical externships at the hospital. With great satisfaction he presided at the graduation in 1954 of the first class to receive the MD degree from the University of North Carolina at Chapel Hill.

As Berryhill viewed the lively medical center around him in March 1973, he could take great pride in all that had happened from that day in March 1947 when the legislature approved the first funding for the new medical center at Chapel Hill until he retired as dean in 1964. An entire medical center had been built almost from scratch (only a medical and public health school building occupied in 1939 and a student infirmary built by the navy during World War II had existed at the medical center site); an outstanding new clinical faculty had been recruited; the existing basic sciences faculty had been augmented; a new medical curriculum had been developed; and residency programs to train physicians in primary and specialty care had been established. Tens of thousands of patients had been served, and an ever-increasing number of physicians and other health care professionals educated at Chapel Hill were bringing their skills to communities throughout the state and nation.

Berryhill might also have remembered with satisfaction his successful attempt, following his retirement as dean, to implement the statewide service challenges of the university president, Edward Kidder Graham, and of the Sanger Report by means of the Division of Education and Research in Community Medical Care, which he directed from 1966 to 1969. These efforts to establish affiliated educational programs with community hospitals in the state provided the foundation for the successful 1972 application by the medical school for federal funding for the North Carolina Area Health Education Center (NC AHEC) program under the energetic and innovative leadership of the founding AHEC director, Glenn Wilson.[28] Today the NC AHEC Program involves all four medical schools and has centers across the state in communities where medical students are introduced to community care, young physicians receive postgraduate education in various primary care specialties, and practicing physicians and other health care providers receive continuing education.

At the conclusion of the formal dedication ceremony, Berryhill joined his many friends, college classmates, and former students at a reception. The *Daily Tar Heel* reporter noted that "Dean Berryhill remembered them all, their classes and the times they had had. He had taught for 43 years. And he still remembered them all," adding, "He is not a man to be fawned over. He is a strong man: the lines in his craggy face are evidence of that. He seemed to grow weary of the endless line [of some 400 well-wishers], but stood, shaking hands, reaching out and greeting the many people whose lives had become entwined with his over the years."[29]

The authors of this work propose to explore three questions about the people and events that transformed health care and medical education in North Carolina during the second half of the twentieth century:

1. What was it about W. Reece Berryhill's upbringing, education, and experiences that gave him a consuming passion "to better the health of the people" of his state by having an academic medical center on the state

university campus at Chapel Hill with "a philosophy of medical education, research, and medical care which will make it a service facility for the whole State"?

2. What explains the success of the state's bold decision in the 1940s to build a university medical center in what was then the small village of Chapel Hill? Although in the postwar years most of the states that built new medical schools or expanded two-year schools did locate them on the state university campus, two states (Alabama and Mississippi) elected to put the clinical school in the state's largest city. Furthermore, more than half a dozen North Carolina communities expressed interest in having the teaching hospital and medical school in their city rather than at Chapel Hill, so it was not a foregone conclusion that the expanded medical school would be on the university campus.

3. How have the nation, the state, and the university performed in the past half century with regard to Governor Broughton's goal in 1944 that "no person in North Carolina shall lack adequate hospital care or medical treatment by reason of poverty or low income?"

PART I

〜

Years of Preparation, 1900–1933

Divide your attentions equally between books and men. The strength of the student of books is to sit still—two or three hours at a stretch—eating the heart out of a subject with pencil and notebook in hand, determined to master the details and intricacies, focusing all your energies on its difficulties . . . The strength of a student of men is to travel—to study men, their habit, character, mode of life, their behaviour under varied conditions, their vices, virtues, and peculiarities. Begin with a careful observation of your fellow students and of your teachers; then every patient you see is a lesson in much more than the malady from which he suffers. Mix as much as you possibly can with the outside world, and learn its ways. Cultivated systematically, the student societies, the students' union, the gymnasium, and the outside social circle will enable you to conquer the diffidence so apt to go with bookishness and which may prove a very serious drawback in after-life.

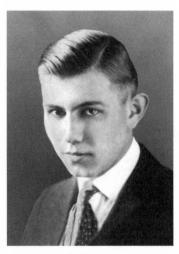

Reece Berryhill, senior at UNC. (1921 *Yackety Yack,* NCC)

—William Osler, "The Student Life," 1905

At the onset [of your medical study] appreciate clearly the aims and objects each one of you should have in view—knowledge of disease and its cure, and knowledge of yourself. The one, special education, will make you a practitioner of medicine; the other, an inner education, may make you a truly good man, four square and without a flaw. The one is extrinsic and is largely accomplished by teacher and tutor, by text and by tongue; the other is intrinsic and is the mental salvation to be wrought out by each one for himself . . . With what I hope to infect you with is a desire to have a due proportion of each.

—William Osler, "The Master-Word in Medicine," 1903

A Childhood in the Rural South

Sunday, October 14, 1900, in Mecklenburg County, North Carolina, was a momentous day for the future of the University of North Carolina and for the health of North Carolinians, although no one could have realized it at the time.

The Sunday-morning edition of the *Charlotte Daily Observer* carried front-page stories of the campaigns of the Democratic nominee for president of the United States, William Jennings Bryan, and of the Republican nominee for vice president, New York Governor Theodore Roosevelt. (Republican William McKinley was to win the presidential election on November 6, but Vice President Theodore Roosevelt became president in 1901 when McKinley succumbed to wounds suffered during an assassination attempt in Buffalo.) An inside story on further experiments testing the mosquito theory for the transmission of malaria was headlined, "The Mosquitoes Are Guilty: They Distribute Malaria Germs."

The front page of the second section of the *Observer* carried the full text of an address given in Chapel Hill two days previously by Francis Preston Venable. The *Observer*'s correspondent prefaced the text with the comment, "President Venable delivered a striking address to the University students this evening, October 12, which is known as University Day." Venable, who had come to the University of North Carolina in 1880 as professor of chemistry and was the first faculty member to have received his PhD from one of the prestigious German universities of his time, had just been appointed president of the university.

Venable used his address to present his credo on the nature of the ideal state university:

The University of a State, when it truly fulfills its duty, should be its chief strength and glory, a light for the people, the fountain-head of their higher life, the source of their uplifting and upbuilding, the bulwark of their liberties. It moulds the leaders of the people. Streams of influence flow from it to gladden the whole land . . . Great movements for the bettering of the condition of the people, for the development of the material resources, for the progress along all lines spring from it.[1]

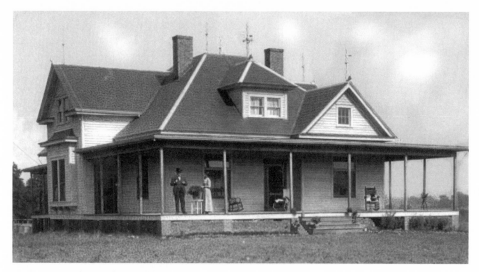

Home in Steele Creek, Mecklenburg County, North Carolina, where Reece Berryhill was born and raised. *(Berryhill Family)*

Two who were to be leaders molded by the University of North Carolina and who were to become staunch proponents of President Venable's philosophy were having birthdays that autumn Sunday, although they would not become acquainted until almost two decades later. Frank Porter Graham, who was born in Fayetteville, North Carolina, on October 14, 1886, was celebrating his fourteenth birthday not far from the *Observer*'s offices at the home of his father, who was superintendent of the Charlotte public schools.

Walter Reece Berryhill was born on October 14, 1900, in the Steele Creek section of Mecklenburg County, southwest of Charlotte, in his parents' home, a site now occupied by one of the runways of Charlotte's Douglas International Airport. His father, Samuel Reece Berryhill, a farmer, and his mother, Eugenia Scott Berryhill, named him Walter for a close friend of his father's and Reece for his father. Reece Berryhill was the oldest of three children in the family. His brother William Scott Berryhill was born in 1904, and another brother, Joseph Oliver Berryhill, was born in 1908.

It is not mere coincidence that these future leaders at the University of North Carolina were both North Carolinians and the products of Calvinistic Presbyterian families with a highly developed sense of duty and a deep respect for education. John Calvin had said, "There cannot be a surer rule, nor a stronger exhortation to the observance of it, than when we are taught that all the endowments which we possess are divine deposits entrusted to us for the very purpose of being distributed for the good of our neighbor."[2] Graham's and Berryhill's lives in the years to come would be a fulfillment of this mandate as they dedicated their considerable endowments to better the condition of their neighbors throughout the state.

Family tradition states that the Berryhill name originated "in Scotland several centuries ago [with] a family named Hill. This family went to North Ireland to become a part of that remarkable people known as the Scotch-Irish. In North Ireland one member of the family was a grower of berries. He became known as berry-Hill, and his descendants . . . came to America at various times during the period [before] 1730."[3]

Another source states, "Alexander Berryhill was the progenitor of the Berryhills of America. He was born in Scotland in 1661. He went to London, England, and married Lady Jane Cartwright, daughter of [the English] Lord Cartwright. One year later they settled in the north of Ireland." Their eldest son, John Berryhill, was born and educated in Ireland, where he became a weaver by trade. After taking an Irish wife, he came to America around 1718, settling in the Carolinas at about the time it was divided into North and South Carolina. Walter Reece Berryhill was directly descended from this John Berryhill, who was of Scots, English, and Irish ancestry. The Berryhills subsequently married with a number of the early prominent families of Mecklenburg County, among them the Alexanders, the Allisons, the Polks, and the Spratts.

Many of the settlers of Mecklenburg County were Scots-Irish—Scots who had first been forced by the English to immigrate to Ulster in Northern Ireland from the early 1600s onward. When the English Parliament started restricting their woolen trade and put pressure on them to give up the Presbyterian Church for the Church of England, large numbers of Scots-Irish migrated to America, starting in the 1680s. The records show that in 1684 six ships with Scots-Irish passengers arrived in Philadelphia in one week. After first dispersing throughout Pennsylvania, many subsequently sought better land and climate by migrating south to Virginia and North Carolina, using an old Indian trading path that became known as the Philadelphia Wagon Road. Smaller numbers of Scots from the Highlands of northern Scotland came directly to North Carolina, arriving in Mecklenburg County via settlements along the Cape Fear River. A third and smaller group of Scots from the Lowlands of southern Scotland came into the ports at Wilmington and Charleston and then migrated northwest to the county.

The Berryhill family was among the early settlers of Mecklenburg County,[4] although it is not precisely known when they first arrived. One of the earlier graves in the Steele Creek Presbyterian Church Cemetery is that of a William Berryhill (1738–1799), who is said to have been a Revolutionary War soldier.[5]

Robert A. Ross, a longtime friend of Berryhill and the first chair of the obstetrics and gynecology department at UNC, also grew up in the Steele Creek community, and his family too belonged to the Steele Creek Presbyterian Church. In a tribute to Ross in 1965, Berryhill elaborated on the connections between the Ross and Berryhill ancestors and their close association with the University of North Carolina:

The relationship between our families actually began two hundred years ago, when two of our ancestors were contemporaries in the then-small and largely Presbyterian school, the College of New Jersey at Princeton. Less than a decade after graduation these two men found themselves in the newly established village of Charlotte, in Mecklenburg County, North Carolina. Dr. Ross's ancestor, one Waightstill Avery, was an able young lawyer; mine, a Presbyterian minister. Both participated in the events leading up to the Mecklenburg Declaration of Independence on May 20, 1775, and were signers of this famous—though somewhat disputed—document. Mr. Avery was the representative from Mecklenburg County in the first State Constitutional Convention held at Halifax in 1776 and is reported to have been the author of the paragraph in the state constitution calling for the establishment of one or more universities for the education of the state's future leaders. In a sense, therefore, he can be called the father of the University of North Carolina.[6]

LIFE IN STEELE CREEK

Steele Creek, named for an early settler, has its origin in a spring on a Mecklenburg County farm and empties into the Catawba River in South Carolina. The settlement in southwestern Mecklenburg County where Reece Berryhill was reared is named for the creek. The primary occupation of the inhabitants was farming, with cotton and tobacco being the cash crops.

We have little documentation of Berryhill's early life, but we can assume that he had a normal, happy childhood doing those things typical of rural boys in North Carolina in the early part of the twentieth century. From comments he made in newspaper interviews many years later, we do have some insight into his daily routine. When he was being interviewed as the *News and Observer*'s Tar Heel of the Week in 1960, he was asked about his plans for the farm outside Carrboro to which he and his wife, Norma, had recently moved. He replied that he wanted some cattle, but not the kind that had to be milked; he had had his fill of that chore as a boy, when he had to milk the cows before going to school and again in the evening.[7] In another newspaper interview the reporter noted, "Even today he can pick blackberries three times as fast as the average person because of his early training in picking cotton."[8]

Berryhill received a staunch Presbyterian upbringing. His parents were members of the Steele Creek Presbyterian Church, and his forebears were among those who established the church about 1760.[9] This upbringing is almost certainly responsible for Berryhill's strong sense of duty and penchant for standing up—and speaking out—for what he considered to be right and proper.

His later consuming mission to use education to better the health of the people of North Carolina can also be traced in large part to the fundamental Presbyterian belief in the importance of education. This conviction manifests itself in the church's well-educated ministers, along with an educated laity who

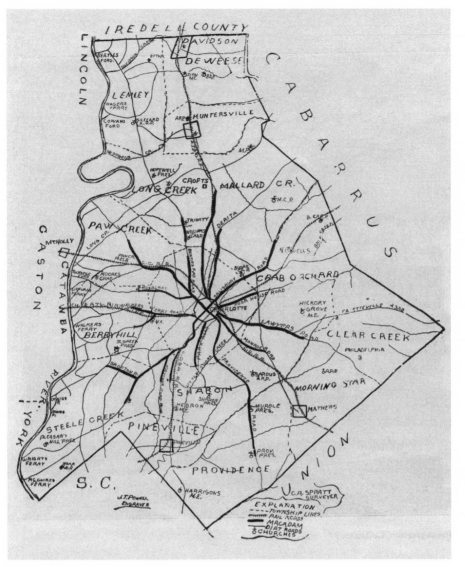

Map of Mecklenburg County, 1902. *(Sketches of Charlotte: North Carolina's Finest City. Vol 4.* Charlotte, NC: Wade H. Harris; 1902. *NCC)*

can read and understand the Bible. This Presbyterian influence was also present in the founding and early years of the University of North Carolina: three of its first presidents, from 1795 to the beginning of the Civil War, were Presbyterian ministers.

An account of the history of the Steele Creek Presbyterian Church elaborates on the place of the church in family life and the Sunday routine:

Well into the twentieth century, Mecklenburg County was largely an agricultural society. A strong part of this society was the church. Because there were few other activities in the rural areas, church attendance was impor-

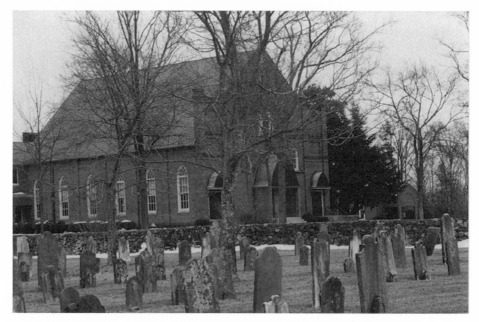

Steele Creek Presbyterian Church, where Reece Berryhill and his family attended church, and where many of his ancestors dating back to the late 1700s are buried. *(Authors)*

tant. Sunday was often a long day. For many years the farm families arose early on Sunday mornings. They milked their cows, prepared breakfast, and packed a lunch. They hitched a team to a farm wagon. Quilts were placed in the bottom of the wagon bed for the children and chairs for the adults. Frequently the families had to leave early in order to arrive at the church for the 10:00 A.M. service. At lunch time they adjourned and spread their lunches on rocks that served as tables. After lunch, they returned to the church for another sermon lasting one hour or more. This was followed by the journey home to repeat the chores of milking and feeding. By the time they reached home many families had traveled fifteen miles or more.[10]

SCHOOLING

The years of Berryhill's schooling in the early 1900s were years of great upheaval in public education in North Carolina. Charles Brantley Aycock (UNC class of 1880), who was inaugurated governor in January 1901, was credited by his biographer with having "inspired the people with visions of the good government which educated voters might create, the economic prosperity which educated workers might produce, and the cultural heights which an educated people might reach."[11] He did this through the Good Schools Program, the first of three "great movements for the bettering of the condition of the people" of North Carolina in the first half of the twentieth century. An average of one school a day was opened in North Carolina during the four years of Aycock's term as governor.

In spite of the good intentions of Aycock and other state educational and political leaders, progress toward achieving universal education was slow, especially for blacks and those in rural areas. The few rural schools that existed at the time typically operated only four to six months a year, while some town schools might have a term as long as nine months. It was not until 1918 that a constitutional amendment passed in North Carolina to require that all public schools have a six-month term. It is thus likely that Berryhill had a school term of six months or less during most of his years in public school.[12]

A report on the progress of education in Mecklenburg County from 1901 to 1907 by the county superintendent of public schools provides some insight into the movement to improve local schools. Only one special tax district existed in the county in 1901; in 1907 that number had ballooned to seventeen. In these districts the apportionment from the state school fund was supplemented by special locally levied school taxes.[13] Not surprisingly in view of the Scottish dedication to education, Steele Creek township in 1906 raised $170.91 to supplement the state's appropriation of $295.50 for a total annual expenditure for the public school in Steele Creek of $473.41. This self-imposed 58 percent supplementation of the state funds by the citizens of Steele Creek Township compared very well with most other districts in the county but could not match the 164 percent supplementation by the citizens of Davidson township, the home of a Presbyterian college, Davidson. The Mecklenburg school report editorialized:

> The good results of the special tax are to be seen on every hand. The schools that have the tax have the longest terms, pay the best salaries, and of course get the best teachers . . . Taxation is not a mark of oppression, but a badge of culture, refinement, and a sign of progress, thrift and industry . . . And when one considers . . . that it costs each individual but a few dollars at most, one is surprised to find any opposition to it in this day of enlightened citizenship.

Berryhill graduated from Steele Creek's Dixie School, where it is likely that he spent all his school years. He did benefit from the new state and local emphasis on good schools. The same 1907 report had a photograph of the old Dixie School building, a somewhat run-down two-story structure, while the new building was a neatly painted, two-story structure with an American flag proudly flying and a cupola holding the school bell.

Although the curriculum undoubtedly had undergone some changes by the time Berryhill completed high school in 1917, the 1907 Mecklenburg County report listed three years of high school (through the tenth grade, the highest grade in most schools at the time) and included courses such as mathematics, history, Latin, science (physical geography, physics, and advanced physiology), and English (including grammar, rhetoric, and American and English literature). The selection of recommended school and home readings for high schoolers included Shakespeare's *Macbeth,* Poe's *Raven,* and Cooper's *Last of the Mohicans.*

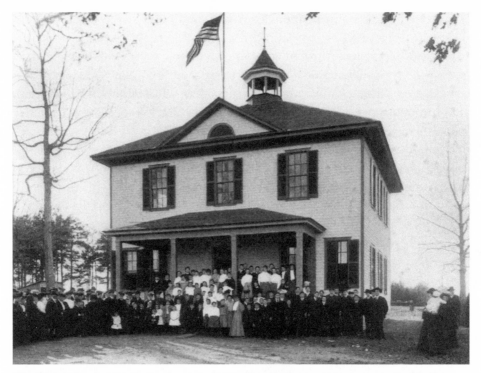

The Dixie School at Steele Creek, where Reece Berryhill attended ten years of schooling and returned for an eleventh year before going to college. (Cochran RJ. *Catalogue of Public Schools in Mecklenburg County, North Carolina, 1901–1907.* Charlotte, NC: Queen City Printing; 1907, *NCC*)

Other readings reflected the predominantly Scottish population of the area and included Sir Walter Scott's *Lady of the Lake* and Jane Porter's *Scottish Chiefs*.[14]

A program for the closing exercises of the Dixie high school on Friday, April 23, 1915, indicates that Reece Berryhill performed a musical piece, "The Land We Love," as part of the Declamation and Recitation Contest. Although he enjoyed classical music in his later years, this is the only documentation we have of his being a performing musician.[15]

PLANNING FOR THE FUTURE

According to Norma Berryhill and several written accounts, Berryhill had planned ever since he was a child to become a minister in the Presbyterian Church. As a consequence he concentrated on the classics while in high school. The transcript of his record shows that he entered college with 2 credits in Greek, 3.7 credits in Latin, and no credits in any of the sciences.[16]

Norma Berryhill said that Reece spent much time with the high school faculty and that they had a major influence on him.[17] During his senior year in high school he came with the debating team to Chapel Hill to participate in an annual high school debating contest that had begun in 1913 through the efforts of Louis Round Wilson and others.[18] This trip was one of the most important of his life, for the faculty at Chapel Hill convinced him that the university—and not Davidson College, where he had planned to go—was the ideal place for him to continue his education.

He returned home dreading to tell his parents that he had changed his mind about Davidson and that he wanted to go to Chapel Hill. Apparently his father embraced Reece's new plans wholeheartedly. His mother gave her blessing only after extracting from him a promise that he would spend an extra year in high school to become a more mature seventeen-year-old and thus better able to withstand the sin-ridden atmosphere of Chapel Hill, as she perceived it.

Heritage and Beliefs

Berryhill's family preserved two essays in his handwriting from this time. Written in the exuberant style of the time, they provide insight into the character and motivation of a complex and driven man who was later determined to achieve his dream of benefiting the people of North Carolina when others had given up in despair.

One paper, signed "W. R. Berryhill, Essay—May 1st, 1916," was entitled "Causes of The Meck. Declaration of Independence."[19] An accompanying program for the Charlotte City Schools Commencement in 1916 had "Reece Berryhill" written beside the Loving Cup award, almost certainly given for this essay, from the Signers of the Mecklenburg Declaration of Independence chapter of the D.A.R. (Daughters of the American Revolution). The essay was rubber stamped in blue ink with "W. Reece BErryhill" [sic] and a second smudged line that was probably his UNC dormitory address. The essay may also have been submitted (perhaps in a modified form) as a paper in one of his courses at UNC, although it has no date, grade, or corrections by a professor.

In "Causes" Berryhill told the story of the Mecklenburg Declaration of Independence, which was said (some forty years after the alleged event) to have been signed on May 20, 1775, more than a year before the Declaration of Independence was signed in Philadelphia. No original document survives, and historians today dispute the existence of the Mecklenburg Declaration. Many think the document became confused with the Mecklenburg Resolves, drawn up in May 1775 in preparation for possible war with Britain.[20] Nonetheless, Berryhill provided a passionate political and religious history of the people of Mecklenburg County and of the principle of individual liberty that "is inseparably connected with the Anglo-Saxon race." He traced the origin of this principle to the people's Anglo-Saxon ancestors on the "bleak shores" of Jutland, where "they lived with nature, and God's teachers, though stern, were the best." He followed their migration to England and Scotland following the downfall of the Roman Empire; their defense of liberty under William Wallace and Robert the Bruce; their adoption of the Presbyterian Reform theology of John Calvin; and their emigration to

America to find religious and political freedom. He quoted George Bancroft as saying, "The first voice publicly raised in America to dissolve all connections with G. Britain came not from the Puritans of New England, not from the Dutch in New York, not from the planters in Virginia, but from the Scotch Irish Presbyterians of North Carolina." Although the Mecklenburg Declaration itself may not have been a historical fact, in his essay Berryhill clearly demonstrated his knowledge of, and pride in, his religious and political heritage.

A second paper in his handwriting is entitled "The New South." Though unsigned, it too has the rubber-stamped impression of his name and his UNC dormitory. This address, by Henry Grady, the young and dynamic editor of the *Atlanta Constitution* in the decades after the Civil War, was so well known in the South at the time that Berryhill did not feel obligated to provide the author's name. Grady first gave it in New York City in 1886 to the New England Society of New York as the first Southerner ever asked to speak to the society. When asked what he was going to say, Grady had replied, "The Lord only knows. I have thought of a thousand things to say, five hundred of which if I say they will murder me when I get back home, and the other five hundred of which will get me murdered at the banquet." His task was complicated by the fact that his fellow speaker was the former Union General William T. Sherman, whose troops had burned Atlanta and much of the Deep South. He handled this by joking that Sherman was "considered an able man in our parts, though some people think he is a kind of careless man about fire." By the end of his presentation Grady had won over the Yankee audience, which "cheered through its tears."[21]

Grady's address is a moving and fervent story of the return home of the Confederate soldiers to a devastated land, and of how they and their descendants rallied to make a New South. He began:

> The picture of your returning armies of the North has been drawn for you by a Master hand . . . they come back to you, marching with a proud and victorious tread, reading their glory in a nation's eyes.
>
> But will you bear with me while I tell you the story of another army, that sought its home at the close of the late war—an army that marched home in defeat and not in victory, in pathos and not in splendor, but in glory equal to yours, and to hearts as loving as ever welcomed heroes home.
>
> Let me picture to you the foot sore Confederate Soldier as buttoning up in his faded gray jacket the parole which was to bear testimony to his children of his fidelity and faith, he turned his face Southward from Appomattox in April 1865: Think of him as ragged, half starved, heavy hearted, enfeebled by wants and wounds, having fought to exhaustion, he surrenders his gun, wrings the hand of his comrades in silence, then lifting his tear stained and pallid face for a last look at the graves which dot old Virginia's hills . . . he begins the slow and painful journey.
>
> What does he find . . . when . . . he reaches the home he left so prosper-

ous and beautiful? He finds his house in ruins, his farm devasted [*sic*], his slaves freed, his stock killed, his barns empty, his money worthless, his social system . . . in its magnificence swept away, his people without law or legal status, his comrades slain and the burden of others heavy on his shoulders . . . besides all this confronted with the gravest problem that ever met human intelligence, the establishment of a status for the vast body of his liberated slaves.

Grady asked, "What does he do, this hero in gray with a heart of gold? Does he sit down in sullenness and despair?"

No, not for a single day. Surely God who has stripped him of his prosperity inspired him in his adversity. As ruin was never before so overwhelming never was restoration swifter. The soldier stepped from the trenches into the furrow, horses that had charged federal guns marched before the plow, and fields that ran red with human blood in April were green with the harvest in June.

Since that time Grady said that the South has

found out that the free Negro counts for more than he did as a slave, we have planted the school-house on the hilltop and made it free to white and black. We have sown towns and cities in the place of theories, and put business above politics.

The New South is enamored of her new work. Her soul is stirred with a breath of new life. The light of a grand day is falling fair upon her face. She is thrilling with a consciousness of growing power and prosperity. As she stands upright . . . and equal among the people of the earth, breathing in the keen air, and looking out upon the expanding horizon, she understands that her emancipation came, because through the inscrutable wisdom of God her honest purposes were crossed and her brave armies beaten.

Grady concluded by calling for a land with "stately and enduring temples, its pillars founded in justice, its arches springing to the skies, its treasures filled with substance, liberty walking in the corridors, [and] religion filling the aisles with incense."

Berryhill's devotion to the Lost Cause of the Confederacy was manifested long after he had made a copy of Grady's address. In the 1940s and early 1950s Berryhill had a large Confederate flag hanging behind his desk in the dean's office. One weekend in the early 1950s, as the student body at the university was undergoing integration, the flag disappeared from the office. The students at the time speculated that some of their colleagues had removed it, but no one dared ask, and its presence in the dean's office was soon forgotten.[22] It is likely that he removed the flag in response to suggestions by faculty members, for it later hung on a wall in his home, according to one of the Berryhills' daughters.[23]

Benefits and Baggage from a Rural Southern Childhood in the Shadow of a City of the New South

When Berryhill left the security of Steele Creek for the challenges of life as a university student at Chapel Hill, he brought with him experiences and character traits that would serve him well in the years to come. He had a genuine interest in people and became a leader among his fellow students. His upbringing had given him the drive and patience that comes from hard work and delayed gratification in a farming community. His firsthand observations of birth, life, and death in farm animals, family, and neighbors would provide a smooth transition into the medical consideration of these same passages, and his sense of integrity would provide him with the moral backbone to pass up temptations that might otherwise have derailed his ambitions.

Like other Southerners of his era, however, Berryhill carried the burden of growing up at a time when the South was still struggling with the devastation of a vast Civil War that during 1861–1865 had laid waste to much of its territory and had killed a total of more than 600,000 Americans on both sides of the conflict. This casualty rate is the equivalent of more than six million wartime deaths in today's US population, or the same as one to two terrorist attacks on the scale of that seen on September 11, 2001, with 3,000 deaths each, every day for four years.

The Civil War had been closely followed by the political and personal tragedies of the postwar years. Abraham Lincoln in his second inauguration address in 1865 had called for a policy "with malice toward none, with charity for all." He was assassinated shortly thereafter, and the Republican Radicals in Congress imposed on the South a Reconstruction policy "that sought to recast the political and social order of the defeated South through direct military control, free elections and state-sponsored economic development."[24] While the Reconstruction effort itself lasted only twelve years, it and the resulting countermeasures by Southern whites affected the South for decades.[25]

At the beginning of the twentieth century, whites across the South reacted with measures that would take another half century even to begin to reverse. White-supremacy political campaigns resulted in the loss by most blacks of their right to vote through a combination of poll taxes and educational requirements. Jim Crow laws were enacted that mandated the segregation of the races in public areas and schools. A federal court ruling in 1896 had upheld state laws that mandated "equal but separate accommodations for the white and colored races," but it would not be until the 1950s that nationwide efforts began to ensure truly equal schooling for all.

Unlike the defeated Germans and Japanese after World War II, the South had no Marshall Plan. As a result, the South and its citizens—black and white alike—struggled for many decades after the Civil War to regain their place in the nation and the world. Gerald Johnson, a journalist and author, observed that the South that had in its earlier days provided the nation with the kind of leadership exemplified by Washington, Jefferson, and Madison was consumed, following the devastation of the Civil War and the chaos of Reconstruction, with "recapturing the leadership of the South itself, trying to sweep back the tide of demagogy, ignorance, stupidity and prejudice that the dynamiting of civilized government loosed upon the luckless country."[26] It also took many areas in the South almost until World War II to eradicate the so-called diseases of laziness—malaria, hookworm, and pellagra—that had chronically sapped the energy of so many Southerners over the years and further accentuated the poverty of those affected.[27] As late as 1938, more than seventy years after the conclusion of the Civil War, President Franklin D. Roosevelt proclaimed that "the South presents right now the Nation's No. 1 economic problem."[28]

Almost a century after the Civil War, the South finally began to catch up with other regions and then began to lead in some areas. Although educational, economic, political, and health changes fueled many of these gains, the post–War World II advances in modern air-conditioning technology played a critical role in making possible the Research Triangle Park, the research universities, the academic medical centers, and the high-tech manufacturing facilities in the "Sahara of the Bozart" (i.e., "Beaux-arts"), as H. L. Mencken described the South in 1917.[29]

Like many others growing up in the South in the first part of the twentieth century, Berryhill would never be able to dismiss these Civil War and Reconstruction stories and experiences from his mind or beliefs. As the years passed, however, he and most Southerners reluctantly accepted the changes that were demanded by the civil-rights movement, mandated by the courts, or enacted into law by Congress. For example, as dean he did not initially support integration of the UNC medical school student body, but he acquiesced once the first black medical student was admitted in 1951 at the insistence of the faculty (not in response to a court order, as in some other Southern schools and universities at the time).[30]

In the words of H. G. Jones concerning another North Carolina leader of this era, "He was, without apology, a man of his time. To attempt to judge our predecessors by the standards of today is to open ourselves to the unmerciful scorn of succeeding generations with standards as yet unimaginable."[31]

In his views on race and on politics, Berryhill was at opposite poles from his future colleague at the university, Frank Porter Graham. Graham, born in 1886, fourteen years earlier than Berryhill, had been raised in an era when the hope still existed that the races could be reconciled and when education was still perceived as the way to counter racial and class conflicts. Graham also grew up in towns where his father was the superintendent of public schools. Some of his earlier memories were of meetings where his father advocated public education before skeptical audiences of "independent farmers and store owners, short on money and long on self-reliance." In response to incredulous questions about his belief in "taxing the rich man to educate the poor man's children" or in "the white man [paying for the education of] the colored children," the senior Graham simply and firmly responded, "I believe in education of all the children, and that's what we have to do."[32] Frank Graham became a Southern liberal who was frequently ahead of his time and suffered for it. He was defeated for reelection to the United States Senate in 1950 in a bitter campaign against an opponent who used Graham's support of blacks and factory workers to introduce racial and class anxieties in white voters.[33] In contrast, Reece Berryhill grew up in the early 1900s in a rural area with farmers who were threatened by the rising ambitions of blacks and in an era when Jim Crow laws, white-supremacy campaigns, and disenfranchisement of blacks were sweeping through the South. Berryhill remained conservative in his political views throughout his life but did not let these skew his public pronouncements or positions.

While being exposed to the negative side of life in the South, both Berryhill and Graham experienced in Charlotte and elsewhere in the state the excitement and potential of the New South. This was a vision of hope and progress—based in railroads, industry, scientific agriculture, and universal education—that the South would be lifted from its depressed and devastated condition following the Civil War and Reconstruction. A 1902 promotional brochure about Charlotte captured the exuberance of the New South with its title: *Sketches of Charlotte: North Carolina's Finest City.* The brochure goes on to describe the city as the "Recognized Cotton Milling Centre of the Southern States . . . It Is the Finest Example in the South of the Thoroughly Progressive, Modern and Rapidly Growing City." A bar chart on the title page elaborated by showing the city's population growth, from 8,500 in 1880 to 15,000 in 1890 and 30,000 in 1902.[34]

In the years to come, Berryhill and Graham would unite their efforts to pursue the dream of a Good Health Movement to improve the health and happiness of the people of North Carolina and the New South.

Undergraduate, Teacher, and Medical Student

After spending his first seventeen years in rural Steele Creek, from 1917 to 1925 Berryhill expanded his horizons. During this time he spent four years as an undergraduate at Chapel Hill, one year teaching in a private preparatory school in Charlotte, another year serving as a principal and teaching in a public high school in Mecklenburg County, and two years back in Chapel Hill as a first- and second-year medical student. He excelled as a student and during this time began to show the leadership skills that would serve him well in his future career. These years also provided him the opportunity to become acquainted with those who would be future political, business, and medical leaders in North Carolina, contacts that would be invaluable when, as dean of the medical school, he sought support for the expansion and subsequent nurture of the medical school. It was also during these years that he met Norma May Connell, his future bride and active partner in helping fulfill his dream of better health for all North Carolinians.

UNDERGRADUATE AT CHAPEL HILL, 1917–1921

When Reece Berryhill arrived on the campus at Chapel Hill in the fall of 1917 as a freshman, he found a university that was on its way from being a cloistered state university with a distinctly local impact to being a university with regional, and eventually national, influence and recognition.[1]

The University of North Carolina had originally opened its doors in 1795 as the nation's first public university. By the time of the Civil War it had the largest student body of any university in the nation other than Yale. It reopened in 1875 after being closed several years during the early, chaotic days of Reconstruction following the Civil War. Under the successive leadership of presidents Kemp Plummer Battle (1876–1891), George Tayloe Winston (1891–1896), and Edwin A. Alderman (1896–1900), state appropriations were gradually increased (but were still far less than those of other leading state universities), the campus underwent some modest physical additions, the faculty was expanded, and the student body increased in number, though it remained predominantly

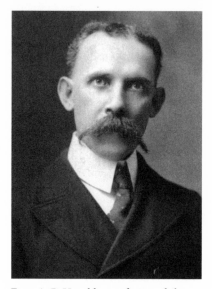

Francis P. Venable, professor of chemistry and UNC president from 1900 to 1914. *(NCC)*

male and North Carolinian. The university during these years—while attempting to remain nonsectarian and nonpolitical—had to fight off frequent attacks from politicians during the rapidly changing political climate in the post-Reconstruction years as well as from the supporters of the private denominational colleges, who did not want to see their tax money sustaining what they perceived as a competing and ungodly university.[2] The university lost federal land-grant funds to the new Agricultural and Mechanical College (later NC State University) that opened in Raleigh in 1889 and saw the beginning of other competition for state university funding with the opening in Greensboro of the State Normal and Industrial School for women (now UNC–Greensboro) in 1892 and the A&T College for blacks (now NC A&T University) in Greensboro in 1893.

A new era for the university began during the presidency of Francis P. Venable from 1900 to 1914. While continuing to teach chemistry, Venable emphasized the teaching and scholarship roles of the university. He restructured its administrative structure, recruited able faculty, and updated the curriculum for undergraduates and the professional schools. The annual state appropriation increased from $25,000 in 1901 to $95,000 by 1913. He was dedicated to the concept of the library as the heart of the university and recruited Louis Round Wilson to help achieve that goal. Through state appropriations and private donations, the campus saw the addition of a number of buildings, including the Carnegie Library (now Hill Hall, the music building); Caldwell Hall, the first structure designed solely for the medical school; a new chemistry building (now Howell Hall); a new student infirmary (now Abernethy Hall); a new biology building (now Davie Hall); a student dining hall (Swain Hall, known to the students as "Swine Hall"); and a three-sectioned dormitory building next to Franklin Street named Battle-Vance-Pettigrew.

Venable's focus was predominantly internal, but Edward Kidder Graham (president from 1914 to 1918) was a champion for education throughout the state and emphasized the role of the university in all of the affairs of the state. He was successful in increasing the state's annual operating appropriation to $215,000 by 1919 and in getting a six-year $500,000 bond issue for new buildings. During his tenure the largest donations ever received by a state university at the time came to UNC through the will of Mary Lily Kenan Flagler Bingham, who died in 1917. These funds were to provide the basis for the Kenan Professorships, which continue today to provide a means of recognizing and retaining distinguished professors at the university and of recruiting others from outside.

Life as an Undergraduate

Coming to Chapel Hill from Charlotte in September 1917 was not the speedy three-hour automobile trip along I-85 North and I-40 East that it is today. An increasing number of automobiles were being seen in the state's communities by 1917, but most intercity roads would remain unpaved until the 1920s, when Governor Cameron Morrison's Good Roads Movement followed Aycock's Good Schools Movement of the early 1900s as the second great movement of the twentieth century to benefit the citizens of the state. Morrison and his supporters successfully obtained bond issues for $65 million and built a system of more than 5,000 miles of modern highways for the state.[3] Prior to that time a trip by auto from Charlotte to Chapel Hill would have been challenging, to say the least.

Berryhill thus came by railroad from Charlotte to Durham and thence to University Station (between Durham and Chapel Hill), with several changes on the way. He made the final change at University Station to the "Chapel Hill Limited," which took him to the depot at Carrboro. There he and his classmates hired a horse-drawn carriage or perhaps a motorized hack to take them and their luggage to the dormitory.

Berryhill's first impressions of Chapel Hill as he rounded the corner from Carrboro would have been similar to those of Robert Burton House (a Carolina student in the class of 1916 who was to become the first chancellor of the university at Chapel Hill during the 1930s):

> As I saw Franklin Street in 1912, it was a dusty red avenue cut through a forest of magnificent trees. The road dipped through a valley [where later students would pass the bus station and Fowler's Grocery] and then rose [to the corner with Columbia], but the trees dominated the scene and obscured any buildings that then existed on that section of Franklin Street. My first impression of Chapel Hill was trees; my last impression is trees . . . It is no wonder that Chapel Hillians are ardent tree worshipers and that the symbol of the place is Davie Poplar.[4]

Of campus customs, House wrote: "Our dress was more conventional then than now [when he was writing in the 1960s]. Everyone wore a coat and hat. Everyone tipped his hat to a professor and received in return a tip of the professorial hat . . . I think it was Frank Graham who started the hatless age on campus in my generation. Frank had a fine shock of hair and a theory that going bareheaded would prevent baldness."

Facilities for UNC students in those days were primitive by today's standards. The dormitories had no hot water. Bathing facilities were located only in some of the buildings. The campus was predominantly male, with only a few female students in the professional schools and a few female undergraduates from Chapel Hill families. According to House, "It was good form to wrap a towel around your middle and, otherwise naked, to go down from your dormitory to the baths. Occasionally ladies would come on the campus. The old cry 'angels on the campus!' was not irreverence or satire. It was simply a warning to gentlemen in undress to duck."

House further observed:

About one-fourth of us were adequately financed [for college] . . . About [an additional] one-fourth were able to get along by strict economy and self-denial. The other half had to take advantage of every sort of job the community offered, and since such jobs were few, they also had to borrow from university loan funds or privately at home. Their education was never far above the bread and butter line. Usually incomplete preparation and incomplete financing coincided in the same person. He was doubly handicapped. And yet, as we stretched out on the academic course like runners in cross-country, it was wonderful to see doubly handicapped students, many of them, forge to the front and finish as leaders. The intangibles of brain and character are the secrets of the "quality education" we talk of so much today.

When Berryhill entered the university in the fall of 1917, his class of 1921 was 360 members strong. Four years later, a little over half that number graduated, "a percentage that would have been very good under entirely favorable circumstances," according to W. LeGette Blythe, the class historian writing in the student annual, the *Yackety Yack,* of 1921. Blythe characterized these four years as "of such intensity and soul-stirring effort that they might have been spread over a half century of ordinary time."[5] During this time America was involved in its first world war; some classmates had gone to fight in France, although most remained and joined the Student Army Training Corps (SATC); and a worldwide pandemic of influenza had stricken hundreds on the campus, with fatalities among students, staff, and faculty.

Looking back at their four years together, the class historian said they found the cause for "the deepest satisfaction" was "not in the number of students that under the most trying conditions have been able to finish with the class. It is, rather, in the fact that through our whole stay here we have been a united class. We very early began to get together, and each succeeding year has strengthened the ties that join us in common brotherhood—that of the Carolina man and the '21 man."

When Berryhill entered the university, it was still with the idea of becoming a minister, and he therefore initially concentrated on English, Latin, and Greek. He later recalled, "I thought all ministers should be well-grounded in the classics, but some time during my sophomore year, I realized my enthusiasm for the ministry was not as great as I thought. I looked around for another way to help people, but I simply cannot tell you why I chose medicine. I don't know." Interestingly enough, in his application to the Harvard Medical School in 1925 he stated that he had wanted to be a doctor since childhood.[6] He certainly saw this

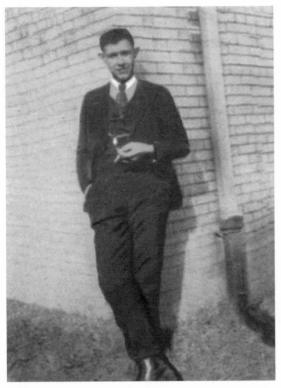

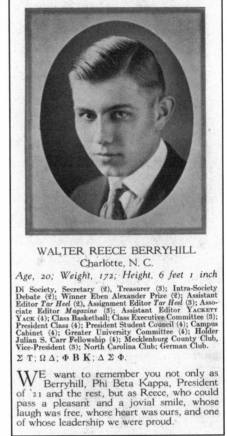

WALTER REECE BERRYHILL
Charlotte, N. C.

Age, 20; Weight, 172; Height, 6 feet 1 inch

Di Society, Secretary (2), Treasurer (3); Intra-Society Debate (2); Winner Eben Alexander Prize (2); Assistant Editor *Tar Heel* (2), Assignment Editor *Tar Heel* (3); Associate Editor *Magazine* (3); Assistant Editor YACKETY YACK (4); Class Basketball; Class Executive Committee (3); President Class (4); President Student Council (4); Campus Cabinet (4); Greater University Committee (4); Holder Julian S. Carr Fellowship (4); Mecklenburg County Club, Vice-President (3); North Carolina Club; German Club.

Σ Τ; Ω Δ; Φ Β Κ; Δ Σ Φ.

WE want to remember you not only as Berryhill, Phi Beta Kappa, President of '21 and the rest, but as Reece, who could pass a pleasant and a jovial smile, whose laugh was free, whose heart was ours, and one of whose leadership we were proud.

Reece Berryhill's senior class photographs and entry in the 1921 *Yackety Yack.* (NCC)

same statement in many medical school applications during his days as dean and must have had a knowing smile each time he read it.

It must have soon been clear to Berryhill that he had made the right choice in coming to Chapel Hill. It was apparent early on that he was to flourish throughout his undergraduate years both scholastically and in extracurricular activities. He was an excellent student, as documented by his election in the spring of his junior year to membership in Phi Beta Kappa. An examination of his academic record reveals that he did much better in English and the classics than he did in modern languages and the sciences. The record further shows that he—like many others before and since—may have studied less in the senior year than he had done in the previous years.

In his sophomore year he was awarded the Eben Alexander Prize for being the outstanding student of Greek in his class, although his career as a Greek scholar had some interesting twists. During the year he found himself the only student in the Greek class as others dropped the course or flunked out. Dr. "Bully" Bernard, the professor of Greek, said to Berryhill, "You're the only person in the class [which was the first class in the morning] and I'm getting to be an old man and don't like to get up early. So why don't you come to my house and we'll

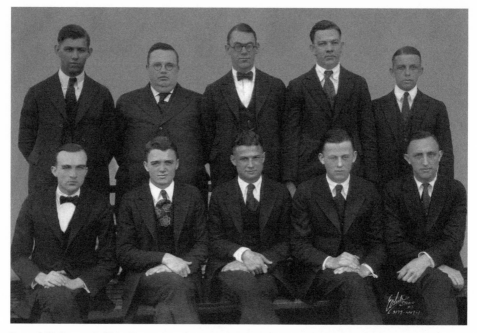

Berryhill *(upper left)* in Sigma Upsilon writing fraternity at UNC. *(Authors)*

hold class there." And so he did. But some time during the year Bernard was a little disappointed that Berryhill was not reading as much Greek as the professor thought he should. He cautioned Berryhill that even though he was the only student in the class and had so far done work that warranted the prize, he would not receive it unless he "straightened up" and improved his work. He must have done just that.[7]

Scholarship obviously did not require all of Berryhill's time. He was active in virtually all of the student organizations, including the *Tar Heel* (the student newspaper) and the student magazine. He was a member of his class basketball team in his junior year, as well as being a member of the German Club and of the Mecklenburg County Club. He held various elective class offices beginning in his sophomore year. During his last year he was president of the senior class and president of the student council. His classmates selected him as the "Best All 'Round" member of the class of 1921.

The stern façade that Berryhill presented to students and colleagues in later years was not formed in his undergraduate time at Chapel Hill. On the contrary, he was deemed by his fellow students to be a thoroughly outgoing and congenial colleague, as exemplified by what was written about him in the *Yackety Yack* in his senior year: "We want to remember you not only as Berryhill, Phi Beta Kappa, President of '21 and the rest, but as Reece, who could pass a pleasant and jovial smile, whose laugh was free, whose heart was ours and one of whose leadership we were proud." LeGette Blythe, a fellow Mecklenburger and an undergraduate classmate of Berryhill's, had great difficulty believing that the Reece

Berryhill he knew in those days was the no-nonsense, serious dean of whom medical students were deathly afraid only two decades later.[8]

Wartime and Postwar Adjustments at Chapel Hill

For almost two years after German armies invaded Belgium in August 1914 to start the Great War (later known as World War I), the university made only sporadic efforts to prepare itself and its students for war. This changed early in 1917, so that by the time the United States entered the conflict in April 1917, the campus was consumed with military activity. A battalion of some 500 students and professors began drilling five times a week. In May 1917, 65 of 161 seniors were allowed to graduate early so they could start US Army officers' training at Fort Oglethorpe, Georgia.[9]

As Berryhill and his fellow freshmen listened to President Edward Kidder Graham's address at the opening of the university on September 13, 1917, they were caught up in the fight for freedom that would radically change the campus over the next year. Graham reminded them of the duty of those at the university in those difficult times: "Our part, if truly conceived and heroically done, is as important, and I dare say as difficult, as that of the men in the trenches. In fact, the vision that they gladly die for, is simply this life of freedom left in trust to us, as trustees of the world's greatest vision, while they fight for its full preservation." In another address Graham described the war as a fight between the American vision of freedom and the German vision of carrying out its policies through the "blood and iron" approach advocated earlier by the despotic Bismarck: "It is now a clear fight to a finish, and without quarter, between national self-government and military despotism, humanity and Germanity, for the liberty of the human race and the whole trend of international and civilized evolution."

Berryhill's freshman year at Carolina saw a continuing buildup of military training and activities on the campus. Some 250 outmoded Civil War rifles were obtained from a donor for drilling purposes, and 50 Springfield rifles were obtained from the Department of the Navy for target practice. At the edge of the campus near Battle Park a system of trenches with barbed wire and machine-gun nests were prepared so that the student battalion could participate in simulated attacks by the enemy. A number of the faculty volunteered for military service or served as consultants to the federal government in areas such as chemical warfare. A Reserve Officers Training Corps (ROTC) program was established in June 1918, and that summer the university sponsored a military training program in Asheville for boys from sixteen to eighteen years of age.

The most profound change in the campus came after August 1918, when the War Department issued General Order 79 establishing Student Army Training Corps (SATC) on more than 500 campuses, including the University of North Carolina. UNC President Graham was designated as the director of the SATC programs on college campuses in five states in the South Atlantic division. With

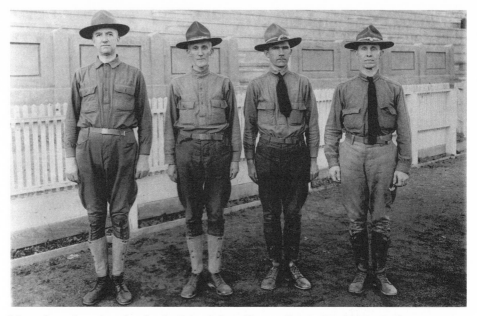

Not only students but also faculty joined the military effort in World War I. Shown at Emerson Stadium are physics professor Andrew H. Patterson, anatomy and physiology professor Charles S. Mangum, engineering and mathematics professor T. Felix Hickerson, and pathology professor James B. Bullitt. *(NCC)*

this program "the University became officially a part of the Nation's Armed Services, and the student-soldier-to-be of 1918, unlike the student-soldier-to-be of 1861, retained his books, donned his uniform, and began his service to his country within the campus walls instead of dropping his books and rushing from the campus to the battle front."

When Berryhill and his fellow students returned to class in the fall of 1918, they found that "the campus has become a military camp, the dormitories are barracks, the dining hall, a mess hall." All student members of the military corps were equipped and maintained as regular members of the armed services. They were subject to military discipline and had a rigid schedule that began with reveille at 6:15 A.M. and ended with taps at 10:00 P.M. Three hours weekly of military subjects were added to the curriculum, as well as eleven hours weekly of military drill.

Many graduates and some undergraduates went on active duty, and many were in France. Most of the remaining eligible college students were organized into four army companies of 160 men each. Berryhill and his classmate Ben Cone, of Greensboro, were privates in a small Marine Corps group commanded by First Lieutenant R. F. Boyd.[10] While other students went to Plattsburgh Barracks, New York, for military training in the summer of 1918, Berryhill and the Marine Corps group went to the Georgia Institute of Technology in Atlanta.

With the signing of the armistice in France on November 11, 1918, and the cessation of hostilities, the SATC was demobilized almost as fast as it had been organized. This was accomplished by December 10. During the remaining ten days before Christmas holidays started, the students and faculty reorganized as a university campus. Class officers were elected, campus organizations were reactivated, and the university prepared for the return of those students who had gone to training camps or overseas.

Berryhill's sophomore year of 1918–1919 was thus one of marked contrasts. In the fall his class had experienced "the nightmare of the S.A.T.C. [and] the old 'Carolina Spirit' that we had learned to cherish the year before was 'nil.' Everything was demoralized and 2nd lieutenants from Maine and Georgia were sent to plague us."

When Berryhill and his fellow sophomores returned in early 1919 after the Christmas holiday, they "were astonished and delighted to find that Carolina was not completely dead in spirit, and at once we set out to build up with the little life that remained a strong and vigorous vitality. Studies were resumed and student activities came in for their place in normal university life. Baseball, basketball, and track started off with renewed life, and the intercollegiate triangular debates were continued." During Berryhill's junior year extracurricular activities at Chapel Hill included a rapprochement between the fraternity and non-fraternity men on campus and "wonderful success in the various intercollegiate contests" with championships in football, baseball, and track and with victories in debating against Johns Hopkins and Virginia.

The senior year began on the previous spring's Class Day, when the president of the graduating class of 1920 "turned over to us the campus with the admonition to transmit it as good and even better than it was when we received it." After "Berryhill [as senior class president of the class of 1921] had given our pledge and had accepted it in the name of the Class of 1921 we marched away from Old Davie Poplar as the masters and guardians of the 'Hill.'" The senior year passed swiftly, and sooner than they wished they were alumni of the University of North Carolina.[11]

The Influenza Pandemic of 1918–1919

In the fall of 1918 the Great War was winding down in Europe, but a new disaster was already striking the world.[12] The first wave of the flu pandemic began in early spring of 1918. Because Spain was a neutral country in the war and had no press censorship, publicity about the flu in Spain convinced others that it began there. The entire outbreak thus became known as the Spanish flu, much to the dismay of the Spanish. Although the first wave of flu in Europe and America was highly contagious and temporarily debilitating, little mortality was associated with it. The second phase, however, which appeared in the late summer and fall, spread rapidly around the world and was both highly contagious and lethal. It was estimated that 20 to 40 million people worldwide were killed by the flu, far more than were killed in the war. More Americans—some 600,000—died from the 1918 flu than died in all of the nation's twentieth-century wars. It was a particularly virulent strain of flu that was more likely to cause deaths in the twenty- to forty-year-old age group, in contrast to the usual seasonal influenza, which was more deadly in the young and the elderly. Those with what appeared to be an "ordinary" case of the flu could develop fulminating respiratory failure due to viral or a secondary bacterial pneumonia, become cyanotic, and suffocate while physicians and nurses looked on helplessly. Recent studies have suggested that the high mortality rate in young and otherwise healthy adults may have been related to the overly vigorous response of their immune system to the invading virus, drowning the patient in a reaction that was supposed to be protective.

One of the first and hardest hit American sites in early September was Camp Devens, west of Boston. Some 50,000 troops were stationed there and the hospital, built to hold 2,000, was soon teeming with 8,000 patients, with some 100 deaths a day. The US Surgeon General sent a visiting team of distinguished physicians to investigate the epidemic. One remembered "hundreds of stalwart young men in the uniform of their country coming into the wards of the hospital in groups of ten or more. They are placed in cots until every bed is full yet others crowd in. Their faces soon wear a bluish cast; a distressing cough brings up the blood stained sputum. In the morning the dead bodies are stacked about the morgue like cord wood." With the horrors of modern war vividly in his mind, this physician was awed by "the deadly influenza virus" that "demonstrated the inferiority of human inventions in the destruction of human life."[13] When the distinguished pathologist, bacteriologist, and former dean of the Johns Hopkins Medical School, William Henry Welch, MD, performed an autopsy on one of the soldiers, another member of the physician team observed: "When the chest was opened and the blue, swollen lungs were removed and opened, and Dr. Welch saw the wet, foamy surfaces with little real consolidation, he turned and said, 'This must be some new kind of infection or plague,' and he was quite excited and obviously very nervous . . . It was not surprising that the rest of us were disturbed, but it shocked me to find that the situation, momentarily at least, was too much even for Dr. Welch."[14]

Thomas Wolfe was in UNC's class of 1920, a year ahead of Berryhill. In *Look Homeward, Angel,* Wolfe's largely autobiographical first novel, published in 1929, the Asheville writer vividly portrayed the tragic impact of the influenza on one North Carolina family.[15] The protagonist, Eugene Gant, was a student at the state's university at Pulpit Hill in the fall of 1918. In October he received a letter from his mother, Eliza:

Daisy has been here with all her tribe. She went home two days ago, leaving Caroline and Richard. They have all been down sick with the flu. We've had a siege of it here. Everyone has had it, and you never know who's going to be next. It seems to get the big strong ones first. Mr. Handy, the Methodist minister, died last week. Pneumonia set in. He was a fine healthy man in the prime of life. The doctors said he was gone from the start.

Not long afterward, Eugene returned to his dormitory room one evening to find a telegram: "Come home at once. [Your older brother] Ben has pneumonia. Mother." Eugene took the next available train from Exeter (Durham) and was met at the Altamont (Asheville) station early the next morning. As the auto speeded home in the dark, he learned of Ben's illness. He had caught the flu, apparently from one of Daisy's children, was "ill and feverish" for a day or so without going to bed, but then was in bed a day or two before the doctor allowed him to get up. After a day he returned to bed with a high fever. By the time Eugene arrived, "Ben had been desperately ill, with pneumonia in both lungs, for over a day."

After greeting his parents, Eugene quietly ascended the stairs to enter the sickroom.

> For a moment Eugene could see nothing, for dizziness and fear . . . Then, under the terrible light which fell directly and brutally upon the bed alone, he saw Ben. And in that moment of searing recognition he saw, what they had all seen, that Ben was dying.
>
> Ben's long thin body . . . was bitterly twisted below the covers, in an attitude of struggle and torture . . . the sallow yellow of his face had turned gray; out of this granite tint of death, lit by two red flags of fever, the stiff black furze of a three-day beard was growing . . . Ben's thin lips were lifted, in a constant grimace of torture and strangulation . . . as inch by inch he gasped a thread of air into his lungs. And the sound of this gasping—loud, hoarse, rapid, unbelievable, filling the room, and orchestrating every moment in it—gave to the scene its final note of horror.

Within twenty-four hours after Eugene's arrival, Ben's struggle for breath and life ended, and "he passed instantly, scornful and unafraid, as he had lived, into the shades of death."

The final edition of the *Journal of the American Medical Association* for 1918 commented on the reversal of priorities for physicians that had suddenly occurred by the end of the year:

> The year 1918 has gone: a year momentous as the termination of the most cruel war in the annals of the human race; a year which marked the end, at least for a time, of man's destruction of man; unfortunately a year in which developed a most fatal infectious disease causing the death of hundreds of thousands of human beings. Medical science for four and one-half years devoted itself to putting men on the firing line and keeping them there. Now it must turn with its whole might to combating the greatest enemy of

all—infectious disease. In this battle there must be no armistice; no peace without victory.[16]

Berryhill and his fellow students felt the impact of the pandemic when more than 500 victims of the flu filled the infirmary and the dormitories after the first case appeared on October 1—the day President Graham had led the ceremony inducting 650 UNC students into the SATC. The student military corps was soon quarantined by William de Berniere MacNider, MD, medical school faculty member and chief medical officer of the corps. On October 7 the newly formed County Board of Health ordered the closure of all public meeting places in order to control the spread of the infection. By the time the influenza was over, the university had lost three students, two women serving as nurses for the students, President Graham, and his replacement, Marvin H. Stacy.[17]

Berryhill escaped the extreme clutches of the influenza, but the experience of this overwhelming pandemic had a lifelong and humbling impact on future physicians and nonmedical persons alike.

University Presidents, Faculty, and Students

Berryhill's class was fortunate in being exposed to an outstanding group of faculty and university leaders during their four years at Chapel Hill. During their freshman year, "We sat in chapel and listened to the counsels of President Graham, Dean Stacy, and our beloved 'Old Pres' Battle, and we shall always love the memory of these three and shall never forget what a privilege we enjoyed in having them with us that first year."[18]

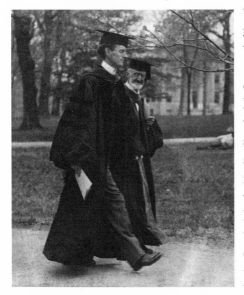

UNC President Edward Kidder Graham and former president Kemp P. Battle in an academic procession in the spring of 1917. Berryhill and his classmates affectionately called Battle "Old Pres." *(NCC)*

In President Edward Kidder Graham students were exposed to a man whose "flower-like frailty of his physique" was contrasted with "the reasoned solidity of his convictions," according to one observer.[19] Louis Round Wilson, university librarian and historian, summarized Graham's unique contribution as university president: "Within a swiftly passing half-decade, in spite of frailness of body and the turmoil of war, he transformed a previously cloistered institution into one fired with the creative spirit of scholarly attainment and beneficent service."[20] At the same time he always reminded the students and faculty that the campus should be "co-extensive with the boundaries of the State" and that the university, "while keeping the standards of university instruction and scholarly research on the highest plane," should be "in warm, sensitive touch with every problem in North Carolina life, small and great."[21] Berryhill's later service to the people of his state would be a lasting testimony to Graham's belief in the role of the university in the state.

Dean Marvin H. Stacy was a North Carolinian who was educated at UNC and Cornell and was appointed professor of civil engineering in 1910. Berryhill and his classmates knew him as the dean of the College of Liberal Arts, which carried with it responsibility for both academic leadership and student discipline. For a brief period after Graham's untimely death, Stacy also served as chairman of the faculty and acting president. According to Wilson, "The faculty found him to be an inspiring academic leader of wide, clear vision, and the students a teacher and guide from whom they invariably received understanding and fair judgment."[22]

Former President Kemp Battle, who had reopened the university in 1875 and who had written the two-volume definitive history of the early years of the university after his retirement, was a favorite of the class. The death of the "Old Pres" on February 4, 1919, shortly following the death from flu of President Graham on October 26, 1918, and Dean Stacy's passing from flu on January 21, 1919, "cast a gloom over the whole campus."[23]

During the class of 1921's last two years, the university was led by Harry Woodburn Chase, a New Englander who had served as a faculty member in the Department and School of Education since 1910. He was appointed president in June 1919 and served until 1930. During this time, "the University, building on the solid foundations laid by his predecessors, completed its transition from college to well-rounded university, a fact which was formally recognized on November 11, 1922, when the University was admitted into the Association of American Universities—an Association which at that date consisted of twenty-four of the leading universities of the nation."[24] President Chase, in a talk during the class smoker at the Carolina Inn just before Christmas of their senior year, reminded the class of 1921 of their unique role in the university's history: "Your class is the connecting link between the old University and the new."

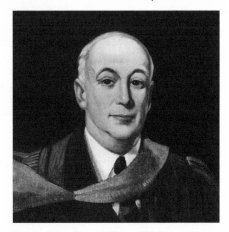

In addition to being exposed to some remarkable faculty and university leaders, Berryhill's fellow students in the class of 1921 proved to be a remarkably talented group of future leaders for the state. The citation for Berryhill's Tar Heel of the Week recognition by the *Raleigh News and Observer* in 1950 enumerated his accomplishments as a student at Chapel Hill and said he "accomplished these things despite the fact he was traveling in some of the fastest company the

Harry Woodburn Chase, UNC president from 1919 to 1930. *(NCC)*

college campus has ever seen . . . [including] among others . . . such Tar Heel leaders of today as W. H. Ruffin, president of Erwin Mills; J. C. Cowan, president of Burlington Mills; W. D. Carmichael, Jr., controller and acting president of the university; playwright Paul Green; editor [of the *News and Observer*] Jonathan Daniels; T. J. Wilson, III, formerly director of the University Press and now director of the Harvard Press; W. H. Bobbitt, superior court judge; and the late J. W. Erwin, former Congressman." As a result, the reporter noted, Berryhill "now has friends in almost every county of the State. As his work requires a lot of travel, these friendships afford him a great deal of pleasure as well as an invaluable assistance in his job."[25] In later years three university buildings would be named for members of the class of 1921: Berryhill Hall on the medical campus, Carmichael Auditorium, and the Paul Green Theatre.

NORMA MAY CONNELL

In the fall of 1919 Berryhill made a trip to Raleigh that would positively affect the remainder of his life. He went there to see Carolina play State in football. Afterward he went over to Peace College to visit Grace McNinch, a friend from Charlotte. It turned out that Miss McNinch was occupied, so he was introduced to Norma May Connell, a student from Warrenton, North Carolina.

She later recalled that they spent their time together seated in the Peace College Chapel—she in front and he behind her in the old-fashioned student desks.

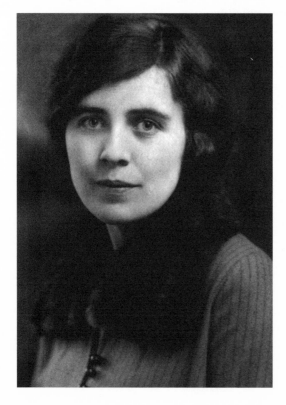

They attempted, with varying degrees of success, to carry on a conversation. Berryhill, in an effort to demonstrate his worldliness, derived from his exposure to Professor Horace Williams, finally asked her if she thought that God was able to fry an egg on a snowball. This apparently blasphemous question from her new acquaintance shocked Connell, the president of the YWCA at Peace and a religious traditionalist.

Nevertheless, an immediate attraction between the two must have developed that afternoon, because they remained in touch and continued to see one another occasionally. When Berryhill returned to Chapel Hill as a medical student in 1923, Connell entered the

Norma May Connell of Warrenton, North Carolina, late 1920s. *(Berryhill Family)*

junior class at the University of North Carolina. They saw one another, although infrequently during his rigorous first year of medical school. During his second year they spent more time together, taking long walks and conversing in the university library, where Berryhill came every day with supper to read the newspapers.[26]

At some point along the way, friendship became romance. They continued to keep in touch while Berryhill was in medical school at Harvard from 1924 to 1926; during his medicine residency in Boston from 1926 to 1929; practicing outside Charlotte in the summer of 1929; and when Berryhill came back to Chapel Hill during the academic year 1929–1930 as a substitute instructor in physiology while the chair of the department recuperated from an illness. After an eleven-year acquaintance and courtship, they would be married in Warrenton in August 1930 and move to Cleveland to begin their life together.

Teaching in Charlotte, 1921–1923

The Elysian undergraduate days at Chapel Hill came to an end in June 1921. By then Berryhill fully realized that he was to be a physician, but he also knew that his plans had to be delayed so that he could fulfill an obligation he had incurred as an undergraduate. Free tuition at that time was "given to candidates for the ministry, to the sons of ministers, to young men under bodily infirmity, to teachers, and to young men preparing to teach," all by an act of the 1887 legislature. Those preparing to teach were obligated "to teach in North Carolina for at least two years after leaving the University."[27]

Berryhill returned to his hometown of Charlotte to hold up his end of the exchange. In 1921–1922 he taught and was assistant superintendent at Major Baird's Academy, a private high school in Charlotte. During 1922–1923 he taught and was principal of Big Springs High School in Mecklenburg County.[28]

While fulfilling his teaching obligations in Charlotte, Berryhill made many friends who much later would be of great aid to him as dean of the medical school at Chapel Hill. He also had the opportunity to see many old friends as well as Norma Connell, who was working before entering UNC in 1923.

Medical Student at Chapel Hill, 1923–1925

Apparently UNC's was the only medical school to which Berryhill applied. Because of his outstanding undergraduate record, his application was undoubtedly approved shortly after being received by Dean Isaac Hall Manning. Upon returning to Chapel Hill in the fall of 1923 he was accompanied by his younger brother, William Scott Berryhill, who was beginning his junior year as an undergraduate.

Much of his time during the two years in medical school at Chapel Hill was spent in Caldwell Hall, the medical school building, completed in 1912 and

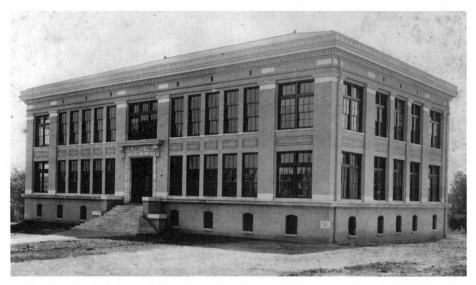

Caldwell Hall, which housed the School of Medicine on the main campus from 1912 to 1939. Berryhill was a student in this building from 1923 to 1925. He taught here in 1929–1930 and then from 1933 until the School of Medicine moved to its new building in 1939. *(NCC)*

named for the first president of the university. The undergraduates seemed to hold the medical school in awe: a large photograph of Caldwell Hall in the 1925 *Yackety Yack* was captioned, "Here are taught the infinite wonders of the human microcosm."[29]

Large laboratories were located in Caldwell Hall on each of two floors and could accommodate about forty students; one lab was designed for microscopic work, while the other provided equipment for experimental physiology, experimental pharmacology, and physiological chemistry. The first floor of a wing on the south side of the building provided a lecture room for about seventy-five students and a library containing some 1,200 bound volumes of medical journals and a number of books on clinical medicine donated by North Carolina physicians. The second floor had a dissecting hall for anatomy instruction. A few small laboratories and offices were available for the use of the eight professors and associate professors whose primary appointments were in the medical school.[30]

Berryhill and his thirty-eight fellow first-year students spent mornings from Monday through Saturday and four or five afternoons a week in lectures and laboratories. Gross and microscopic anatomy consumed the lion's share of the 720 hours of work required in the first year. Berryhill's transcript shows that during the first year of medical school in 1923–1924, he received an A in bacteriology with a P (passing) in applied anatomy, gross anatomy, histology, embryology, pharmacy, and neurology.[31] The "neurology" course was "a special laboratory study of the gross and microscopic anatomy of the cord and encephalon . . . with numerous prepared dissections of the human brain." This study was followed by a dissection of a brain by a group of four students and then by "a practical examination [to test] the student's ability to locate the various tracts and nuclei."[32]

By the second year his class had been diminished to thirty-six students. In the second year he received an A in physiology, immunology, pathology, pharmacology, minor surgery, hygiene, and toxicology, while receiving a B in physiologic chemistry and physical diagnosis.[33]

The intensity and variety of the instruction Berryhill and his fellow medical students received is illustrated by the 250 hours they had in bacteriology and immunology. A new associate professor, Daniel Allan MacPherson, PhD, a native of Rhode Island who had studied at Brown University, the University of Chicago, and the Rockefeller Institute, taught both courses. As later described by MacPherson, the "facilities were spartan by present standards consisting of a small office, a class laboratory and a sterilizer cubby hole in the second floor of old Caldwell Hall . . . The dirt floor basement served as animal quarters for experimental and class rabbits, guinea pigs and three sheep . . . The sea of mud then prevailing on unpaved Cameron Avenue in wet weather led the students to wear army hobnailed boots. The cacophony of sound on the old wooden floors when classes changed was deafening."[34]

The bacteriology course was five afternoons a week in the third quarter of the first year. As described in the university catalogue for 1923–1924, "The major portion of the course is devoted to the detailed study of the pathogens. Unknown mixtures are used to test the student's ability to differentiate organisms of the various groups. Practical applications of bacteriology in the diagnosis of disease are stressed by the examination of sputa, pus, feces, and blood. Animal inoculations are made to demonstrate the processes of infection and the differentiation of certain organisms."[35]

The immunology course was three afternoons a week in the first quarter of the second year. According to the catalogue course description,

Practical training is given in the production and use of agglutinins, precipitins, lysins, and complement fixing antibodies. Vaccines are prepared, and their use demonstrated. The preparation and standardization of antimicrobic and antitoxin sera is studied. Anaphylaxis and allergy are produced in animals, and methods of diagnosis and desensitization practiced. The student is required to prepare his own materials, and to inject and bleed animals himself. Special attention is given to the use of these principles in the diagnosis of blood stains; blood grouping; typhoid fever; typhus fever; diphtheria; tuberculosis; hay fever; gonorrhea; and syphilis. Unknown specimens test the student's ability to use the reactions.

A former student remembered, "Dr. MacPherson repeatedly emphasized that bacteriology was 'the most important course' for would-be physicians—saying that infectious disease was the physician's chief problem." Other students, who had transferred elsewhere for their clinical years, later commented that their instruction in bacteriology and immunology at UNC under Dr. MacPherson was equal to, or far superior to, the instruction their classmates had received in some very well recognized medical schools.[36]

Clinical instruction was minimal in the second year because of the small population of Chapel Hill at the time and the lack of a medical facility other than the small student infirmary. Minor surgery, a course of four hours a week in the winter quarter for a total of 44 hours, included lectures on "the method of the treatment of wounds, the dislocations, fractures, and some of the more common surgical conditions." The laboratory sessions allowed the student to learn the techniques of bandaging and provided the "opportunity to practice some of the amputations and resections of joints on the cadaver." The course on physical diagnosis occupied a similar number of hours in the final spring quarter. This

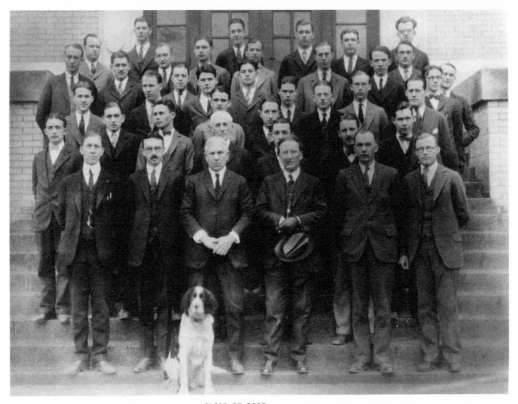

CLASS OF 1925

MEMBERS: C.W.Ashburn, C.H.Ashford, P.L.Barnes, W.R.Berryhill, C.A.Boseman, J.A.Bradley, E.H.Brown, E.E.Covington, S.W.Davis, H.F.Easom, R.L.Felton, Jr., J.R.Grigg, J.O.Haizlip, J.C.Holloway, J.H.Hunt, A.H.London, Jr., T.D.MacRae,Jr., J.McG. McAnally, C.M.McCoy, W.J.Martin,Jr., E.B.Mewborne, C.G.Milham, J.L.Miller, T.Mitchell, L.T.Morton, Z.B.Newton, R.B.Nye, D.P.Ross, T.W.Ross, P.F.Smith, W.G.Smith, H.V.Staton, R.T.Stimpson, W.T.Tice, J.H.Wall.

Faculty and members of the medical school class of 1925. Berryhill is third from the right in the top row. *(NCC)*

was described as "a brief course in the methods of physical examination, largely of the normal person. As far as possible, abnormal heart and lung cases will be submitted for examination."[37] Berryhill supplemented the clinical instruction at UNC by working summers "with two of the leading internists in Charlotte."[38]

In medical school Berryhill continued his outstanding undergraduate record in both scholarship and leadership. During his second year he served as president of the medical student body (the Whitehead Society).

Just as he had been exposed as an undergraduate to some of the giants of university history, Berryhill as a medical student learned from, and became friends with, some of the giants of medical school history. These included Isaac Hall Manning, MD, professor of physiology and dean; Charles Staples Mangum, MD, professor of anatomy; James Bell Bullitt, MD, professor of pathology; and William de Berniere MacNider, MD, Kenan Research Professor of Pharmacology.

Medical school did not permit the wide variety of extracurricular activity that engaged him as an undergraduate. He did have time, however, to see more of Norma Connell. Also, during both of his first two years in medical school Berryhill was a member of Phi Chi,[39] a medical fraternity that had been founded at Louisville Medical School in 1893. Although he was undoubtedly loyal to his fraternity, when he was dean in the mid-1950s his membership did not sway his judgment about a Phi Chi matter. Two Phi Chi members were selected to approach the dean and ask him to approve their plan to secure a fraternity house "outside of the jurisdiction of the university authorities so that our efforts at entertaining, rest, and relaxation would in no way be inhibited." They met during a break in classes with Dean Berryhill, whom they described as "very cordial." As he sat behind his desk, they presented their plan, emphasizing that they would not live away from the school and hospital, but rather use this facility on weekends as a place to "socialize and be together." Dean Berryhill listened intently, his ever-present cigarette dangling from his lower lip. When they finished their presentation, he got up out of his chair and walked to one side of the room. He then did an about-face and, looking straight at the two students, said:

> This won't wash and I will tell you why. The University, the faculty of this Medical School and your parents have invested much time and effort on your behalf. They all admire you and look forward to your success as physicians. What you have presented is a ticket to disaster and we cannot participate in such folly. I have walked in your shoes and can understand your wishes. But you must remember that this School's responsibility and mine as its administrator is to continue to provide a proper atmosphere for you to complete your medical education. This idea does not fit into that mold. Good day, gentlemen. It has been a good session for us all.

So the embryonic plan for a Phi Chi "party house" in the 1950s was stillborn.[40]

When Berryhill left Chapel Hill in the spring of 1925, he was faced with an exciting but somewhat daunting prospect. Rather than returning to the comfort of his home community, as he did upon graduating in 1921, he would be moving to faraway Boston and entering the world-famous Harvard Medical School.

Harvard, UNC, and Western Reserve

The years 1925 to 1933 were crucial years for Berryhill both professionally and personally. After growing up in a rural community and spending the first twenty-five years of his life in North Carolina, he had the opportunity to live and work in two large cities—one in New England and one in the Midwest. His clinical education and further maturation as a physician occurred at one of the outstanding medical schools of his time—the Harvard Medical School and the Harvard Medical Service at Boston City Hospital. Furthermore, he had a valuable introduction to academic medicine in three settings: observing the workings of the Harvard Medical School and its affiliated hospitals in Boston from the perspective of a student and then as an intern; teaching physiology for an academic year as a temporary instructor at his alma mater at Chapel Hill; and serving in his first regular position as a faculty member at the Western Reserve University Medical School in Cleveland. It was also during this time that Berryhill and Norma Connell were married in 1930 and that their first child, Jane, was born in 1933.

MEDICAL STUDENT AT HARVARD

During Berryhill's second year in medical school at UNC, he applied for admission to the third-year classes at both the Harvard Medical School and the University of Pennsylvania Medical School and had transcripts of his grades sent from the university to both.[1]

The medical schools in Philadelphia were very popular with UNC transfer students, and Berryhill and several of his classmates were accepted at the University of Pennsylvania for the last two years of their medical education. Norma Berryhill later said that as he neared the completion of his second year at UNC, however, Berryhill became increasingly concerned because his Pennsylvania-bound classmates were partying so much. Worried that this would interfere with his performance in medical school, he took the problem to Dean Manning, who was sympathetic. After some discussion, the dean asked Berryhill if he would like to go to Harvard. Berryhill reacted positively, whereupon Dean

Manning proceeded to see if he could arrange for his transfer. Within a few days he informed Berryhill that he had been successful: Berryhill was accepted for admission to Harvard as a third-year student.[2]

According to Berryhill's records at Harvard, he was highly recommended. In a letter dated April 8, 1925, to Assistant Dean Worth Hale at Harvard, Dean Manning wrote: "I am very glad you will give us one place in your third year class. I have no hesitation in recommending W. R. Berryhill who has a Phi Beta Kappa record in our university and has done equally high-grade work with us in medical school." Berryhill's Harvard transcript also quotes MacNider as having said that Berryhill was "among the best students I have taught for the last 25 years."[3]

Berryhill's application for admission to the junior year at the Harvard Medical School had been received there two months earlier, but apparently had not been acted upon until Dean Manning's letter was received. In his own handwriting, Berryhill had this to say about why he wanted to study medicine:

It is often a difficult matter to choose one's life work, and then perhaps still more difficult to know, after the choice has been made, just why one decided upon that particular profession.

The most worthwhile reason . . . [for] studying medicine is simply this—I have never wanted to do anything else. Even as a boy my imagination never had me doing anything except "being a doctor," and later I came to feel that I could only be satisfied in studying and practicing medicine. So in the first place, I want to study medicine because I know it is the one thing in life, in the continued study and practice of which, I shall be personally satisfied.

Medicine, with all its as yet unknown and undiscovered fields, offers the possibility of exploring these unknown branches, a potential adventure as thrilling as any in history. Then, too, it stimulates the ambition to find out the *truth* about so many things about [which] we have now only a vague idea.

In the study and practice of medicine one is assured of a life that will never become monotonous, for with the constant uncertainties, the unexpected-ness, the infinite varieties of disease, and the ever increasing discover[ie]s in medical science, each day will hold some new adventure.

Finally, every one wishes to do something worthwhile in life in aiding humanity, and to have that feeling of personal happiness that comes from the knowledge of having helped others. Medicine offers this opportunity, and trite as it may sound, the ideal of service influenced me to choose medicine as a profession.

As noted in the previous chapter, Berryhill's decision about medicine had actually occurred after he started college. His assertion of a longtime interest in medicine was an embellishment, but one practiced by many medical school applicants before and after him.

Another letter in Berryhill's file at Harvard was from James B. Bullitt, MD, chair of pathology at UNC, who wrote on May 15 in response to Dean Hale's inquiry concerning the clinical pathology training Berryhill had at UNC:

In our two year medical course we do not give a course in Clinical Pathology. Some of the content of such a course is covered in our courses in Bacteriology, Serology, Pathology and Physiological Chemistry; e.g. the examination of tuberculous sputum, the typing of pneumococci, the typing of blood, the ordinary chemical examination of urine, the study of malarial blood. However the amount of time devoted to such procedures is not as much as would be required in any really good regular course in Clinical Pathology; moreover some things covered in such a course, such as intestinal parasites, are barely touched upon in our courses . . . Mr. Berryhill is a capable man; he has had good preliminary training; he is very industrious and thoughtful. He made a high record in his academic work and he has done equally well in his first two years of medical work. I am confident that you will find him well worthy of entrance into your third year class, although it will be necessary for him to make up some of the work that you give in the second year but which we do not give."

To another inquiry from Dean Hale concerning course content at UNC, Dean Manning responded on July 16: "Our course in physical diagnosis is given

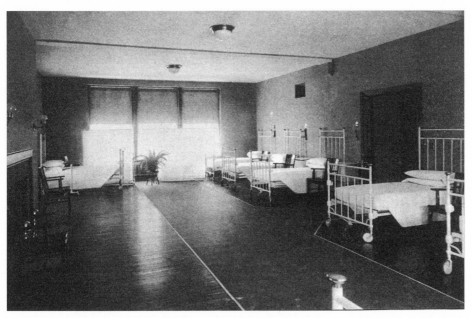

A ward at Huntington Memorial Hospital, where Berryhill and other students transferring into the third year at Harvard sharpened their skills in physical diagnosis and clinical pathology during the summer of 1925. (Parkins, *The Harvard Medical School and Its Clinical Opportunities*, 1916)

largely on the normal, four hours a week for ten weeks. The professor who gives this course is also Physical [?Physician] Director of the University and he has the class do quite a little work in connection with his general work."

Berryhill recalled years later:

> It was necessary to report to Boston for the summer months [of 1925] in order to become better prepared in physical diagnosis and clinical pathology. This was not an unusual requirement for students from the two-year schools at that time. Along with several other transfer students from two-year schools, I spent a profitable and enjoyable summer at the Huntington Hospital [a cancer hospital founded in the early 1900s] under the superb instruction of Dr. Raphael Isaacs, who was assisted by several medical residents.[4]

In spite of his busy schedule as a medical student at Harvard, Berryhill wrote regular letters to Norma Connell. She said later that he liked it so much, "he thought he had landed in Heaven." He was also pleasantly surprised to see how well prepared he was in comparison to other students. Norma related an interesting sidelight on Berryhill's years at Harvard. MacNider, who had many contacts in Boston, had written a number of letters of introduction to Harvard professors on Berryhill's behalf. Years later, after her husband's death, Norma found these letters untouched among his belongings. Evidently he had wanted to be successful on his own, without outside help.[5]

Harvard Medical School

Harvard Medical School opened in 1783 as the third medical school in the United States, following the establishment in 1765 of what is now the University of Pennsylvania Medical School and in 1768 of what is now the Columbia University College of Physicians and Surgeons. In those days the medical curriculum consisted of a year or more of didactic lectures, followed by apprenticeship with local physicians in practice.

Harvard Medical School was initially located on the Harvard campus in Cambridge, Massachusetts, but the school moved into Boston in 1810 to be closer to the Boston hospitals.[6] In spite of its nominal affiliation with Harvard, the medical school remained "a proprietary institution run by a few families, its leaders supporting the interests of themselves and their relatives and friends," until the time of Charles William Eliot, who served as Harvard's president from 1869 to 1909. Eliot himself initially described the medical school as "a sort of trading corporation as well as a body of teachers."[7]

Eliot helped start the trend toward making medical schools an integral part of a university almost four decades before the Carnegie Foundation's 1910 report advocated such a status for all medical schools. Eliot's initial efforts were vigorously opposed by many among the medical school faculty, who valued being identified with the parent university but did not want someone else setting

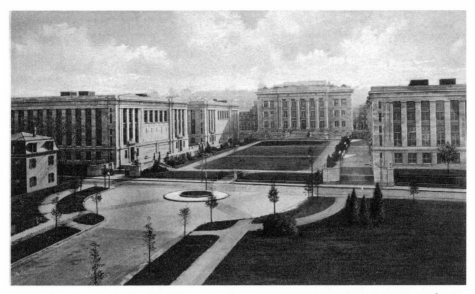

The Harvard Medical School Quadrangle, about 1916. *(The Harvard Medical Library in the Francis Countway Library of Medicine)*

standards for them. Eliot was joined in the movement to advance the quality of medical education by presidents of other universities, such as Pennsylvania, Michigan, and Johns Hopkins, as well as by the American Medical Association in the early 1900s. This gradually led to defined academic requirements for admission (eventually a college degree in some medical schools); a graded two-year basic-sciences curriculum with hands-on laboratory experiences; a two-year hands-on clinical curriculum taught primarily by university-appointed physicians; and written examinations. Thus, when the Carnegie Foundation and Abraham Flexner did their landmark survey of medical schools in the United States and Canada in 1910, they were not promulgating new standards but were instead insisting that all medical schools adhere to the standards that had already been put in place by these pioneering university medical schools.[8]

Two decades prior to Berryhill's arrival in Boston in 1925, the Harvard Medical School, still under the farsighted influence of Eliot, moved into the five marble-covered buildings on Longwood Avenue that have been called "The Great White Quadrangle" and that have served to this day as the school's icon. In a stirring dedicatory address in 1906, Eliot proclaimed:

> I devote these buildings and their successors in coming time to the teaching of the medical and surgical arts which combat disease and death, alleviate injuries, and defend and assure private and public health; and to the pursuit of the biological and medical sciences, on which depends all progress in the medical arts and preventive medicine.
>
> I solemnly dedicate them to the service of individual man and of human society, and invoke upon them the favor of man and the blessing of God.

Berryhill spent most of his time during his two years at Harvard as an extern or acting intern on the clinical services at the affiliated hospitals. The Harvard Medical School buildings, however, served as a focus of his activities because they housed the dean's office, the lecture halls, and the medical library. The adjacent Vanderbilt Hall, a dormitory and eating facility for medical and other health-sciences students, did not open until the fall of 1927 (just after Berryhill had graduated), so he had to make other arrangements in the community for his room and board.

Unlike the Johns Hopkins Medical School, which opened in 1893 several years after the completion of its own university teaching hospital, Harvard did not own a university hospital when Berryhill arrived in 1925 (and does not own one to this day).[9] The new location of the medical school on Longwood Avenue did put the school almost equidistant from its two major teaching hospitals at that time, Massachusetts General Hospital (opened in 1821) and Boston City Hospital (opened in 1864). Medical students could easily commute to these hospitals on the Boston trolleys. Furthermore, the move provided abundant adjoining land, and a number of other affiliated hospitals and medical institutions migrated to the area over the years to provide a large complex of buildings available for patient care, teaching, and research—all within walking distance of each other.

As a third- and fourth-year medical student Berryhill was exposed to numerous patients and many outstanding physicians in the Harvard-affiliated hospitals. It is likely that before leaving for Boston he consulted a small red-bound volume available in the UNC Zoology Department and entitled *The Harvard Medical School and Its Clinical Opportunities*.[10] This book, compiled and edited in 1916 by Leroy E. Parkins, "A. B., Fourth Year H.M.S." (Harvard Medical Student), provided a photograph of the quadrangle and a brief history of the medical school, along with photographs, brief histories, and summaries of the clinical opportunities available at the seventeen affiliated Harvard hospitals at the time. One panoramic photograph shows the myriad of affiliated hospitals that had already been built in the previous decade around the new medical school buildings, including Peter Bent Brigham Hospital, the Children's Hospital, and Collis P. Huntington Memorial Hospital. A statistical table for the affiliated hospitals revealed that the Boston City Hospital had 60 interns and 1,236 beds, and had 9,697 house (inpatient) medical cases and 11,196 house surgical cases in 1915. The other major affiliated teaching hospital, Massachusetts General Hospital, had 28 interns and 334 beds and had seen 2,793 house medical cases and 4,036 house surgical cases. The total for all of the affiliated hospitals at the time Parkins wrote was 3,968 beds with approximately 25,000 medical cases, 25,000 surgical cases, and more than 575,000 outpatient department visits. After the rarity of patients for clinical study in Chapel Hill, Berryhill was in awe at the wide variety of case material available in Boston.

Berryhill took third-year externships in medicine, surgery, obstetrics, and pediatrics, receiving a C on all except for a B on pediatrics—not a bad record in the days before grade inflation for a young man who was new to the city and the medical school. In the fourth year he took externships in surgery, obstetrics, and pediatrics, in all of which he received a B. His acting internship in medicine on the Harvard Service at Boston City during his fourth year was noted on his Harvard transcript as "Special Medicine—B.C.H." with a grade of B. He obviously did an outstanding job in view of his later appointment to the house staff there.

The evaluations of Berryhill by the attending faculty physicians varied but generally commented positively on his personality, hard work, and attitude with patients. Dr. Wearn in medicine commented early in his third year that Berryhill was a "good student, slightly above average [who was] improving steadily." Dr. Cheever, his surgery attending in the latter part of the fourth year, did comment, "[Berryhill] acts as though he were not in good physical condition which gives the impression that he does not approach his work with enthusiasm . . . He did whatever was required of him in his ward work, but he made no particular impression on me." This comment may have simply reflected the Bostonian stereotype of Southerners but more likely was due to Berryhill's exhaustion after serving as an acting intern on the Medical Service at Boston City Hospital and his lack of interest in surgery.[11]

Berryhill later recalled that during his junior year at Harvard he "became impressed by the high level of teaching, patient care, and the general philosophy of the senior staff members of the Fourth [Harvard] Medical [Service] at BCH [Boston City Hospital] and the Thorndike Laboratory. [He] was especially impressed by Dr. Francis W. Peabody, professor of medicine and director of the laboratory."[12] Peabody, a member of an old Boston family and an MD graduate of Harvard in 1907, had trained in both clinical medicine and medical science at Massachusetts General Hospital, Johns Hopkins Hospital, the University of Berlin, and the Rockefeller Institute. Peabody returned to Boston in 1913 and gradually rose through the ranks to become professor of medicine at Harvard in 1921. He was appointed the first director of the Thorndike Memorial Laboratory, established in 1921 as a clinical research laboratory at Boston City with a bequest honoring William H. Thorndike, MD, a visiting surgeon at the hospital from 1866 to 1884. The laboratory was housed in the new Thorndike Building, which was completed in 1923. It contained a clinical research unit (the first in Boston) to accommodate up to seventeen patients, two floors of laboratories, and an animal house. Peabody also served as chief of the Fourth Medical Service at Boston City Hospital from 1922 to 1927. He set the spirit of the laboratory and of the service with his belief that "the treatment of a disease must be completely impersonal; the treatment of a patient must be completely personal."[13]

Berryhill, like many other physicians of his day, was imbued with Peabody's view that "the secret of the care of the patient is in caring for the patient," a philosophy that received wide attention when it was published in the *Journal of the American Medical Association* in 1927 in an article entitled "The Care of the

Patient."[14] This essay and three others by Peabody were published in 1930 in a small volume, *Doctor and Patient: Papers on the Relationship of the Physician to Men and Institutions.*[15] Berryhill gave his mentor and former teacher, MacNider, an inscribed copy of this book, for which MacNider thanked him in a letter: "I have wished so many times that I might have known Peabody. He is the only man we have produced in this country who had the spirit of Osler and who could have taken his place."[16]

Unfortunately, Peabody became ill during Berryhill's junior year at Harvard and was discovered to have an abdominal malignancy. Prior to Peabody's death in October 1927, however, Berryhill and his fellow house staff at Boston City Hospital were privileged to be invited on Sunday afternoons to his home, where they discussed many medical topics of current interest. Berryhill later wrote, "These sessions permanently impressed us with his greatness and his lasting contributions to medicine."[17]

House Officer at Boston City Hospital

By the summer of 1926, prior to starting his senior year, Berryhill had decided to seek an internship in medicine in Boston, although he had a fallback strategy of applying for internships at Touro Infirmary in New Orleans, Presbyterian Hospital in New York City, and Rochester General Hospital in Rochester, New York. In a letter of reference to Rochester, Assistant Dean Worth Hale said about Berryhill: "His instructors here speak of his pleasant personality and they have found him an industrious worker. His attitude with patients is excellent. I think without doubt Mr. Berryhill is an unusual man and will make an exceedingly valuable house officer. I can recommend him to you warmly."[18]

His first choice for an internship in Boston was a position on the highly competitive Fourth Medical Service at Boston City. His senior clerkship on this service was not scheduled until January 1927—just before interviews began for the internships in all the hospitals—and he feared that he would be disadvantaged if he had not had his clerkship by that time. When one of the interns developed severe nephritis in the fall of 1926, however, Berryhill was asked to be a substitute intern on the service. He later said:

> I shall never forget the subsequent thrill when Dr. Perrin Long, the senior house officer, told me that I have been awarded the first of the five house officer slots. He asked me to complete my senior clerkship in medicine and also to carry out the duties and obligations of a beginning intern. During this period as the pup [the most junior of the interns] I spent as much time as possible, both day and night, with patients . . . [His fellow house officers were] a tremendously able group . . . [who] were among the ablest and most conscientious men I have ever seen.[19]

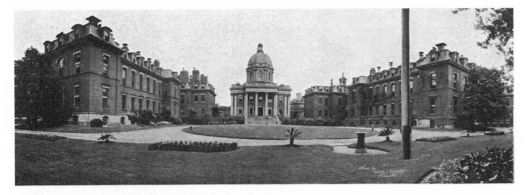

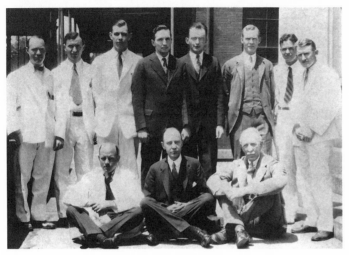

Boston City Hospital. (Parkins, *The Harvard Medical School and Its Clinical Opportunities*, 1916)

(left) Harvard Fourth Medical Service at Boston City Hospital, 1928. *Seated, left to right:* Drs. J. Wearn, G. R. Minot, and E. A. Locke. Dr. Berryhill is standing third from the left. (Finland, *The Harvard Medical Unit at Boston City Hospital*, vol. 1, 1982)

Berryhill spent twenty months as an intern in medicine at Boston City Hospital. At a time when there were no resident physicians on the house staff, his last few months as a senior house officer provided him with the experience and responsibility equivalent to that of the chief resident on a medical teaching service today.

Edwin Locke, MD, was appointed acting director of the Thorndike Laboratory and Fourth Medical Service in the summer of 1927, prior to Peabody's death. George R. Minot, MD, was appointed permanent director of Thorndike Laboratory, chief of the Fourth Medical Service, and professor of medicine at Harvard in April 1928. Joseph Wearn, MD, like Berryhill a native of Mecklenburg County in North Carolina, was appointed associate director of the Thorndike, but soon left to become professor and chair of the Department of Medicine at Western Reserve University.

Minot, like Peabody, was a Bostonian and a graduate of Harvard University and Harvard Medical School. He developed an early interest in hematology. His studies on feeding liver to patients with pernicious anemia to produce regeneration of the red cells and marked clinical improvement led to his receipt in 1934 of the Nobel Prize, which he shared with his clinical colleague W. P. Murphy, MD, and pathologist George H. Whipple, MD, who had done the preliminary studies in animals. An editorial about Minot's accomplishments, published in the *Journal of the American Medical Association* some years later, concluded with the observation, "Minot was a survivor of the superb cultural tradition of the 19th century Harvard who exploited his training in medical science with enviable skill; in so doing he discovered the cure of a disease, even though his monocular microscope, a few cover glasses and glass slides, and a bottle of Wright stain were the only tools that seemed necessary."[20]

Berryhill's exposure in Boston to physicians such as Peabody and Minot—who combined outstanding patient care with inspiring teaching and successful clinical research—provided a standard for the physician faculty members he would recruit in the early 1950s to lead the expanded medical school and the new NC Memorial Hospital at Chapel Hill. Writing years later, Berryhill summarized his experiences as a house officer at Boston City Hospital:

> Dr. Peabody's death resulted in some loss of morale among the house staff and the fellows at the Thorndike Laboratory, but the new leadership—different in many ways and yet wise and imaginative—developed strength in the group that contributed much to the quality of patient care, teaching, research, and scholarship through this difficult period.
>
> Almost continuously the wards of the Fourth Medical Service presented an extraordinary number of patients with various exciting illnesses. We lived through a mild epidemic of typhoid fever. There were malaria patients, patients with acute rheumatic fever, others with various stages of rheumatic heart disease, and many elderly people with cardiovascular, pulmonary, and gastrointestinal illnesses. There were interesting and difficult neurological diseases, which Dr. Stanley Cobb with his able associates and the senior resident, Houston Merritt (a former undergraduate student at the University of North Carolina and a graduate of Johns Hopkins), were most helpful in diagnosing and treating . . .
>
> In 1928, Maxwell Finland (Harvard Medical School 1926), who had completed his internship on the Second Medical Service, became the pneumonia fellow . . . for the entire hospital. He was a wise and valuable teacher and investigator in infectious diseases, their treatment, control, and prevention. He and Bill Castle in their respective fields and in their wise direction of the Second and Fourth Medical services . . . have superbly carried on the Peabody-Minot tradition in medicine.

Although he worked hard "on this very extraordinary service," Berryhill also remembered "times for relaxation and fun on weekends occasionally, on holidays, and in the farewell parties for interns finishing their period of service." He added:

In the evening we could sometimes relax with colleagues on one or more of the services at Boston City Hospital. There were graduates of my alma mater and natives of my home state who were in other Boston hospitals—the Peter Bent Brigham and the Massachusetts General, among them—who frequently got together for a weekend dinner, Southern style, or in typical Boston restaurants, with a little bourbon saved up for an evening of relaxation.[21]

Practice in Charlotte and Teaching at Chapel Hill

Berryhill's term as a house officer at Boston City Hospital ended in March of 1929. He returned home to Charlotte, North Carolina, with the intention of practicing internal medicine with the two older internists he had worked with during summers while in medical school. This plan did not materialize due to the illness of one of the internists and the depression, which was affecting the southern states even before the stock market crash in October of 1929. Instead, Berryhill "entered practice with a very able physician in a small textile town [Belmont] close to Charlotte and spent a very happy summer there."[22]

A major contribution to his happiness that summer was Norma Connell, who had returned from working in New York City and graduate study in guidance counseling at Columbia University to be dean of girls at Charlotte's Central High School. They were now able to see each other frequently, in contrast to the situation when she was a student in New York and he was a house officer in Boston. Neither one of them had much money at the time, and he came down to New York to see her only once, although she received at least five letters from him each week.[23]

During the summer Berryhill was approached by President Chase at UNC to come to Chapel Hill and teach the physiology course while Dean Isaac Manning recuperated from a gallbladder operation. (Convalescence from a cholecystectomy then could be many months rather than the days with the current laparoscopic surgery.) Manning also called to persuade Berryhill to accept the offer. When Berryhill protested that he didn't know any physiology, Manning convinced him that the best way to learn the subject was to teach it. After visiting Manning in Chapel Hill, Berryhill accepted a temporary position as acting assistant professor of physiology at a salary of $3,600. Acting Dean Charles S. Mangum wrote President Chase to confirm the appointment and added, "I consider Dr. Berryhill fully qualified to undertake the work and am confident that the standards of the school will be maintained in the department of physiology."[24]

Berryhill left the practice in Belmont and returned to Chapel Hill in September 1929, where he taught at the medical school for six months during the academic year 1929–1930.[25] Several years later, in a letter to MacNider from Cleveland, Berryhill described this time teaching in the medical school as "the happiest year I have ever spent."[26]

Joseph T. Wearn, MD (1893–1984) was—like Peabody and Minot—another physician who had a major impact on Berryhill's development as a physician and a medical educator. A cousin of Berryhill's, Wearn was born in Charlotte in 1893 and graduated from Davidson College in 1913. He received his MD degree from Harvard in 1917, had a residency in Boston, and served on the medical faculty at both Pennsylvania and Harvard before becoming professor and chair of medicine at the Western Reserve University School of Medicine in Cleveland in 1929. He later served as dean of the Western Reserve School of Medicine from 1945 to 1959, during which time the innovative Western Reserve medical curriculum was implemented. This approach to medical education emphasized teaching medicine in an integrated approach using committees of faculty to teach the basic and clinical aspects of an organ system (such as the cardiovascular or nervous system), rather than the traditional approach of a series of usually uncoordinated courses in a particular discipline (such as anatomy, biochemistry, and physiology). The curriculum also introduced students to patients in the first year, instead of, as was usual, the end of the second year or the beginning of the third year. Wearn's important contributions to the Western Reserve School of Medicine were recognized with the dedication of the Joseph T. Wearn Laboratory for Medical Research in his honor in 1961.[27] His contributions to Berryhill's career and to the evolving UNC School of Medicine were recognized in 1953 when he was asked to give the keynote address at the dedication of the new medical center at Chapel Hill.

While Berryhill was teaching physiology at Chapel Hill during 1929–1930, Wearn called and asked him to be his first chief resident in medicine at Lakeside Hospital in Cleveland. Berryhill accepted the offer with enthusiasm. Wearn did not need Berryhill's services until the new residency group arrived in July 1930, so Wearn asked him to go to Thomasville, Georgia, to care for Perry Harvey, a prominent citizen of Cleveland, who had experienced a "coronary" while vacationing at his winter home in Georgia. This was the beginning of a relationship with the Harveys that would be very meaningful to the Berryhills both during and after their years in Cleveland.[28]

Marriage and Living in Cleveland

Norma Berryhill once said, "Reece . . . never asked me to marry him. It just evolved and we set a date."[29] On another occasion she recalled with amusement, "After saying he wouldn't marry me until he could support me, we got married in the depths of the Depression. We would have gotten along very poorly if I hadn't had a job."[30]

A month after starting his residency in Cleveland, Berryhill returned by train to North Carolina for their marriage on August 2, 1930, at the home of Norma Connell's family in Warrenton. They had a 9:00 A.M. wedding in the garden to minimize the August heat and so they could catch the only train to Norfolk later that morning. A number of family and friends attended, including Berryhill's mother and brother; Frank Porter Graham, the newly appointed president of UNC; and Luther Hodges, a future governor of North Carolina. William Mac-Nider, Berryhill's mentor and former professor, wrote in early September, "I had a most happy time at your wedding. It was full of naturalness and simplicity and enveloped in love."[31]

After reaching Norfolk, Berryhill and his new bride boarded a ship for Boston, where he introduced her to some old friends. After a few days they took the train to Cleveland to begin their married life together.

The Berryhills initially lived very near the hospital in a small, roach-infested apartment on Cornell Street, very close to Lakeside Hospital. During their last year in Cleveland they moved farther out, where they had "a very tiny cottage . . . with space for a garden and several nice trees . . . [but] the air [was] not as pure as that in North Carolina."[32]

Norma worked with delinquent girls as a caseworker in a social agency downtown. Although they lived close to the hospital, she had long, cold rides on the streetcar to get to work and then to visit her clients in various parts of the city. Finally, out of her savings she bought a Ford Roadster for about $400. She and Berryhill used that car until well after they returned to Chapel Hill.

On Sunday afternoons when Berryhill wasn't on call, they enjoyed antiquing. Because of the depression, many rural families had had to sell their possessions in order to purchase food. Real bargains were thus available in the barns outside the city—the equivalent of today's yard sales. The newlyweds could not afford anything expensive but found some much-needed chairs, as well as some smaller items, such as a teapot that she treasured for years.

The Berryhills' first daughter, Jane Carroll, was born in Cleveland on January 14, 1933. Berryhill wrote to MacNider on March 24: "Norma and Jane are fine. The young lady is growing and gaining in weight very rapidly. She still looks and behaves very much like her father but ever so often there is an Irish outburst of temper which shows that she is also partly Connell."[33] In August the proud father wrote MacNider, "The baby now has two teeth and weighs twenty-one pounds. I am anxious for you to get a peep at her."[34]

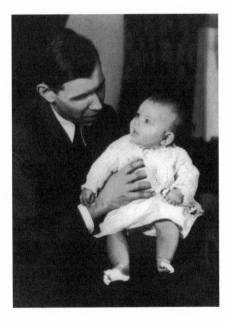

Reece Berryhill with daughter Jane, 1933. *(Berryhill Family)*

Norma Berryhill later recalled the paradoxical and unfortunate initial reception that Wearn and Berryhill got when they arrived in Cleveland. After enduring the southern stereotype as a student in Boston, Berryhill found that they were viewed by many of the Clevelanders on the hospital staff as Boston Yankees who were taking positions the locals considered theirs. In contrast to their reception by the hospital staff, however, the hospital trustees and the Harveys treated them graciously. Norma said that this experience impressed upon her and her husband the importance of welcoming new students, residents, and faculty to the medical community. When Berryhill's position as dean later gave them the opportunity, their hospitality became renowned.

In spite of the cold winters and the initial cool reception by some, Norma remembered years later that she "enjoyed Cleveland greatly." She found her job stimulating, although it could be difficult and disheartening working with teen-age girls who could not find jobs during the depression. She and Reece did make many friends, among them many old-time and wealthy Cleveland supporters of Western Reserve who invited them to their homes for social events. When the Harveys departed Cleveland to winter in Georgia, they left their season symphony tickets with the Berryhills, who otherwise could not have afforded to attend the concerts.

Although Wearn was older and the "chief," Norma and Reece Berryhill became close and lifelong friends of Joe and Susan Wearn during their three years in Cleveland. Afterward the Wearns visited Chapel Hill on occasion, and the Berryhills visited them at their summer home in Maine and at their winter home in South Carolina.[35]

Cleveland, Western Reserve Medical School, and Lakeside Hospital

Cleveland evolved as an industrial city and a Great Lakes port on the shores of Lake Erie. The Cuyahoga River ran through the center of town. Western Reserve University began in 1826 as Western Reserve College in a community some twenty-five miles southeast of Cleveland and assumed the title of university when it moved to Cleveland in 1882. It was named for a region in northeastern Ohio known in the early days of the country as the Western Reserve of Connecticut. The state later sold the land for settlement, but the name "Western Reserve" remains in use to this day. The merger in 1967 of Case Institute of Technology and Western Reserve University led to the current name of Case Western Reserve University.

The School of Medicine of Western Reserve was started in 1843 and moved with the university in 1882 to the Cleveland site later known as University Circle. This 550-acre parklike area became the site of a number of university, medical, and cultural institutions during the past century.

Cleveland's Lakeside Hospital, which had its origin in the mid-nineteenth

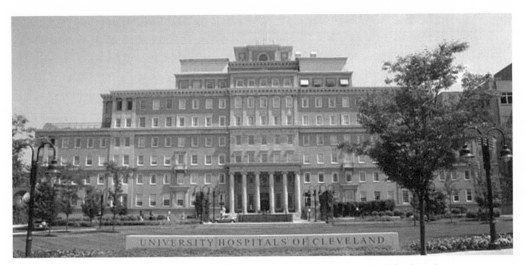

University Hospitals of Cleveland. *(Web site: www.case.edu/visit/tours/health/uh.jpg)*

century, became the exclusive teaching hospital for the Western Reserve School of Medicine in 1895. In 1925 the Lakeside, Babies and Children's, and Maternity hospitals joined to form the University Hospitals of Cleveland, and in the next several years they occupied new buildings in the University Circle area adjacent to the new medical school building, which was occupied in 1924. The new general hospital unit of 316 beds—still known as Lakeside although it was now located some four miles from the shore—was the last of the three new hospitals to open its doors to patients in February 1931. Berryhill thus spent his first seven months as chief resident at the old Lakeside Hospital, which was opened in 1898 on the north side of Lakeside Avenue along the lakefront. He spent the balance of his residency and his two years as an instructor in the new Lakeside Hospital, now known as University Hospitals of Cleveland.

Berryhill was followed as the chief resident in medicine in the summer of 1931 by Frank Miller, MD, another former member of the Harvard Fourth Medical Service house staff at Boston City Hospital. Berryhill was then appointed instructor in medicine and was asked to develop an allergy clinic in association with Roger Egeberg, MD. Berryhill also assumed the responsibility for teaching clinical pathology to second-year medical students at Western Reserve. He continued these duties until his return to North Carolina in the summer of 1933.

While at Western Reserve, Berryhill participated in a study on "calcification of experimental intraabdominal tuberculosis" that appeared in 1932 in the *American Review of Tuberculosis*—his only experimental medical research publication.[36] The senior author, Tom Douglas Spies, MD, was also at Lakeside Hospital and was in the Department of Medicine at Western Reserve. He had previously shown that calcification of acute military tuberculosis and of chronic pulmonary tuberculosis in rabbits could be produced by giving large amounts of vitamin D–containing preparations. Many workers in the field of tuberculosis felt that "the calcified tuberculous lesions found in the natural course of the disease represent a less dangerous focus for further dissemination than the noncalcified areas." Spies and Berryhill extended these studies by producing intraabdominal tuberculosis in guinea pigs with a "highly virulent strain" of the bovine tuberculous bacillus. The infected animals that also received large doses of a vitamin D preparation did not survive longer than the nontreated infected animals, but they did have calcification of many tubercles. In conclusion, the authors "suggested that a diet high in vitamine D might be beneficial in intraperitoneal tuberculosis," thus supporting clinical observations that "heliotherapy and . . . the administration of codliver oil to patients with chronic tuberculous peritonitis" was therapeutically beneficial.

An Encounter with the Tubercle Bacillus

Tuberculosis had been a common occupational hazard of medical students and house officers for centuries until the latter half of the twentieth century. A number of students and residents had to interrupt their medical training for prolonged recuperation in the pre-antibiotic era, and some never returned to medicine.

Berryhill joined this group sometime after he and Norma moved to Cleveland, when he caught a "terrible cold." Tubercle bacilli were discovered on sputum examination, and he was hospitalized for a time, followed by a period of recuperation. He returned home to North Carolina, where "his mother nurtured him and fed him." Under this regimen he made a rapid recovery and was back at work in Cleveland after being out for about four months. Norma, who had become accustomed to living alone in a big city during her time in New York City, kept her job in Cleveland and remained there while he was away.[37]

Berryhill wrote MacNider in July 1932 concerning a visit to Cleveland by Henry A. Christian, MD, a distinguished professor of medicine at Harvard and former dean of the Harvard Medical School. Christian examined him and found "no signs of activity and decided that it would be perfectly safe for [him] to go back to work."[38]

This experience with tuberculosis enhanced Berryhill's understanding of what his patients and students were going through when they had similar trials. For example, Julian W. Selig, Jr., a member of the third-year medical class, was admitted with acute poliomyelitis to North Carolina Memorial Hospital in October 1956. The student—who later became a successful psychiatrist in Norfolk, Virginia—remembered years later that he "did not have any type of relationship with Dr. Berryhill any different from the other students. Yet he visited me frequently, usually early AM on his way to his office—and often with flowers he had grown. His visits were always brief—and never intrusive. He always assured me the medical school wanted me back."[39] While attending a meeting at the

Broadmoor at Colorado Springs in November, Berryhill hand-wrote the student a four-page letter:

My dear Julian,

I am terribly sorry not to have had a chance to see you these pass [sic] 10 days—the momentum around the school seems to get faster and faster each day—or perhaps it's only because I am getting older.

I hope your progress is continuing in a satisfactory manner . . .

We are all here for a meeting of the Assoc. of American Medical Colleges which concludes next Wednesday. I shall drop up to see you as soon as I get home.

Best wishes always. Remember to keep you[r] chin up. I'm sure you'll be a more understanding doctor even 'tho this is a hard way to acquire this price-less ingredient of a *really* successful physician.

On this point I can speak from experience because many years ago—when a Resident in Medicine—I came down with tuberculosis. Just as you are do-ing I spent many weeks in bed—thinking and speculating about the future. And then out of a clear sky 10 years ago there was a recurrence and I went thru the same process, only this time fortunately Streptomycin had just been developed.

You see I have full understanding of what you are going thru. At the same time, knowing the fiber of which you're made, I do not have concern over your adjustments emotional and otherwise.

Affectionately
Reece Berryhill[40]

This and many other episodes revealed the compassionate physician and wise counselor behind the stern, no-nonsense façade that most medical students saw.

PART II

Physician, Teacher, and Dean:
Chapel Hill, 1933–1952

Here in Chapel Hill among a friendly folk, this old University, the first state university to open its doors, stands on a hill set in the midst of beautiful forests under skies that give their color and their charm to the life of youth gathered here. Traditions grow here with the ivy on the historic buildings and the moss on the ancient oaks. Friendships form here for the human pilgrimage. There is music in the air of the place. To the artist's touch flowers grow beautifully from the soil and plays come simply from the life of the people. Above the traffic of the hour church spires reach toward the life of the spirit. Into this life, with its ideals, failures, and high courage, comes youth with his body and his mind, his hopes and his dreams. Scholars muster here the intellectual and spiritual resources of the race for the development of the whole personality of the poorest boy and would make the University of North Carolina a stronghold of learning with out-posts of research along all the frontiers of the world. Great teachers on this hill kindle the fires that burn for him and light up the heavens of the commonwealth with the hopes of light and liberty for all mankind.

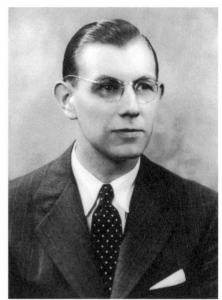

W. Reece Berryhill, MD, physician and teacher, late 1930s. *(Berryhill Family)*

—Inaugural address of UNC President Frank Porter Graham,
University of North Carolina, November 11, 1931

When the historian comes, fifty years from now, to deal with the Southern Renaissance, he will have to say, as he can say in all truth, that its primary impulse came from, and its greatest influence was the University of North Carolina. This little City of Chapel Hill has become indeed the Capital of the Southern Mind.

—Mark Ethridge, editor, *Louisville (Kentucky) Courier-Journal and Times*, 1939.
Quoted in William de Berniere MacNider, *The Good Doctor and Other Selections
from the Essays and Addresses of William de Berniere MacNider*, 1953

CHAPTER 4

University Physician and Medical School Faculty Member

$\mathcal{N}$orma Berryhill recalled that she and Reece had always intended to return to North Carolina from Cleveland; they kept in such close touch with events in the state that "it was almost like we had never left." They did not need a subscription to a North Carolina paper because many family members and friends sent them newspaper clippings. It took only a day or two for these to arrive in Cleveland, thanks to the priority then given the US mail on the nation's vast network of trains.[1] These indirect contacts with the state were supplemented with a number of return visits to the state by Norma, Reece, or both during their three years in Cleveland, from 1930 to 1933.

Berryhill's correspondence during this time with William "Dr. Billy" Mac-Nider, MD, chair of pharmacology at UNC, provides valuable insight into Berryhill's desire to return to the South from Cleveland and into their relationship as former student and mentor.[2] Their letters covered a wide variety of topics, from people and events in Chapel Hill and the state to the flowers then in bloom, academic medicine, and personal issues. On one occasion MacNider excitedly told Berryhill of some of his recent experimental work in reversible liver injury from ethyl alcohol in dogs and asked for his help: "The next time you have a case of chronic alcoholism with a large liver I wish you would try the phenoltetra-chlorphthalein liver test and see if you can confirm my experimental finding in that there is an initial plasm[a] concentration of the dye which may be delayed for even an hour or more in its disappearance from the plasm[a]."[3] In another letter Berryhill told how he was anticipating a coming visit to Chapel Hill to see MacNider: "There is nothing so far that I have been able to discover which so restores my confidence and self-respect as a visit with you, and from the spiritual benefits that I always derive from such a talk, you will more than likely have to put up with me for many years to come."[4]

When the Berryhills did return to Chapel Hill in 1933—Reece's first time in Chapel Hill with a wife and child—they established their first homes and rapidly became a part of the university and wider communities. He became increasingly busy with his clinical duties as the university physician and with his teaching duties as a medical school faculty member responsible for the clinical teach-

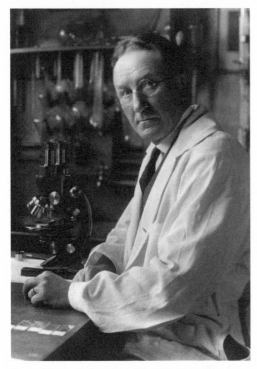

Dr. William de Berniere MacNider, professor and chair of pharmacology; dean of the School of Medicine from 1937 to 1940. *(Med. Illustrations, NCC)*

ing of the second-year medical students. These years from 1933 until he became dean in 1941 also gave him an introduction to university administration and further expanded his wide range of contacts at Chapel Hill and throughout the state.

North Carolina Seen from a Distance

The three years that the Berryhills spent in Cleveland were ones of profound—and generally regressive—changes in North Carolina and the nation following a decade of prosperity.

The prior decade, the Roaring Twenties, had seen significant positive changes in North Carolina, including a new statewide highway system, the establishment of minimal school terms of six months, and tax reform. Under the presidency of urbane New Englander Harry Woodburn Chase, the university progressed steadily from a good provincial university to one that was increasingly recognized nationally. Academic standards were raised so that, in Chase's words, the university would "not shrink from measurement by national standards." These efforts led the university to membership in the prestigious Association of American Universities (a recognition previously afforded only one southern university, the University of Virginia). During Chase's tenure the faculty increased from 78 to 225, and the annual state appropriation went from $270,000 to $1,343,000. Chase instituted programs that were to have a major impact on the university's future, including the Institute for Research in Social Science, the University of North Carolina Press, and various new departments. A major building program funded by the state and some private funds provided a number of much-needed buildings, including an impressive library (later named Wilson Library), a chemistry building, a music building, a law school building, classroom buildings, and dormitories. Polk Place, the portion of the campus between South Building and Wilson Library, was completed essentially to its present status during this time. The beauty of the campus was enhanced by the Morehead-Patterson Bell Tower and Kenan Stadium, both funded by donations from loyal friends of the university.[5]

But the era was also a time of religiously based challenges to academic freedom. In the mid-1920s a movement gathered steam around the nation and in

North Carolina to prohibit the teaching of evolution by any teacher paid with state funds. Chase provided leadership in defeating this measure in the 1925 legislature after a bitter statewide campaign.[6] A similar bill was introduced in 1927 but failed to pass. In the meantime, Tennessee was in the national spotlight over the trial of John T. Scopes for teaching evolution in a public school.[7]

Prohibition of the manufacture and sale of alcoholic beverages had gone into effect in 1920, a year following the ratification of the Eighteenth Amendment to the Constitution and the passage by Congress of the National Prohibition Act (also known as the Volstead Act) to enforce a ban on alcohol consumption. As one historian later observed, "Because the Congress and the state legislatures . . . were reluctant to appropriate enough money for more than token enforcement—and because the opportunities for disregarding the law through smuggling, distilling, fermenting, and brewing were legion—Prohibition always represented more of an ideal than a reality."[8]

During Prohibition Berryhill and MacNider made several references in their correspondence to the therapeutic value of a drink at the end of a busy day. On a gloomy winter day in Cleveland in December 1931, Berryhill wrote, "Sometimes I get terribly discouraged about this business of trying to do or find out anything. In such times that most indispensable drug, alcohol, is very comforting and very valuable." He concluded the letter by wishing MacNider "a very happy Christmas" and hoping that "there will be plenty of the good North Carolina rye" available.[9]

On another occasion, in July 1932, Berryhill wrote MacNider, "Thank God North Carolina has now a wet senator. I never expected the Methodist-ridden state to rise up in arms and do that."[10] Prior to returning to Chapel Hill in the summer of 1933, Berryhill wrote MacNider about their trip to Canada, Maine, and Boston: "Thank you so much for arranging to get the material [a five-gallon keg of bootleg whiskey for $15] for the winter. We had loads of it in Canada and it was very nice to be able to get it in an open and sort of self-respecting fashion."[11]

Prohibition led to a decade of bootleggers, speakeasies, and at least the perception of an increasing crime rate and disrespect for the law. Florence R. Sabin, the noted anatomist and teacher at the Johns Hopkins Medical School, observed in 1931, "The prohibition law, written for weaklings and derelicts, has divided the nation, like Gaul, into three parts—wets, drys, and hypocrites."[12] This failed experiment in enforcing morality through a constitutional amendment was repealed in 1933 by the ratification of the Twenty-first Amendment.

When Chase resigned from the university in February 1930 to assume the presidency of the University of Illinois, the state had already borne the brunt of a farm recession and was beginning to feel the full impact of the Great Depression, with its bank closures, unemployment, and decline in public revenues following the stock market crash on Black Tuesday, October 29, 1929. Governor O.

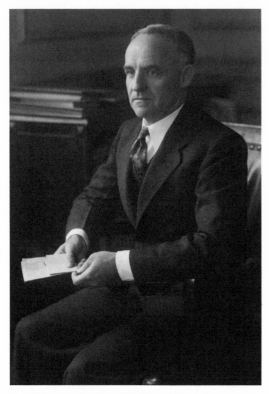

Frank Porter Graham, UNC president from 1930 to 1949. *(NCC)*

Max Gardner recognized the increasing importance of the university in the life of the state when he noted, "The election of a president of this university is of more importance to North Carolinians than the election of any governor or any senator at any time."[13]

Frank Porter Graham, a UNC faculty member in history, was a very reluctant candidate to follow Chase for the presidency of the university. After accepting the challenge, however, he devoted his characteristic energy and vision to the task. He was appointed in June 1930 but was not inaugurated until Armistice Day, November 11, 1931. In his seventy-eight-minute address to a crowd of some 5,000 in Kenan Stadium he resisted the temptation to dwell only on the current budget difficulties, instead laying out a plan for the future of the university.[14]

Graham anticipated the development at Chapel Hill of an academic medical center that would be an integral part of the university. In his inaugural address he discussed the role of the professional schools in the university:

> We need not only the specialized knowledge and the integrated way of life [of the undergraduate and graduate colleges] but also specialized ways of making a living ... The vocational and professional schools came in America largely outside the universities on account of the gaps in the university structure ... In time the joint processes of specialization and synthesis in all fields of knowledge resulted in the incorporation of all professional schools ... within the framework of the university.
>
> The university needs the professional schools with their specialized knowledge, equipment, and skill, their high standards of scholarship, their spirit of work, thoroughness, and excellence. The professional school, assimilated into the organic structure of the university, needs the university with its wide variety of skills, interest, and contacts; its general resources, and wholeness of view. Consider the reciprocal contributions of Osler, Welch, and Hopkins, the Pound group and Harvard.[15]

Berryhill, in a letter to MacNider a few weeks later, observed that Graham's speech "seemed to me to be a very clear-cut analysis of the University problems and hopes." While Berryhill and Graham were to disagree on some social and political issues in the future, they were in complete agreement about the inter-relationship of the medical school and the university. In an address in 1950 on the advantages of locating a medical school on a university campus, Berryhill would argue:

> If medicine is in truth a learned profession and not a trade and if it has finally become, after a long and somewhat devious course, a university discipline, then it is logical to believe that a school of medicine whenever possible should be an integral part of a university, physically and spiritually . . .
>
> It is axiomatic that progress in medicine is dependent on close association with the basic sciences which serve as its foundation. This has perhaps been best stated by Dr. Alan Gregg . . . "the physics and chemistry of today become the physiology and pathology of tomorrow and the clinical medicine of the day following." A scientific environment which would permit and encourage such a coalescence cannot be provided easily or adequately away from close physical relationship with the total scientific resources of a university . . . without staggering cost and duplication which no institution can afford . . .
>
> In summary . . . we believe it is possible for a medical school as an in-tegral part of a university, even though it is located in a small community, to have all the educational advantages available in such an environment—administrative, scientific, humanistic, and cultural—and at the same time to secure maximal results in its medical training program both in its own hospital and by the utilization of the facilities and the well trained potential teaching talent in other hospitals of the region (see Appendix K).[16]

The difficulties facing the university and its new president in the early 1930s were both financial and political, but a speaker at Graham's inauguration had astutely observed that "the spiritual leadership of this man is the moral equiva-lent of an unimpaired appropriation."[17] Graham considered it part of his mission to remind the public at every opportunity that depressions are temporary, but that education is a permanent source of material and spiritual prosperity for the citizens of the state. And, he observed, "Budget-making in a depression tests what we really believe in."[18]

In 1932 Graham had to deal with a 25 percent cut in the university's approved appropriation, which brought the actual appropriation to only some 40 percent of the 1929 peak appropriation.[19] This necessitated an across-the-board cut in faculty salaries, but his leadership was such that a professor later commented that Graham was "the only university president I know who can announce a cut in salaries and receive a standing ovation."[20] The faculty's loyalty to the univer-sity and to Graham was demonstrated in his first nine months in office, when he could count "more than twenty persons who had received offers from other universities, sometimes for as much as three times what they were making at Chapel Hill, but who had refused such offers because of their loyalty."[21]

MacNider detailed the impact of these cuts on one faculty member. He wrote that Berryhill's invitation for a long visit with them and the Wearns in Cleveland was "simply out of the question. We now have a 30% cut in salary, and a 40% cut is just around the corner, which means that if a body's life insurance is to be continued, and if they are to approach paying their bills, they will have to stay at home and be contented. I think I can do this with a microscope and a garden and the eternal presence of God, as manifested in nature."[22] It was not until the 1937–1938 fiscal year that President Graham could report on "the general budgetary recovery of the University and restoration of the salaries from the 68% basis to 93.5%."[23]

Faculty members were not the only ones in the university community affected by the Depression. Graham was quoted in the 1932 *Yackety Yack,* the university annual, as noting that "in this most critical year in the life of the University in the present century the student body has stood like a rock in the storm." With many students "faced with the necessity of going back to bankrupt homes and jobless towns, the student body started off the emergency loan funded with two thousand dollars. With [the University] budget cut to a destructive point they put into the budget a saving spiritual power." In the 1933 annual Graham observed, "The students, faculty, townspeople, alumni, and friends rallied to the University with their meager financial resources and their great reserves of spiritual power." The new student loan fund grew to $110,000 with a generous donation from Mrs. Jessie Kenan Wise as well as many other smaller donations. The fund permitted students to stay and continue their education in 1932 and to return in 1932–1933.[24] The funds supplied by another member of the Kenan family—Mary Lily Kenan Flagler, whose fortune had established the Kenan Professorships at her death in 1917—provided critically needed salary and expense monies during the Depression to help keep some of Chapel Hill's outstanding faculty.

According to a student's account in the 1933 *Yackety Yack,* in 1932–1933 the medical school also underwent "the trials and pitfalls which have been common to the University." He stated that the appropriations fight had been especially bitter in reference to the medical school, where "suggestions of the suspension of this department of the University have brought forth the most favorable defense of the school, tending to show its high standing among the nation's medical schools, its almost unbelievably low maintenance cost, and the accomplishments of its sterling faculty."[25]

In March 1933 Berryhill wrote MacNider that he had been "following the appropriations fight [for the university] in the state legislature with much fear and trembling and while I suppose it is too much to hope for an average sized appropriation, I do hope that the yokels will not be able to get through such a ruinous budget as has been proposed in the past week. I know it must be very trying and disheartening to Frank and to all of you there. It certainly is to all of us away from Chapel Hill." Later in the letter, Berryhill expressed his hope that "the coming of spring ought to do something to put a kinder feeling into the hearts of some of the legislators toward the University."[26]

One of the results of the state's financial crises was the plan to administratively consolidate North Carolina State College at Raleigh, UNC at Chapel Hill, and the Woman's College at Greensboro. Graham again very reluctantly accepted the presidency of the Consolidated University in late 1932 out of a sense of duty to the state and the university.

In a letter to MacNider in July 1932, Berryhill said he hoped MacNider would write him "something about the University Consolidation Plan because I am unable to make out a great deal from what I have seen in the papers and naturally I am very much interested, particularly in the way it may affect any of the departments in what, to me at least, will always be THE University."[27] It was not until 1938 that President Graham could confirm "the settlement of the major issues of consolidation within the University framework to serve the needs of all the people of North Carolina."[28]

The advice between mentor and former student was a two-way street. In January 1932 MacNider, then fifty-one years old, asked Berryhill's opinion concerning an offer he had received to become the chair of pharmacology at Jefferson in Philadelphia. Berryhill responded, "I am awfully glad that the honor has come to you because it's one we all here recognize is certainly due you." Two pages of advice followed. "There is, of course, considerably more national prestige attached to the chair of pharmacology in one of the leading medical schools in the country than the place you now have and as we have discussed so often before it is certainly true that a professor south of Washington is never accorded the things that are due him," he told MacNider. Berryhill pointed out other advantages to a move but said, "I am not at all certain that it is the best thing for you to do . . . with so much longer classes and with the administrative work to do." He also interjected that he had "always hoped that you would accept the place at Duke," because he could still live in Chapel Hill and would be associated with "an institution with infinite possibilities and one that is likely to attain some national prominence while you are still connected with it." Berryhill observed that MacNider's leaving would "probably ring down the curtain on the [medical] school [at Chapel Hill]," but he concluded by saying, "If you want to go to Philadelphia for God's sake don't let anybody tell you it is your duty to remain at the University."[29] MacNider replied to Berryhill a few days later. "The position at Jefferson did interest me considerably," he wrote, but "it would be difficult for me to make an adjustment at this stage of the game to city type of life. So that, after thinking it over, I decided to turn the call down."[30] Neither did he accept an appointment as chair at Duke, although he was a member of the original faculty at the Duke University Medical School in 1930–1931 as Visiting Lecturer in Special Pharmacology and subsequently taught at Duke part time while maintaining his professorship at UNC.[31]

Paradoxically, one of the most vicious political threats to the university's academic freedom during this time came in 1932 from Presbyterians, the same denomination that in the eighteenth century was instrumental in establishing the university and that had furnished three of its first presidents. Ostensibly in response to visits on the university campus by Bertrand Russell, the British philosopher, and Langston Hughes, the black American poet, "one hundred prominent citizens of North Carolina" sent a petition to the governor insisting that he halt "further predatory acts by so-called modern educators."[32] In a letter to MacNider in September 1932, Berryhill stated that he had been "terribly depressed" about the move against the university, one "originating chiefly I suspect among the damn bigoted and narrow-minded Presbyterians in my own and adjoining counties." He hoped this would "go up in smoke as all similar movements in the last twenty years have done but at a more or less critical time like this I cannot help but feel somewhat distressed." He added, "Walter Hines Page's statement about the [South's need for some] first-class funerals is particularly applicable to the signers of that petition and I should be delighted to officiate as an honorary or active pall-bearer at any or all of such funerals. There is no one who has any more deep or abiding sense and love and loyalty to North Carolina and especially to the University as I feel and such idiotic protests from the people in the state who refuse in spite of everything to be intelligent simply rile me to death."[33] MacNider reassured him in his next letter that "the mess about teaching here at the University will soon blow over."[34]

Berryhill, however, was so worked up over this petition that he wrote on September 16 to the Reverend W. M. Currie, the minister of the Belmont Presbyterian Church, where he was a member during his brief stay in Belmont in 1929. He stated that he had been "terribly disappointed to see your name among" the signers of the petition against the university. After writing and discarding several letters, he said, he had "cooled down to such a point that I am simply writing this now to ask you to forward my church letter [church membership] immediately to me here." He added:

> I have always looked forward to perhaps coming home and leaving the letter where it is but your action in signing the petition, which in my mind has identified you and other members of the church there with the unprogressive, intolerant and unseeing people in the state, makes it impossible for me to have any further connection with the Presbyterian Church—either there or in general.
>
> I only hope you have not failed to see the deeper significance behind this appeal . . . and that is, the fight on the part of the industrial forces against the more enlightening, humane and intelligent policy of the university leaders in the sociological and industrial field, and this fight to gain the attention and sympathy of the people is being camouflaged under the head of that bug-bear to the masses, Atheism and Communist Russia . . .
>
> I have heard the men whom you condemn in your petition. I have read

the book of Freud's. I do not accept them any more than I accept the things you say in your sermons or the doctrines of the Presbyterian Church or the Bible itself. Both you and they have thoughts that are worthwhile, but not everything you think or say. The book of Freud's is a standard reference book in all worthwhile psychology and psychiatric courses and it has helped many people to get an insight into their difficulties.

The University has meant more to me and taught me more about the meaning of life and has equipped me better to deal with life and has made me happier and taught me to think more clearly and sanely than my association with any minister of any church, with the possible exception of that one in Chapel Hill of which Dr. W. D. Moss is the minister, and he, interestingly enough, has for a long time been almost excommunicated by the hierarchy of the Presbyterian Church. It seems to me that your church opposes many things that make for enlightenment, tolerance and freedom and I cannot longer be associated with that sort of an organization. I would much prefer to be religious in my own way . . .

I hope that you do not take this personally . . . I trust that if I see you again we shall continue to be friends . . . but for Heaven's sake, study in an unprejudiced manner the principles that are involved in the state at the present. I think you have as wonderful an opportunity to do intelligent work in the textile community in which you live as any person I know by promoting a better understanding of capital and labor . . .

You are wasting your time and energy in fighting against the principles for which the University stands for they can no more be separated from our modern life or from the fundamental principles of Christianity than the heart can be taken out of the body, and long after you and I have gone and been forgotten the University and the things it stands for will continue to be the source of enlightenment to the state just as it has been for one hundred and forty years. I believe the Trustees' answer to this petition will be the election of Frank Graham to the presidency of the greater university—thus re-affirming their confidence in and approval of his policies.

A few days later Berryhill sent Currie a copy of the *Chapel Hill Weekly* "containing a summary of the editorial comments from the various state papers on the petition which apparently originated around Belmont." He thought "it might be of interest to you to see what supposedly unprejudiced minds in the state thought of the ridiculousness and absurdity of such a stand . . . Those of us who try to see clearly and who have hopes for the future of the state are decidedly encouraged by the intelligent comments from so many editors in different parts of the state." Currie returned the newspaper along with the church letter stating that Berryhill was "a member in full and regular standing . . . and that at his own request he is dismissed to unite with the church of his choice, to which church he is cordially commended." In a cover letter Currie said he didn't want to meddle "in someones [*sic*] affairs but let me urge you to place this letter with some church body whose Christian ideals and ideas are in keeping with your own."

The exchange between Berryhill and Currie apparently ended with a letter from Berryhill on November 8 in which he elaborated on his criticism. He reiterated that he thought "the camouflaged reason for the last petition against the university" was "the labor situation in the textile mills." Unsaid was the fact that Frank Graham had been active in supporting the mill workers in their conflicts with the mills, including those involved in the bitter 1929 strike at the Loray Mill in Gastonia, where a police chief and a striker lost their lives. Berryhill criticized the ministers and other leaders in the involved communities for not "working out a new social order." He felt that "the old expression, 'God is always on the side of the management' is particularly applicable to the mill situation in the south." He urged them to "influence both sides in the right direction. Each undoubtedly has his rights but the rights should not always be on the side of the mill owners."[35]

This exchange with Currie reflected Berryhill's youthful sense of justice and fair play. Like many young persons before and after him, he would become more conservative in his outlook over the years. Also in the coming years he would inevitably be spending more time with the political leaders and mill owners than with the mill workers as he marshaled support for the teaching hospital and medical school that would ultimately benefit all North Carolinians—mill workers and owners alike.

PLANNING FOR A CAREER DURING THE GREAT DEPRESSION

Berryhill wrote to MacNider in the spring of 1933 that "especially this year there has been so much turmoil and strife and uncertainty here and elsewhere that it has sort of got under my skin, I suppose, and I have stopped writing entirely."[36] His gloom was a reflection of the despondent state of millions of Americans at the time, a sense described by distinguished historian William W. Leuchtenburg:

> Like a manic-depressive patient, noted one writer, the nation had moved from the unstable euphoria of 1929 to the depression of 1932 which was characterized by panic, utter hopelessness about the future, an inability to initiate or sustain any activity, and a mood of apprehension . . .
>
> "Yes, we could smell the depression in the air," one writer remembered of "that historically cruel winter of 1932–3, which chilled so many of us like a world's end . . . It was like a raw wind; the very houses we lived in seemed to be shrinking, hopeless of real comfort." The interval between Roosevelt's election in November 1932, and his inauguration in March 1933, proved the most harrowing four months of the depression. Three years of hard times

had cut national income [by] more than half; the crash of five thousand banks had wiped out nine million savings accounts.[37]

Cleveland and Western Reserve Medical School were not immune to the financial uncertainty and suffering that the Depression was bringing to North Carolina and the nation. According to Norma Berryhill, the medical school there, a private school, was "having a very hard time because of the Depression. There were rumors around that the school just wouldn't be able to make it. The banks were closed and the people who had been the chief supporters had lost a lot of money."[38]

All these events complicated Berryhill's planning for his career. One possibility for the future would be the private practice of his specialty of internal medicine. This prospect was not bright in Cleveland owing to the large number of doctors there and to the fact that "a person had to be almost dead before he would go to see a doctor" during the Depression years.[39] In one letter to Mac-Nider, Berryhill said he loved "the teaching and the little bit of research that I've only started" but speculated that, if a position at Duke didn't become available, "I shall go back south and go into private medical practice."[40]

Another possibility would be a continuing appointment at Western Reserve. As an instructor for only two years, Berryhill had little seniority at the medical school, although he was a friend and close associate of Joseph T. Wearn, MD, the chair of medicine. Even if Berryhill had been offered a position at Western Reserve, he hinted in his letters to MacNider that he didn't like the atmosphere there in the clinical services. His relations with Wearn and the next in charge were "pleasant and cordial," but he knew "that eventually the day will come when my self respect will compel me to resign." He told MacNider, "I have been too strongly molded by you and Francis Peabody to be very happy under the present set up . . . where one feels so hopelessly out of place."[41]

Nonetheless, in a January 1933 letter MacNider said that Joe Wearn had commented to him that Berryhill had "done the best job of anyone connected with the department." He believed Wearn would be offering Berryhill a position there doing "exactly what you want—a teaching position, time for investigation and time to build up a limited amount of consultation work. Such an arrangement, I should think, would be about ideal. The only trouble is that it happens in the Middle West instead of in the South." MacNider advised Berryhill to talk with Wearn about a future position.[42] Apparently Wearn was interesting in having Berryhill stay on the faculty, for in tentatively accepting the position in Chapel Hill later in 1933, Berryhill said that Wearn was holding his position there open until he heard from UNC.[43]

Still another possibility was to return to North Carolina with an appointment at the new Duke University School of Medicine and Hospital, which had opened in Durham in July 1930. As early as December 1931, Berryhill brought up Duke in a letter to MacNider.[44] He asked MacNider how much time he had spent at Duke during the fall and then added, "I certainly hope that they will be an outstanding school some day and I think perhaps I made a mistake in not trying to get in there as resident or something several years ago because I feel sure that both of us would be happier and much better satisfied living in North Carolina. Please don't misunderstand me for I am not unhappy here but I think you can understand our feelings in preferring to be in the south, especially in that part of the south that is near Chapel Hill."

MacNider replied on January 6, 1932: "My work at Duke does not commence until the spring quarter, and I am ashamed to say that I have seen practically nothing of these people since the school year commenced last September. I can well understand how you and Miss Norma feel about living in North Carolina, and especially near Chapel Hill. So far as I know, we only live once, and if possible I reckon this should be made as pleasant as we can make it." He went on to say that it was good Berryhill had not applied to Duke for an internship, because "with the advanced training which you have had, with the splendid piece of work you have done at Lakeside [Hospital], according to Joe Wearn, you would be in a position to secure something more worth while, both in terms of finances and responsibility at Duke than you would sometime ago." MacNider added that he would soon be seeing Duke's medical school dean, Wilbur Davison, and would talk with him about Berryhill, if Berryhill had no objections.[45]

A year later MacNider said he didn't know "what to say about the situation at Duke. I fear they are going to get into a horrible mess. From what I have understood, [Harold Lindsay] Amoss [the first chair of medicine] was asked to resign without a hearing, more than likely on insufficient grounds . . . if this is a fact, I would very certainly hesitate to recommend or suggest anyone for a position there."[46]

Returning to Chapel Hill

The final career possibility Berryhill considered was to return to Chapel Hill in a position at the university. In May 1932, MacNider wrote Berryhill a letter elaborating on the university physician position that, a year later, would be the means by which Berryhill was recruited back to Chapel Hill, where he would remain for the rest of his life. MacNider stated that he was speaking confidentially and that "the whole question is entirely in the air. I have had several talks with Frank [Graham] about this and he is greatly interested in working out a real health organization at the University, not only in terms of actually treating sick students, but in terms of obtaining very worth while physical examinations of all of the students and getting some insight into their family background which might throw some light on their predisposition to various physical disturbances, and especially to disorders of a mental character." He warned that this was some time off, but he would keep Berryhill informed as things developed.[47]

MacNider reported to Berryhill in January 1933 that Eric A. Abernethy, MD,

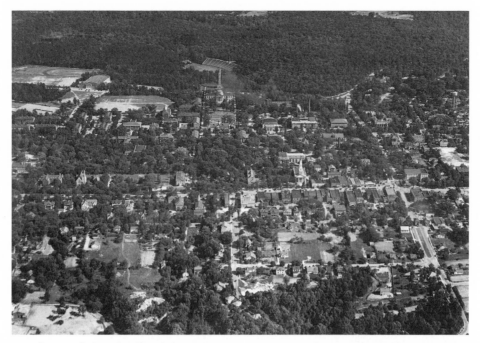

Aerial view of Chapel Hill and the UNC campus in 1932, at the time Berryhill was considering a return to UNC. Note the wooded area in the upper right where the medical center would later be built. *(NCC)*

the director of the university infirmary for the previous fourteen years, had resigned about two weeks previously and that temporary arrangements had been made to provide physician coverage for the students in the infirmary. Foy Roberson, MD, a graduate of UNC and of Jefferson Medical College, was appointed director of the infirmary and would be coming over from Durham daily. MacNider spoke with Graham, and a permanent Infirmary Committee was appointed, made up of Manning (chair), Mangum, and MacNider. It was the hope of the committee that a full-time university physician could be appointed for the next fiscal year beginning in July 1933 and that a younger assistant physician could also be appointed, but nothing was certain.[48]

The next month MacNider reported, "There is no telling what is going to happen here. It may be that for a year or more we will have to sit tight in terms of developing the medical side of the University, but . . . with Frank's great interest in it, we may be able to do something by September. I will keep you informed."[49] Berryhill replied, "I am delighted that men like you and Frank are interested in what seems to me a most important aspect of university life and organization and I shall be very much interest[ed] in following the development of the splendid idea." He added, "Your letters always have the effect of restoring my self-respect which at times is at a very low ebb even though I fully realize your judgment is biased in my favor."

In a letter dated May 15, 1933, MacNider provided Berryhill a more realistic appraisal of the university physician position he had discussed in such glowing terms earlier: "I do not know just how you would feel about the type of position which will be available July first for someone here at the University. In a certain sense, of course, it would mean at least temporarily your changing from academic medicine. Not knowing what is ahead of you in the Medical School at Western Reserve, I am not in a position to advise you about this." MacNider suggested that it might be four years before the university's health service could be developed "in a rather ideal fashion." In the meantime, "all we can do now is to select an excellent type of University Physician. There is no reason, however, if this individual likes his work and is of the right type, why he should not in several years head up the health service here at the University. This in turn would have a more academic flavor, and would be a rather pleasant type of experience, I should think." He advised Berryhill to visit and talk with Graham and Manning, the medical school dean, about the proposed position, for which several others were also being considered.[50]

Berryhill came to Chapel Hill in May to discuss the position of university physician with Graham, though he missed seeing Dean Manning and apparently MacNider as well. Graham offered him the position, and in a telegram to Graham on May 26 he accepted, subject to the conditions they had discussed in their meeting and as outlined in a letter dated May 27. He wanted to start on September 1 rather than on July 1, owing to commitments in Cleveland, and Graham granted his request.[51]

On June 7, 1933, MacNider wrote enthusiastically to Berryhill: "I cannot even approach telling you and Norma how happy I am that you are to be here in Chapel Hill, connected with the University in the fine capacity of University Physician. I do not know of anything that has given me deeper joy."[52]

Later in the month Graham wrote Norma and Reece a personal letter "to confirm what they [Dean Manning and Mr. House] have said officially and to express my great personal happiness at the prospect of both of you being in our community and in our life, I hope, permanently." He said, "We are overjoyed that you are coming here, personally and institutionally," and added:

> You are just the sort of human beings that we want in this place to help us save, restore and go forward. You have resources of mind and spirit that will mean much to me I know.
>
> Reece, you have the training, equipment, the experience, the skill, and the attitudes that will mean great things to our students. Your personality will communicate an influence that will be immeasurable.
>
> Norma, it will be like old times to have you here in the community again touching in a beautiful way the lives of our people here.

Graham expressed his regret that "we do not have the equipment and auxiliaries that we want Reece to have in his work but we will come to those things soon. We want everything that he wants and will put into effect his desires as immediately as possible."[53] Although the letters in Berryhill's UNC personnel files do not mention the prospect of an expanded medical school and teaching hospital at Chapel Hill, Norma remembers Graham saying that Berryhill "could teach and looked forward through the years to the time when the Medical School could be expanded to a third and fourth year and a teaching hospital could be built."[54]

Homes in Chapel Hill for a Growing Family

After a busy summer finishing up things in Cleveland while trying to keep up with events in Chapel Hill concerning the infirmary, the Berryhills took a ten-day road trip in August through Canada, Maine, and Boston to see Norma's family and friends while Norma's sixteen-year-old sister kept their six-month-old baby, Jane, in Cleveland. They returned to Cleveland to finish packing and to sign a lease for a house in Chapel Hill. The furniture left Cleveland for Chapel Hill by truck while Berryhill and Norma's sister left Cleveland by auto. Norma and Jane took the day-and-a-half train trip from Cleveland to Warrenton, where they all met for a few days of visits with Norma's relatives the Connells. The family arrived in Chapel Hill on the morning of September 1, 1933. The furniture didn't arrive until several days later, but they were able to get established in their new home before the university opened for the fall term.

Reece, Norma, and Jane settled in the house they were renting from Dan Grant in the Gimghoul area, east of the campus, at 246 Glandon Road. It had no insulation, and Norma remembered it as "terribly, terribly cold . . . In the dead of winter I would have to do a thawing job before I could get water or heat enough to fix any lunch."

The Berryhills next moved into a smaller, "very, very comfortable" house in the same neighborhood at 733 Gimghoul Road.[55] This house is across the street from the present Chapel Hill home of Reece and Norma's younger daughter, Catherine "Cat" Berryhill Williams, who was born on October 13, 1935, two years after the Berryhills returned to Chapel Hill. Cat later said she was a birthday present for her dad, who had turned thirty-five the previous day. Since there were then no obstetrical facilities in Chapel Hill, family legend has it that she was "born in Duke Gardens on the way to see their obstetrician, 'Daddy' Ross, at Duke Hospital." She said that she has no recollection of that home, but her older sister had pleasant memories of sitting on the porch with their mother while waiting for their father to return home from work at the medical school.[56]

After a couple of years the Berryhills purchased their first home, a 100-year-old house on two acres between West Franklin and West Rosemary Streets. MacNider had been born in this house in 1881. The house had most recently been owned by a fraternity that went broke during the Depression, so the Berryhills were able to purchase it at a bargain price. Norma described it as a "big, rambling house" with a full basement, five bedrooms, and three baths. An avenue of southern maple trees came from Franklin Street to the front entrance, while

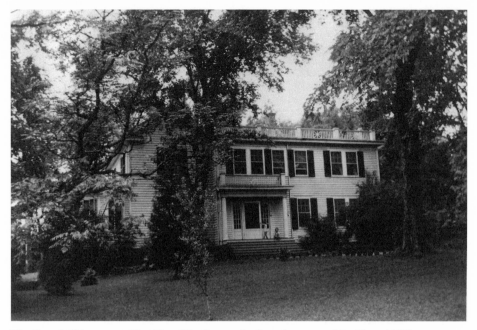

The Berryhill home on West Franklin Street, the first they owned in Chapel Hill, c. 1939.
Daughters Catherine and Jane are on the porch. *(Berryhill Family)*

a driveway and garage were on the Rosemary Street side next to Fowler's Food
Store. They lived in this house during the early years of Berryhill's deanship
and raised their two girls there. Cat Berryhill said that her fondest Chapel Hill
memories were of this "wonderful, big house."[57]

Jane Berryhill remembered this house as the site of an important maturing
experience for her. It was during the war, and she was about ten years old. Her
father suggested that she could help the war effort by growing flowers and taking
them in her little red wagon up to the Carolina Inn two blocks away. She pleaded,
"Daddy, I don't know how," to which he replied, "Yes, you do." So she did as he
told her, and later she recalled, "Day by day, week by week my responsibilities
grew, but hopefully so did my maturity."[58]

The Berryhills sold the West Franklin Street house and land after the war to
the neighboring Fowler's Food Store, which later built Chapel Hill's first super-
market on the site. The Berryhills had an option to lease the house until their
new home was built, but the long delays in building their home owing to the
postwar shortage of building materials forced them to move temporarily for
a year to Graham Court Apartments near the Carolina Inn and then for two
years to the university-owned Horace Williams House on East Franklin Street.
They tried to buy this house, but the university refused to sell. While very disappointed at the time, they were later glad because otherwise they would not have
had their beloved home in the country.

The Berryhills knew they wanted to live in the country. During the war years
they purchased from Miles Andrews a seventy-two-acre farm just south of Carr-

boro on Smith Level Road. Before their new home was completed, Berryhill was quoted in a 1950 interview as saying he dreamed of having some "white faced" cattle on the farm and that he and his wife were preparing for that day by planting permanent pasture for "the cattle-to-come." He laughingly added, "I want only the cows you eat, not those you drink"—he recalled milking the cows on his family's farm at Steele Creek before and after school "without any aid from those fancy milking machines."[59]

William N. Hubbard, Jr., a student in the two-year class of 1943, recalled, "One of the joys [of being a medical student] was the occasion when the students were invited to The Farm. Hogs had been slaughtered that fall, and Dr. Berryhill showed off the box in which the fresh hams were being salt- and sugar-cured before smoking." Good food and good fellowship were enjoyed by all, with Norma providing "the calm, kind and considerate presence that we all loved."[60] A reporter in 1950 elaborated, "Oftentimes, students follow their dean to his farm. It has become a common sight to find Dr. Berryhill seated on a stump catching his breath from hoeing or plowing, with several medical students perched on other stumps around talking to him."[61]

By the time they got around to building their home, Berryhill was busy with the hospital construction and with faculty recruiting, which left most of the planning and supervision to Norma. She wanted to renovate a log cabin on the site for their home but lost the argument to her husband when lightning struck and burned the cabin down. She apparently won most of the other arguments about the design, however, and they moved into their new home in 1951.[62] It was a house with white siding, located on a ridge looking westward. Adding to the gardens and yard through the years, they made the house a warm

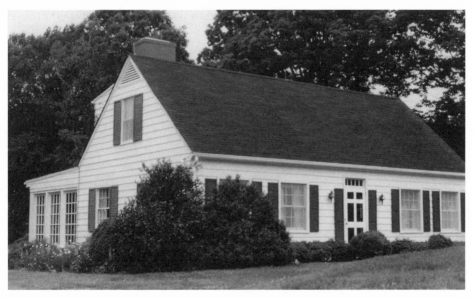

The Berryhill country home outside of Carrboro. *(Berryhill Family)*

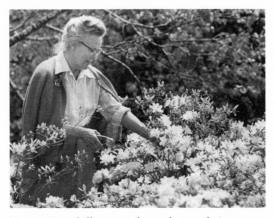

Norma Berryhill among the azaleas at their country home, 1960s. *(Berryhill Family)*

and welcoming home for their family and numerous guests. Both Norma and Reece enjoyed working in the garden and sharing their flowers and produce with acquaintances.

Cat Berryhill remembers well the move to the country home in 1951: "Dr. Womack, the new chief of surgery, and his family were to move in the university's Horace Williams House temporarily until they found a house in Chapel Hill. We were still packing when the moving truck come to the house with the Womacks' furniture from Iowa. Because the floors in the new house weren't finished we had to stay with friends in town for a short time before we could move." She recalled that the only thing she detested about the new house was that she had to ride the school bus from Carrboro to Chapel Hill High School, which was then located on West Franklin Street, where University Square and Granville Towers are now located.[63]

Norma's determination to design and supervise the building of their country home was paralleled by her determination to protect it, as attested in an article on the front page of the *Chapel Hill Weekly* for September 10, 1948:

> A tractor and much valuable corn were burned in a fire at the Berryhill farm outside of Carrboro last Saturday afternoon . . . The blaze started, it is believed, when the tractor, which was providing the power for a corn-shucking machine, backfired and ignited the shucks in a pile of corn . . .
>
> In addition to the loss of the tractor and the corn pile, a nearby compost heap and numerous farm tools were partially destroyed. A holly hedge and an apple tree were ruined.
>
> The fire was extinguished with the aid of five fire extinguishe[r]s and water from a 300-gallon tank which Mrs. Berryhill obtained in Carrboro. Persons who aided in putting out the fire were Mrs. Berryhill; George Pendergraft and his father; John Blackman, another neighbor; Fire Warden Fitzgerald from Hillsborough; Clayton Rogers and Mr. Baldwin of the Chapel Hill [F]ire Department. Through their efforts, the spacious barn nearby was saved.[64]

The same episode demonstrated Berryhill's integrity. When he learned of the fire, he had the keys to the state automobile in his pocket. Yet he went around the medical school to find someone whose car he could borrow, because he would not use the state car for personal reasons.

One of the younger faculty members who joined the surgery department in 1952 added this about Norma's activities on the farm:

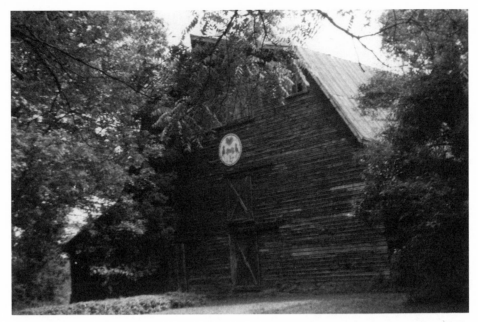

The barn that was on the country-home property when the Berryhills bought it. *(Berryhill Family)*

Norma had a career of her own that few people knew about. She raised cattle on their land. It was grass, not grain, fed cattle (she was ahead of her time on low fat). On more than one occasion we purchased a quarter or side of beef from her. Also on more that one occasion she invited our children to the farm to see the cattle, explained to them what she did and allowed you to pick the steer you were to purchase. At that time Fowler's food store also packed and stored the beef for Norma's customers. I am sure she had a hand in making this arrangement.

Family Life

According to Jane Berryhill, she and her sister never felt neglected for lack of attention from their father. "He wasn't there physically a lot of the time, but I knew he was there." She especially treasured times when the two of them were together alone, such as when she and her father went to Charlotte to visit her paternal grandmother, "the sweetest, dearest lady, so gentle, so loving." She felt that her father's mother was the origin of "the calm side of Daddy, the reassuring, loving" side.

Asked what the most important things were that she remembered about her father, Jane replied, "From a daughter's point of view it was the immense sense of security, love, and constant dedication to what ever he was doing. Tenaciousness may not be the right word, but that's the word that comes to mind."

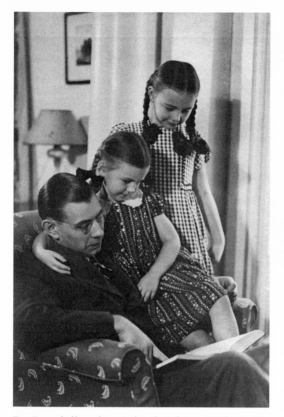

Dr. Berryhill reading to his daughters, Catherine, age five, and Jane, age seven, c. 1940. *(Berryhill Family)*

He would discipline them, Jane said, just by looking at them in the eye. "Never said a word, just looked me in the eye. I knew . . . He expected the best of everyone . . . he was understanding, but he had his expectations. But I understood that because I saw how hard he worked."

Berryhill would immediately put on music when he came home, especially the classics such as Beethoven and Bach. Jane remembered, "It was soothing to us because often by the time he got home in my early years it was almost time for us to go to bed. So we went to sleep every night to this marvelous music." In addition to the music, Berryhill enjoyed "the yard, the flowers, and the vegetables." Said Jane, "I think one of his brightest joys was the produce and the flowers." He would get up early in the morning to see that everything was picked at its best—the vegetables for their meals or for friends and flowers for friends or hospital patients.

Jane said that her father always made holidays very special. "I think Thanksgiving was a very, very special time because he was always so thankful for so many things in life. I [also] remember going out with him to cut down Christmas trees. He was very proud of picking the right one and setting it up for mother and making it perfect . . . The most wonderful memories I have of holidays are during the Christmas times because in those days we had so many friends of their age group with whom I had grown up. He loved hearing the Christmas carols and singing and we'd all go to one person's house or another to gather around singing. Daddy always said he couldn't sing but he enjoyed listening."

Jane never heard her father tell an off-color joke, and others would not tell one in his presence. Although he would not take the Lord's name in vain, he was known to use an emphatic "damn" or "hell" as the occasion demanded.

Jane summarized her feelings thus: "Frankly, I worshipped my father. Truly worshipped him. In the days that began my real memories of this—Franklin Street, the medical school, and the war—there was planning and all this activity and Daddy would be out so at late meetings, going to the legislature and doing all this . . . Almost every night when he was not home when I thought he should be, I would go downstairs and sit in his chair until he came home."[65]

When the children were young they all went to church at the Presbyterian Church (now the University Presbyterian Church) on East Franklin Street across from the university campus. Jane said her father went every Sunday that he wasn't out of town or working. After the arrival of the new and controversial minister, the Reverend Charles M. Jones, she started to detect a change in her father's attitude. Eventually Berryhill resigned from the church's session in protest and stopped attending the services. Jane said that was when she "began gradually to leave the Presbyterian Church, because I thought, if my father [was] unhappy," something was wrong. "At that age I didn't understand it wasn't the Presbyterian Church, it was that person."

Social Life in Chapel Hill

Social life during the Depression and war years in Chapel Hill was fairly simple. The Berryhills did not play bridge, but Norma enjoyed morning Coca-Cola parties or coffees, and they both went to dinner parties at the homes of friends. They actively participated in the life of the university community, attending most of the Playmakers productions and never missing a football game or a commencement.

Although their circle of friends and professional colleagues expanded during the years, in the early years they remained close to the MacNiders. Once, though, there was a sharp encounter between "Dr. Billy" and Norma. They had had a discussion about women's relationships with the university and why UNC was not approved by the American Association of University Women (AAUW), and MacNider had apparently said something that greatly upset Norma. The breach was healed when he sent her some flowers from his garden, and Norma relented in a handwritten note:

> *Dear Bill—*
> Last night when Reece gave me your message I was ready to write a note and sign it "go to hell" but after living in the same room all morning with those sweet, lovely, pink, buds that you brought.
>
>

Love

Norma[66]
>

One unexpected break from the Berryhills' routine occurred not long after they returned to Chapel Hill. Berryhill had taken care of a man who managed a Georgia plantation for a prominent member of Western Reserve's board of trustees in Cleveland. When the patient returned to his native Scotland to recuperate from a long illness, he became worse, and his Scottish physicians told him he was dying. The board member paid the way for Berryhill and Norma to go check up on him. On very short notice they set sail on a German liner, the *Bremen*.

Norma wrote "Dr. Billy and Sally" (Dr. and Mrs. MacNider) from the ship thanking them for the candy and telegram that were in their cabin when they boarded. She added, "This is the most pleasant experience—never have I heard of such food—venison, pheasant and everything else . . . We started out in a big way but have decided we better curb ourselves and live a simple life and we might stay on our feet longer . . . Reece hasn't shown any too much of his Presbyterian traits . . . [he] is asleep at the moment and I am off to the bar alone." She added that they felt safe with "our Jane there near friends. Do keep an ear to the ground for an S.O.S. from her."[67] By the time they arrived in Scotland, however, the patient was doing well, and as it turned out, he lived for many more years. This unexpectedly happy turn freed the Berryhills to enjoy a two-week-long grand tour of Scotland and England.[68]

Norma stayed busy in the community with many volunteer efforts. She was a founder and first president of the University Women's Club, which became a very active group with a monthly "occasion" ("as a club we don't meet—we have occasions"). She also joined in various other activities such as book clubs and an investment club. In the early 1950s, after the hospital opened, Norma "did twist a number of arms to get the University Women's Club to have meetings early in the year when the legislature was in session and then invite the legislators' wives here." After lunch the club would give the wives a tour of the hospital. "We did that for a couple of years, and then other sections of the University saw what a good idea it was, so they sort of took over the idea" and took the wives on tours of other areas of the university.

Norma particularly enjoyed the investment club. The twenty members contributed $10 (later $20) a month, and the group invested in the stock market. Not only did this give Norma a relatively risk-free way to learn about the stock mar-

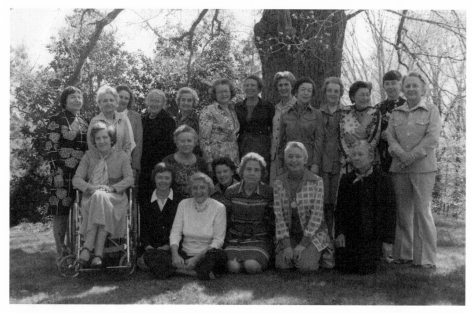

Norma Berryhill (kneeling, middle row, second from left) entertaining medical faculty wives at the Berryhill country home, c. 1952. (Berryhill Family)

ket, it also provided her an opportunity to meet new women in the university outside the medical school. "For years, I made a little money myself but I soon discovered that my trust officer could make more than I could, so I let him have it. But I go and I enjoy [the investment club because] academically I enjoy the stock market."[69]

Once Berryhill became dean, Norma would often give pre-football-game luncheons at their home for medical alumni, members of the legislature, and other friends of the university and the medical school. Norma also entertained wives of students, residents, and faculty at their home. Cat Berryhill says that in those days, before funding was available to support such entertainment, she dreaded these events because she and her older sister had to wash a lot of dishes after everyone left. She was particularly upset when her sister Jane left for college—it meant Cat had to shoulder the burden by herself.[70]

University Physician

The student infirmary in which Berryhill was to work as the university physician from 1933 to 1941 was located in what is now Abernethy Hall. This was the third infirmary built by the university for sick students. The first, completed in 1858, was a small cottage on the corner of East Franklin Street where Spencer Dormitory is now located. Called "The Retreat," it was replaced in 1895 by the second infirmary, which in turn was replaced by Abernethy Hall in 1907. Abernethy Hall served the health needs of the student body until the Navy Hospital, built in

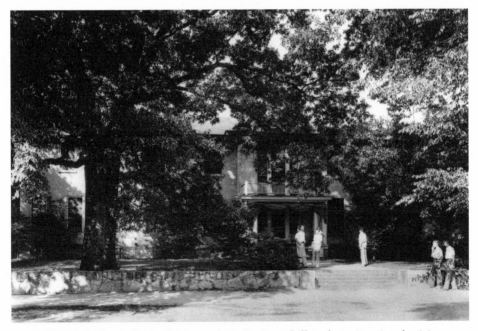

Abernethy Hall, the student infirmary, where Dr. Berryhill as the university physician cared for ambulatory and hospitalized students from 1933 to 1941. *(NCC)*

University Physician and Faculty Member   91

1942 for the Naval Pre-Flight School, was occupied by the student health service in 1946. That infirmary, located just behind MacNider Hall on what is now the medical campus, served the students until the current building, the James A. Taylor Student Health Service Building, opened in 1980 adjacent to the south side of Kenan Stadium.[71]

Built in 1907, Abernethy Hall, a two-story gray brick building on South Columbia Street diagonally across from the Carolina Inn, was named for Eric A. Abernethy, MD, a practicing physician in Chapel Hill who served in World War I and then became the full-time university physician from 1919 to 1933. The original building contained four wards, a dispensary, an operating room, and various supporting rooms. An east wing addition in 1924 doubled the capacity of the original building. A south wing was added in 1939, while Berryhill was university physician. Based on his requirements, this addition provided space for teaching physical diagnosis to second-year medical students, improved laboratory facilities for patient care and teaching clinical pathology to medical students, and additional beds, including single rooms for critically ill students.

Because of the small size of the village and the university, until Abernethy's appointment in 1919 most physicians caring for students were in practice in the town or were full-time medical school faculty members. William Peter Mallett, MD, a beloved town physician and MacNider's maternal grandfather, served the students from 1857 until his death in 1889. Medical School Dean Richard White-head and Charles S. Mangum served as the physicians for the infirmary around the turn of the century. From 1907 until after World War I, Drs. Mangum, Manning, and MacNider each served the students for a three-month period during the nine-month school year, while Abernethy cared for the summer-school students. After Abernethy returned from military service in France, he became the first full-time university physician. Foy Roberson, MD, of Durham served temporarily from then until Berryhill assumed the post in September 1933.[72] During the late 1930s and early 1940s, Roberson served as surgical consultant for the freshman and varsity football squads.

As Berryhill was preparing for the move to Chapel Hill, he wrote MacNider, "I feel very humble about undertaking the responsibility of that infirmary job. I hope you will let me talk to you freely about the various problems that come up and that any time you think that I may be making a mistake or, if you ever have any suggestions, you will please feel perfectly free to tell me about them." He felt "that there is a very worth while work to be done there" but acknowledged that it would take some time to get everything working well. He added that he felt "the infirmary committee [Manning, Mangum, and MacNider] will be very helpful, sympathetic and patient."[73]

Notwithstanding his apparent sense of inadequacy about the new position, Berryhill had been exposed to some of the problems of providing health care for students and hospital employees in Cleveland. In his response, written in September 1931, to a request by Dr. A. B. Denison of the Western Reserve University Health Clinic, Berryhill had provided a detailed and thoughtful two-page analysis of the existing arrangements for the care of student nurses and others by Lakeside Hospital and by the university health service. As chief resident in medicine Berryhill had had a year of experience with taking care of nurses and others in a system where responsibility was often split between the hospital and the university depending on the nature of the illness, the time of day, and the status of the patient. Residents set aside an hour a day for sick calls, but they were still being called day and night to treat the nurses and others. Wrote Berryhill: "The present arrangement is now too time-consuming for the resident physician or any member of the hospital staff to take care of adequately and at the same time fulfill his hospital duties. Neither the clinical experience nor the meager salary warrants a member of the hospital staff continuing this job." He recommended the appointment of a part-time hospital personnel physician, who would be responsible for examining new employees and for treating illnesses among the hospital staff. The infirmary "should be enlarged and should be run by the hospital rather than by the university . . . In spite of the name, University Hospitals, the three hospitals here are still not integral parts of Western Reserve University, and I see no particular advantage in placing the hospital personnel under the care of the university health service." These jurisdictional problems would be similar to ones he would later experience as dean concerning the administrative boundaries between the hospital and the university concerning the care of university students and hospital staff.[74] Berryhill continued to be involved in the discussion of this organizational problem while in Cleveland, but he left before the new organizational structure was implemented.[75]

In negotiations with President Graham and Dean Manning concerning the position as university physician, Berryhill gave a preview of his future administrative and negotiating skills. He conditions for acceptance included a technician and equipment in the infirmary for basic blood and urine examinations, throat cultures, and X-rays. He also wanted "laboratory space properly equipped to continue my own research in bacteriology and immunology." He "heartily endorsed" the suggestion that the position be "more or less full-time," but asked for permission to have a consulting practice because "the opportunity of seeing a few difficult medical problems on the outside would add considerably to the enjoyment of the position."[76]

MacNider had seen the list of requirements Berryhill had negotiated and "thought these were just right." MacNider also gave his younger colleague some practical advice: "I would be careful to have a very clean-cut business understanding about it in terms of the physical development of the University Infirmary. Of course Frank [Graham] will do anything in the world that he can, and there is never any necessity of having any written statement from him about anything; but Frank, like the rest of us, may slip out sometime, and in such an event you want to know very definitely where you stand." He cautioned that these requirements "should be put in on the University basis [presumably he

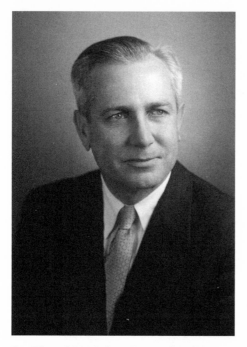

Dr. Edward M. Hedgpeth served with Berryhill as assistant university physician and then as university physician for a number of years. He was chair of the medical school admissions committee from 1949 to 1966. *(Wootten-Moulton Collection, NCC)*

meant in the annual appropriations] and not on a make-shift basis."[77]

During the fall of 1933 Berryhill worked alone as the university physician, although he had two registered nurses to assist him. Edward M. Hedgpeth, MD, who had completed the two-year school at Chapel Hill in 1929 and obtained his MD from the University of Pennsylvania in 1931, returned to Chapel Hill in early 1934 to join Berryhill as the assistant university physician. Hedgpeth became the associate university physician in 1938 and university physician in 1941 when Berryhill became dean.[78] By 1937–1938 three full-time physicians staffed the infirmary; the following year the staff increased to four physicians, and by 1940–1941, Berryhill's last year as university physician, the infirmary staff had increased to five physicians. Between 1933–1934 and 1940–1941, the infirmary nursing staff increased from two nurses to four.

The 1940–1941 UNC catalog described the infirmary, which by that time had been under Berryhill's direction for eight years:

> In order to provide proper attention for the student during sickness the University employs five full time physicians and maintains a well-appointed infirmary. The infirmary is equipped with all necessary conveniences and comforts, and with a modern X-ray unit and a laboratory for diagnostic purposes under the direction of a full time technician. It is under the immediate supervision of the University Physician, and is provided with four experienced nurses. At the discretion of the University Physician a student may be admitted to its wards, and for such services as may be rendered by the staff no charges are made. But should any additional service (consultation, special nurses, operations requiring the attendance of a trained surgeon), recommended by the attending physician and approved by the patient or guardian, be necessary, the student will be required to pay for such service.

MacNider did take Berryhill up on his request for questions or suggestions at any time about the infirmary. In response to a letter from MacNider about the cost of some so-called cold capsules to be sold to students, Berryhill replied, "I had no idea the actual cost of the materials would be so little." He documented this with an enclosure showing the cost of the four ingredients ("atropine sulphate, aspirin, caffeine cit, and powd. cascarin"), the six capsules, and one bottle. The total was less than four cents for six capsules. Berryhill said, "Of course, if codeine is added—as in most of ours with about ¼ gr. [grain] per capsule—the cost would be more, but even then the charge of 75 cents for 6 is just plain damn Robbery. Considering all the overhead & service charges, as is also the charge of 75 cents for 6 oz. Calamine lotion."[79] His calculation gave Berryhill insight into a costing practice that has been a growing problem for hospitals and patients ever since, as hospitals disguise their real costs with low daily room charges and make up the difference with inflated charges for drugs, laboratory and radiological procedures, and the like.

The students viewed Berryhill as a serious and concerned physician. One student, a freshman during Berryhill's first year as the university physician, recounted that he had almost lost a fingernail when it was caught in the swinging door at the grocery store where he worked to pay his university expenses. This occurred on a Saturday, so he bandaged it and then went to the infirmary on Monday. "I was so scared. Dr Berryhill took that finger, took a scalpel, looked at it and all of a sudden he took that thing off. I don't remember that it hurt much . . . Everything was very businesslike." Berryhill then gave him a little lecture, insisting that he come in immediately if he had red streaks going up his arm.[80]

Another student was an undergraduate freshman when he first met Berryhill at the infirmary. "With every student visit he seemed always thorough but very austere. He was not given to many words but, on the other hand, he answered any question that the somewhat intimidated student might have . . . He gave the impression that if he prescribed a certain action he expected it to be carried out and, if there was any doubt, he would keep the student in the Infirmary to see that it was."[81]

John F. Lynch, a future medical student, described his first encounter with Berryhill in the winter of 1937 when he was an undergraduate sophomore at UNC, "a young country boy" who at the time had never touched alcohol. He was seldom sick, but one Monday morning he had "a little fever and felt terrible." He went to the infirmary in Abernathy Hall across from the Deke House and "with time I was called to see Dr. Reece Berryhill. After a brief exam I was dressed down, told I had no problem and to get out. Needless to say, I thought Dr. Berryhill might be the biggest S.O.B. I had ever seen. In retrospect, . . . he probably thought I was hung over . . . With this start you may be surprised to know that Dr. Berryhill became one of my lifelong heroes. He was a major supporter of mine always, and I consider him one of my very closest friends. He was . . . this to me as he was to many of our classmates, colleagues, and friends. This just proves that first impressions can be very, very wrong!"[82] In this case both Lynch and Berryhill—who could be very impatient with complainers—were guilty of wrong first impressions.

Berryhill and his physician colleagues published two papers in the *North Carolina Medical Journal* based on their experiences with the students at the UNC infirmary. The first, published in October 1943, concerned primary atypical pneumonia of unknown etiology. This was a review of 400 cases (350 in university students and 50 in private practice) that had been seen between 1935 and 1943. These cases differed from the "typical" pneumococcal pneumonia (caused by the bacillus *Streptococcus pneumoniae*) in that they had minimal pulmonary findings on physical examination while showing definite evidence of a "pneumonic process in the lungs" by X-ray, a normal or only slightly increased white-blood-cell count, no demonstrable bacterial agent as a cause, a lack of response to sulfonamides, and a low mortality but frequently a prolonged convalescence. "This latter feature," wrote the authors in a justification of their study, "together with the high and possibly increasing incidence and virulence of the disease, both in the civilian population and in the personnel of the armed forces, makes this one of the most important of the acute infectious diseases involving the respiratory tract at the present time."

Berryhill, as the lead author, had presented the paper at the North Carolina Medical Society meeting a few months previously. The active debate on the nature of the disease that followed his presentation was documented in the published abstract of the discussion. Several speakers, including James B. Bullitt, MD, chair of pathology at UNC, felt strongly that this disease was not the same as the "flu-pneumonia" seen in the deadly 1918 influenza pandemic. A physician from High Point postulated, "There are a group of diseases, caused by closely related viruses and clinically indistinguishable. Until we are in a position to do a lot of exhaustive and expensive research and ferret out the causative agents we cannot be sure that we are dealing with the same entity."[83] Today the syndrome known as primary atypical pneumonia is usually caused by *Mycoplasma pneumoniae,* although other agents such as *Legionella pneumophilia* and *Chlamydia pneumoniae* can cause a similar syndrome. All these agents are bacteria, not viruses, but they were unknown at the time of Berryhill's paper due to the difficulty of isolating and identifying them.[84]

In February 1944 Berryhill was the second author of a *North Carolina Medical Journal* article by Hedgpeth and four other colleagues. They presented twenty cases of spontaneous pneumothorax occurring in UNC students from 1937 to 1943. The students were all young males between eighteen and twenty-one years of age with the exception of one female student. The authors noted that "it has been generally accepted that tuberculosis is the most common cause of spontaneous pneumothorax . . . in many instances a provisional diagnosis of tuberculosis is made and the patient is subjected to unnecessarily long periods of hospital or sanatorium care when there are no findings to support the diagnosis of tuberculosis other than the presence of the collapsed lung." They believed not all of their cases were associated with tuberculosis, even though a few of the patients were lost to long-term follow-up. In contrast to collapsed lung caused by tuberculosis, their cases had "a benign, usually afebrile, course, with complete recovery in a few weeks."

Paul P. McCain, MD, of Sanatorium, North Carolina, in the printed abstract

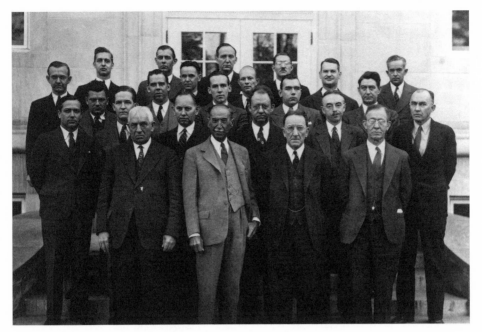

School of Medicine and Public Health faculty, 1940. *Front row, left to right:* Drs. Isaac H. Manning, Milton J. Rosenau, William de Berniere MacNider, and James B. Bullitt. Dr. Berryhill is at the left on the top row. *(NCC)*

of the discussion at the state medical society meeting, complemented Hedgpeth on his "splendid presentation of the subject" and said it was "a good sample of the careful medical attention that is being given to the students at the University." He added, "It has been my pleasure to follow pretty closely the work of the medical service at the university for several years, and it seems to me that it is the best of any student health service of which I have knowledge."[85]

Teaching Responsibilities

Berryhill emphasized his desire to teach in his May 1933 letter to Dean Manning concerning his appointment as university physician: "My plans and training since the year [1929–1930] I spent as your substitute in the Physiology Department have been in the direction of academic clinical medicine. It is a rather sudden jolt to depart from that path, particularly as regards teaching and the daily contact with a large amount of clinical material. I asked President Graham if in the future—I realize it is out of the question at the moment—some arrangement could be made for actual teaching work."[86]

In his autobiographical sketch for the Boston City Hospital volume, Berryhill elaborated on this theme: "President Frank Graham . . . invited me to Chapel Hill as university physician and director of the student health service, with responsibilities for improving the quality of medical services for the students of the University, as well as for improving the introductory courses in clinical medicine to better prepare the medical students for transfer for their clinical years and to plan and work for this Medical School's expansion."[87]

Berryhill later described the changes in clinical instruction for medical students in the 1979 history of the school:

The university's decision in 1933 to reorganize the Student Health Service under the direction of the writer with a full-time staff who were also members of the medical school faculty, coupled with the increased time provided for instruction in introductory clinical medicine in 1934 were essential developments in improving the quality of instruction in these important areas of the curriculum of the two-year school.

Gradually, over the period 1935–1950, the quality of the clinical instruction greatly improved. This was accomplished through attracting additional full-time clinical staff for the Student Health Service and having them assume the major responsibility for organizing and directing the teaching. Valuable assistance was provided also by the able clinical teachers in various specialties at the Watts and Rex Hospitals and at some of the state hospitals, especially the North Carolina Tuberculosis Sanatorium at McCain [formerly Sanatorium, NC] and the Dorothea Dix Hospital [at Raleigh].[88]

The changes effected after Berryhill's arrival are mirrored in the course listings in UNC's annual catalogs. In contrast to a brief listing in the 1933–1934 medical school section for physical diagnosis as "four hours a week, winter quarter" for a total of forty hours in the two-year curriculum, the 1934–1935 medical school catalog had a numbered course with an allocation of seventy hours:

231. PHYSICAL DIAGNOSIS.
A course in the method of history taking and physical examination with lectures, demonstrations, and practical exercises.

At the beginning emphasis is placed on the physical signs in the normal subject. The class is divided into groups for practical exercises on and demonstrations of the clinical material in the University Infirmary, in the wards and out-patient department of Watts Hospital (Durham), and in the State Tubercular Sanitorium [sic]. Each student has twenty practical exercises of three hours each. *Seven hours a week, spring quarter.* Associate Professor Berryhill and assistants from Medical Staff of Watts Hospital.

The 220-bed hospital and clinics at Watts were to provide "clinical material for the courses in Physical Diagnosis and Clinical Pathology, and afford opportunity for attendance upon autopsies and the study of fresh pathological specimens." This same catalog also listed a new course, "Introduction to Obstetrics," consisting of 10 one-hour lectures in the winter quarter of the second year taught by Robert Alexander Ross, MD, of Durham, lecturer on obstetrics, who in 1952 would become the professor and first chair of obstetrics and gynecology at UNC.[89]

Berryhill accepted this teaching assignment with enthusiasm, but it posed considerable logistical challenges. The infirmary never had enough patients to assure an adequate number and variety of illnesses for the course. Berryhill thus spent much time each spring arranging for the students to see patients at Watts, McPherson (ear, nose, and throat), and Lincoln Hospitals in Durham; at the State (mental) Hospital in Raleigh; and at the State Tuberculosis Hospital in Sanatorium. He then accompanied them to the sites for most of the sessions.

In the spring of 1936, Berryhill had half of the approximately thirty-five students going to Watts on Monday and Thursday afternoons, with the other half going on Tuesday and Friday afternoons. He arranged for various physicians to spend an hour with the small groups of students "going over the cases and demonstrating physical signs."[90] He or Hedgpeth also accompanied the students for one session at the State Tuberculosis Hospital. Berryhill wrote Paul P. McCain, MD, the medical director, about their needs: "So far we have had very few pathological chests for the students. I should like if possible for them to listen to chests that have definite signs of consolidation, of fluid and cavitation and pneumothorax as well as to hear a lot of rales and bronchial breathing of which so far they have had very little."[91]

Although physical diagnosis was an essential course for the students if they were to be successful when they transferred elsewhere for their clinical years, the university had a very limited budget to support it. To the physicians who helped instruct the students, Berryhill wrote: "I am sorry that gratitude is the only form in which we can remunerate the people who help with this work at the present time." On some occasions Dean House did write on behalf of the university to thank those outside physicians and institutions who helped with the course.

The financial limitations and logistical challenges at the time are highlighted in a letter dated June 1935 from Berryhill to Robert B. House, the dean of administration under President Graham. Berryhill began: "According to the terms of my appointment as an Associate Professor in the Medical School the sole remuneration is traveling expenses in connection with the [physical diagnosis] course." He explains that the total expenses of $99.72 (sixty trips for a total of 1940 miles at five cents per mile or $97, plus $2.72 for telephone calls and postage) are much more than the previous year because the number of hours had doubled, resulting in four round trips a week to Durham and one trip to the State Tuberculosis Hospital during the spring quarter. The total number included additional trips to select the patients before the students went over as well as to confer with the medical staff. "In other words," Berryhill explained, "it has been necessary to play a game of politics with the people at both [Watts and Lincoln] Hospitals in order to make better facilities for teaching our students in terms of using the charity and clinic patients at these two hospitals."[92]

Berryhill did tell House that considerable progress had been made in improving the physical diagnosis course: "We have been able this year to offer a course in Physical Diagnosis which compares very favorably with those given in medical schools situated in larger cities," but Berryhill reminded him that "the future of the Medical School depends entirely upon its ability to modernize the curriculum and keep pace with the present tendencies in medical education."[93]

A statement by the medical school advisory committee (Mangum, MacNider, and Berryhill) dated May 4, 1936, documented the need for further enhancement of clinical teaching for the second-year medical students.[94] The curriculum had been revised to provide more hours for physical diagnosis, clinical pathology, and a proposed new course in the principles of surgery. Although the course in physical diagnosis had been taught the past three years at Watts, "the attitude of the majority of the staff at the hospital is one of indifference, if not actual hostility, toward the teaching of students in the hospital." This situation changed over the years, for in his 1979 history of the medical school, Berryhill stated that "the Watts Hospital supplied the chief clinical resources without which the courses in clinical medicine and surgery would never have been adequate. To this institution, its staff, its administration, and its trustees the university owes a lasting debt."[95]

The committee also recommended that a Department of Clinical Medicine be established to function like a Department of Medicine in a four-year school— that is, to care for ill students, operate a charity medical service, be responsible for teaching all the clinical courses in the medical school, and conduct clinical investigations.[96] MacNider had said he was going to recommend to President Graham that Berryhill be made professor and chair of the proposed new Department of Clinical Medicine. Berryhill wrote MacNider several days later to urge that MacNider not suggest him for the position, for two reasons: "First, the appointment of a person to that position should be made after a committee has surveyed the field just as other University appointments should be made. The mere fact of the presence here of one individual does not mean at all that that person is the best fitted for the position we had in mind . . . In the second place, because of the friendship that exists I think your motive might be misunderstood." Berryhill added a handwritten note to the typed letter: "I know and you know that I am not the person to be a prof. of medicine in terms of a Real University. I would simply be 'rattling around'—as Peabody used to say."[97] In his reply MacNider thanked Berryhill for his "thoughtful and at the same time very characteristic note." He continued, "In my judgment you never 'rattled around' in your life. Your movements are those of poise, dependent upon understanding and judgment. There is no question in my mind but what you are the proper person to be made Professor and Head of the Department of Medicine at the University. I am willing to admit there may be an element of emotion in this decision. How could it fail to be? But nevertheless this is my judgment based on reason extending over not a few months but some years." MacNider did go on to concede that he had always insisted that "Heads of Departments . . . should be selected in terms of competitive merit by a committee." He said he was going to ask Graham to appoint such a search committee (one that didn't include

Berryhill). In the end, though, nothing came of the recommendation for a new department or for a search committee.[98]

The commitment to the expanded physical diagnosis course and the workload at the infirmary led Berryhill to ask Dean House to relieve him and Hedgpeth of the responsibility for teaching a course in the Department of Physical Education in the winter quarter of 1936–1937. They had "neither time nor mental energy to prepare five lectures a week after seeing from one hundred to one hundred and sixty boys a day as we have been doing recently over here." Berryhill added that he hoped some help could be obtained in the infirmary for the spring quarter because he would be teaching physical diagnosis fifteen hours a week in the medical school.[99] In his response House stated that he fully understood their situation and would make other arrangements for the course in question. He also appreciated Berryhill's need for help in the infirmary during the spring quarter and asked Berryhill for suggestions and a cost estimate.

Later that fall House made available $500 to the medical school to help the situation with regard to clinical teaching for second-year medical students and physician coverage for the infirmary. House further demonstrated his sensitivity to the dilemma in which Berryhill found himself when he urged him in December 1936 "to keep teaching within the sphere of things that you are going to do. No matter how discouraging the situation may look in advance, I believe it is possible to find someone to relieve you at the Infirmary for enough time to allow you to teach." He concluded, "You certainly from the very beginning have been considered as a member of the teaching staff, as well as University Physician."[100]

At the conclusion of the physical diagnosis course in the spring of 1937, Berryhill sent his request for reimbursement of his travel expenses to Dean Mangum at the medical school. He also suggested that, since some funds were left over, $45 be paid to Edwin Robertson, MD, a young physician in Durham, who had taught the class for two hours a week for four weeks at Watts Hospital. After the reimbursement of Berryhill's travel expenses and the $45, Berryhill noted, a small balance would remain from the original $200 allocated to this course, and he applied for it: "I would appreciate it so much if you could feel free to recommend to Mr. House that the balance be paid to me on account of I have not in the four years I have taught this course received any remuneration other than the actual traveling expenses incurred in the course. I can't very well ask the Administrator myself to do this and I should prefer to remain out of it, but if the money is available for that purpose and if I have done about nine-tenths of the work then it seems a fair request for me to get the remainder of this rather than turning it back into the general pot of the state."[101]

By 1938 the university had obtained appropriations from the State and a Works Progress Administration (WPA) grant from the federal government to make the proposed addition to the infirmary and to construct the new medical school and public health building. In 1938 Dean MacNider commented on it in

Yackety Yack: "This building will be placed as a key building on a large plateau in a southwesterly direction from the University Library, which will make possible in the future the development in this location of other buildings of a medical order."[102]

Berryhill's attempts to improve clinical teaching for the second-year medical students before they transferred continued until Memorial Hospital opened in Chapel Hill in 1952 and the four-year curriculum was implemented. In an article for *Yackety Yack* in 1942, the student writing the medical school section commented on the fact that "the clinical courses are now receiving more time and emphasis in the curriculum. This is largely possible through the cooperation of Watts Hospital in Durham, which provides a source of invaluable clinical and pathological material."[103]

Berryhill and His Students

A student who completed the two-year school during World War II remembered, "Patient contact for medical students was hard to come by in Chapel Hill so Dr. Berryhill acquired a Model A Ford of uncertain age, which—along with a small bus—took students to Durham."[104]

A student who graduated from the two-year school in 1942 said that Berryhill "taught a course in physical diagnosis so it was from him that we learned percussion, palpation and auscultation, and the rest. This is an endeavor that required patience with many students and he had it. By this time in our relationship I, along with most of the students, looked on him as a kind, concerned father figure."[105]

The lessons learned in those physical diagnosis sessions with Berryhill made a lasting impression: "I well remember him presenting a black man with diffuse pulmonary densities and a perforated nasal septum who carried a diagnosis of Boeck's sarcoid, noting that the perforation aids the differential diagnosis. I fear I will go to my grave before I see the second instance, although I have carefully inspected the nasal septum of each patient with sarcoidosis."[106] Another student from the two-year class of 1950 said, "To this day I think of him occasionally when auscultating a chest because he taught physical diagnosis and would not let us get away with saying we heard something when we did not."[107]

That same student said that "over the years Dr. Berryhill became a very dependable and trusted friend," but his "first experiences with him were not that comfortable. Without knowledge of his ancestry, I saw him as a dour Scot with an occasional fleeting glimpse of good humor. New medical students held him [in] a position close to the Almighty." One experience reinforced this view: "Sometime in the first year I was summoned to his office. We had no grades and I did not know how we stood. I saw the summons as the likely end of my medical career. On entering I found him writing at his desk. Without looking up he pointed to a chair and I sat on it. For about fifteen minutes I waited and my life passed before my eyes. Finally, he said, 'Lewis, do you like being in this medical school?' I replied, 'Yes sir, Dr. Berryhill, I really like this school.' He said, 'Great. You are in the top 10 percent of your class. Keep it up.' I don't even remember leaving the office with my reprieve." Yet, he added, years later, when his first wife died, Berryhill "was among the first to show up and he came back the next day to the funeral on a cold, blustery winter day."

Berryhill's diagnostic acumen was demonstrated to James H. Scatliff, MD, the second chair of radiology, not long after he arrived at UNC in 1966. Berryhill started experiencing abdominal pain one evening after dinner. By the time he came to the emergency room about midnight he had a boardlike acute abdomen. He insisted that he had a perforated duodenal ulcer, but the initial X-rays did not reveal the telltale sign of air under the diaphragm. George Johnson, MD, the attending surgeon, called in the new chief of radiology. After taking flat plates in several positions, the air was finally seen, and Berryhill was taken to the operating room for a repair of his perforated ulcer.[108]

THE NEXT CHALLENGES

Having proven his skills as a clinician, teacher, and university faculty member in his first career in the 1930s, from the 1940s to the early 1960s Berryhill would have an opportunity to pursue his second career as a medical school dean and a leader in a great movement to improve the health of all North Carolinians.

CHAPTER 5

Dean of the Two-Year School of Medicine

During the mid- to late 1930s, Berryhill was highly visible to all UNC students as university physician and to the second-year medical students as their instructor in physical diagnosis and clinical medicine. Behind the scenes he was serving in a number of capacities that were to prepare him for his future academic administrative responsibilities. He was a member of several medical school committees in the 1930s and then served as an assistant dean to Dean MacNider from 1937 to 1940. His leadership of the medical school began in 1940–1941 when he served as acting dean. From 1941 to 1952 he served as dean of the two-year medical school while actively planning for and implementing the expansion to a four-year school with a teaching hospital at Chapel Hill. With these experiences he was able to make a smooth transition to his service as dean of the four-year, MD-granting medical school from 1952 to 1964.

MEDICAL SCHOOL ADMINISTRATION

In September 1933, shortly after Berryhill's return to Chapel Hill, Isaac Hall Manning, MD, professor and chair of physiology and dean of the medical school since 1905, resigned as dean "because of an unfortunate incident which resulted in President Frank P. Graham's overruling the dean's decision with respect to the admission of a student" who was Jewish and not a resident of North Carolina. Berryhill, Blythe, and Manning, in the 1979 history of the school, elaborated on this incident:[1]

> All Jewish students who were residents of North Carolina and who met the entrance requirement had always been admitted to the School of Medicine, and for the most part the school had encountered relatively little difficulty in transferring them to the four-year schools. However, beginning in the 1920s there was an increasing number of Jewish students from the East who attended this and other universities with two-year medical schools and applied for admission to these schools. The difficulty of transferring these out-of-state residents to four-year medical schools, even those in areas of which

they were natives, became a serious problem. Experience at this school had shown that it was unrealistic to expect that more than ten per cent of the class (four students) could be out-of-state Jewish students if transfer of all was to be accomplished.

The student in question had applied in the summer of 1933 for admission after four qualified Jewish students had already been accepted for the fall of that year. None of them withdrew in September, so after Manning consulted with most of the medical faculty, the student was rejected. He appealed to President Graham and had a petition signed by prominent alumni in Durham, the hometown of the student's wife. Graham determined that the student could not be refused admission because of "racial prejudice," overruled Manning, and admitted the student, at which point the dean resigned. As a follow-up to the episode, it was noted that the student, "while passing the required work in the first two years with a very low grade average, was not accepted for transfer by either of the two four-year schools to which application was made."

Frank Graham was true to his convictions and reacted to what he perceived as anti-Semitic prejudice. For Dean Manning (and later for Berryhill as dean of the two-year school), however, this was a pragmatic issue. A person with two years of medical school and no MD degree was of no help in addressing the health care needs of the people of the state. In the face of the severely limited budgets in the Depression and in respect for the time and effort of their faculty, they felt they had to react to the anti-Semitic quotas of the northeastern medical schools by themselves imposing quotas based on their experience over the years in successfully transferring Jewish students to these MD-granting schools.

It is noteworthy that Manning, after his resignation, was a leader in persuading the state medical society to adopt a voluntary prepaid hospitalization insurance plan for the citizens of North Carolina. The resulting nonprofit Hospital Savings Association of North Carolina was chartered in 1935 with an organizational grant of $25,000 from the Duke Endowment. Manning served as president of the board until 1941, after which he was medical director and chairman of the board until his final illness and death in 1946.[2] Manning's support for the hospital insurance plan was not without controversy, even among his fellow faculty members. MacNider wrote in response to a question from one of his former students, "On principle I did not care to find myself in the position of actively opposing one of my colleagues here in the University." He went on to say that he thought competing organizations might be healthy (the Hospital Care Association had been established in 1933 in Durham), but that the medical society's acceptance of money from the Duke Endowment to help start the plan was "most dangerous": "The Duke Foundation wants this type of hospitalization [insurance] so that they can dictate, and they will dictate, I believe, what sick people should do, and therefore what doctors should do. I am perfectly certain that the hos-

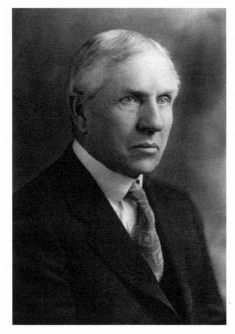

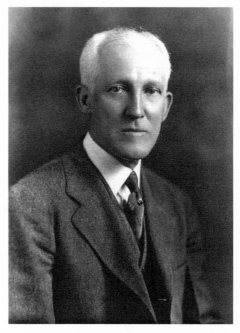

Dr. Isaac H. Manning, dean of the School of Medicine from 1905 to 1933. *(NCC)*

Dr. Charles S. Mangum, dean of the School of Medicine from 1933 to 1937. *(NCC)*

pitalization [insurance] is the first step to controlling the freedom of physicians through socialized medicine. In my judgment nothing could be more inimical to the medical profession than this."[3] The Hospital Savings Association, based in Chapel Hill, and the Hospital Care Association, based in Durham, were both recognized by the national Blue Cross organization in 1938. They merged in 1968 to become today's Blue Cross Blue Shield of North Carolina, which by 2005 had 2.9 million members.

Charles S. Mangum, MD, who had been professor and chair of the Department of Anatomy since 1905, succeeded Manning as dean in the fall of 1933. In response to the incident that had resulted in Manning's retirement, Mangum in 1934 appointed the school's first faculty committee on student admissions. The members of the committee were Drs. James Bullitt, Critz George, and Reece Berryhill, with Dean Mangum serving as chairman.[4] Berryhill became chair of this committee in the 1937–1938 school year and served for several years. Edward Hedgpeth served as chair from 1949 to 1966.[5] This important committee still functions, although the dean no longer is an active member or chair.

Mangum's most lasting contribution to the university came about because of his longtime interest in public health. In cooperation with the state board of health he secured the funds to develop a Division of Public Health in the School of Medicine in 1936. Milton J. Rosenau, MD, who had recently retired as the dean of the Harvard School of Public Health, was recruited as the director of the Division. The new Division incorporated the nationally recognized Department of Sanitary Engineering, which stayed in Chapel Hill when the rest of the UNC

School of Engineering was consolidated with the one at North Carolina State College. Herman G. Baity, ScD, former dean of the UNC School of Engineering at Chapel Hill, remained in the Division as professor of sanitary engineering.[6]

In addition to its "basic work in this field," the Division of Public Health was designated by the United States Public Health Service as the public health teaching unit for a district composed of nine states and the District of Columbia. The Division began by offering sixteen-week courses twice a year for physicians serving as health officers.[7] Undergraduate and graduate degrees were later added to the initial offerings of short courses for health officers. Rosenau was successful in recruiting faculty and in building the program in Public Health. In 1940 the Division became the School of Public Health, and Rosenau served as the first dean.[8] Today it is widely viewed as one of the three leading schools of public health in the nation, along with those at Harvard and Johns Hopkins.

In spite of these accomplishments, Mangum apparently was neither skilled nor interested in the administrative tasks of a dean. According to MacNider in a memorandum for the file dated June 1936, "Mangum is a fine type of kindly person . . . without much . . . determination, and without much knowledge of [modern] medical education . . . [who] had a definite tendency, perhaps out of the freedom of his heart[,] to talk freely and make unwise statements." These characteristics, according to MacNider, were causing the medical school to run "with difficulty and dissatisfaction on the part of the members of its Faculty and the Administrative Boards of the Medical School."[9]

President Graham recognized these problems and, apparently without pressure from the medical faculty, appointed in 1936 a special dean's committee for the medical school, consisting of Dean Mangum, Berryhill, and MacNider. Dean House's letter to the three outlined Graham's charge to the special committee, which included dealing with "the current problems of the Medical School, as well as . . . plans for the future." House elaborated, "So many vital elements are unsettled with regard to the whole Medical School situation at the present that President Graham wanted Doctors MacNider and Berryhill constantly in touch with them and acting with Dean Mangum on them in the interest of the Medical School and the University as a whole."[10] Mangum had earlier told House that

> the appointment by you of an advisory committee to the dean of the medical school, to confer with and advise me in all administrative matters related to the budget, the personnel, the development, and expansion of the school, should have beneficial results. Decisions reached, after study and discussion by such a group should coordinate and crystallize the opinions of all the medical faculty, and result in well thought out and constructive recommendations. I know that the members of the staff whom you have appointed to this committee are devoted to the best interests of the medical school and I shall welcome all the assistance that they can give me.[11]

According to MacNider, this "very abnormal and atypical" situation meant that

> requests from all Departments, processes of expansion of the School, the policies of the School come before this Committee and are then transmitted with recommendation to the Dean of Administration, Mr. R. B. House, and President Graham . . . It means that there is a Dean and then two other individuals to supervise the activities of the Dean. In my judgment as much as such [a] Committee was needed, Dean Mangum should have resigned when the suggestion of this Committee was made to him by the President. A Dean in his activities as well as a President in his has to shoulder the organization which he is supposed to run and survive it, develop it, or sink with it.[12]

In spite of MacNider's concerns, the situation provided Berryhill with an invaluable introduction to medical school administration.

DEAN MACNIDER AND ASSISTANT DEAN BERRYHILL, 1937–1940

In 1937 poor health forced Mangum to resign as dean and as chair of the Department of Anatomy. He died in September 1939 after having served the university and medical school for more than thirty years.

President Graham appointed a faculty committee to make recommendations to him concerning the new dean. It unanimously recommended that the advisory committee of the faculty appoint MacNider dean, even though MacNider had previously asked the committee not to consider him. He told Graham, "It has been the ideal of my life to accomplish something both definite and outstanding in terms of scientific research for the University, the state, and the South and . . . I did not care to permit such an administrative position to in any way interfere with this ideal."[13]

Graham would not take no for an answer, and MacNider had intense negotiations with him in regard to the resources necessary for the continuing development of the medical school. In addition to several new faculty positions, the president pledged to attempt to increase the medical school faculty salaries to a level corresponding to those in the law school for comparable positions. As MacNider reminded him in a memorandum to the file on this issue, "The maximum salary in the Law School for a full professor is apparently $6000 with salaries for similar positions in the Medical School being $4500 as a maximum."[14]

In these discussions MacNider also made it clear that he had no intention of decreasing his research. In a letter to Graham dated May 29, 1937, MacNider accepted "with the proviso and understanding that I am at liberty to resign from the post, the Deanship, at any time should I find that it interferes with my research work."[15] Graham replied the same day that he accepted these conditions because "this research work is too important to the University and the world of science to be interfered with."[16]

A junior faculty member in the medical school wrote to congratulate Graham on his appointment of MacNider as dean: "Dr. MacNider's ability to think clearly, his intimate association with the best minds in medicine, and his understanding of a properly constituted department, a school, and a university will in time prove the wisdom of your choice." The faculty member recognized that when MacNider and Graham were at odds "the majestic storms of the turbulent Atlantic became in comparison somewhat pale," but he had confidence that MacNider's devotion to Graham would compensate for any such disagreements. He concluded with thanks for Graham's "active interest in the well being of our Medical School. It increases our enthusiasm and gives us all a renewed determination to do more work and better work."[17]

One of MacNider's conditions for accepting the deanship was the appointment of a faculty member as assistant dean, whose salary would be supplemented by $500 annually. MacNider had Berryhill in mind for the assistant deanship but Berryhill had major reservations. He wrote MacNider in June 1937 as he was leaving town for a vacation:

> I want to talk with you when I get back. The Assistant Dean situation worries me. I honestly do not want the place or the title. I think that the University has over done this thing on deans. We have entirely too many of them. I don't feel that I could take the money when you aren't getting any. [MacNider had refused a raise when he became dean, but he wanted Berryhill to have the extra $500 allocated by Graham for the assistant dean.] If you would only let me be chairman of the Admissions Committee or some sort of semi-official capacity and at the same time allow me to work for and with you as a member of the Medical School faculty I feel certain I could do more of what I think you want me to do and at the same time be much happier.
>
> Many things have worried me this past year. There hasn't been any one thing, rather it is an accumulation of things over the three years plus a certain amount of unhappiness in my work which with the end of the year always becomes more acute. Just now I need to get away for awhile. Things may not look so hopeless and so confused when I get back.

In a postscript to the letter Berryhill—who had become the physician for both students and many townspeople—gave a follow-up on his examination that morning of the MacNiders' daughter, Sally Foard, apparently to rule out appendicitis. Berryhill also reported on a patient in town who was accumulating more postoperative abdominal fluid and again becoming jaundiced. He said that Hedgpeth would be checking her while he was away, but suggested that MacNider might also stop by when he had time.[18]

MacNider replied several days later in a letter sent to Cleveland, where the Berryhills were staying:

Your dear, fine letter made me unhappy solely for one reason, because I could see that you are unhappy and I feared that this unhappiness might permeate through your vacation and mar a period which you so richly deserved to be one of peace and joy.

For more than a month I have heard that I was the cause of some of this worry and concern on your part and I want you to consider that this is cleared up. I realized that you do not care to be an assistant administrative officer in the Medical School and I can understand this both in general and in terms of certain particular and personal things which you have mentioned to me. So I hope you will just forget this and consider it all off and when you come back we can talk about some other person. You have such strength of character and fineness of understanding that I wanted to borrow some of this to help me through a few years of this burden, but I know full well that I will have this and have it frequently whether you have any designated title or not, and, in turn, I will feel free to lean on it and draw from it. So please be at ease in this connection.[19]

Berryhill's period of "peace and joy," however, was fairly short-lived. Arnold King recalled that he was in Frank Graham's office not long after MacNider had been appointed dean. MacNider telephoned Graham to say he was "tired of being a God damned dean . . . I want out." Graham encouraged him not to resign, saying, "I'll send you an assistant dean first thing tomorrow." Graham then called Berryhill at the infirmary and "told him to report to MacNider tomorrow morning at 8:30, to be his assistant." Berryhill protested that he "didn't want to be an assistant to anybody [and] there was nobody to run the infirmary." Graham replied that Ed Hedgpeth "has been there for years . . . [and is] as good a doctor as you are. I'm putting him in charge there, and you are now Assistant Dean of Medicine."[20] Once again Graham demonstrated how hard it was for anyone to say no to him once he had made up his mind. Although Berryhill assumed his new duties as assistant dean in 1937, he didn't relinquish the title of university physician to Hedgpeth until he became dean in 1941.

MacNider appointed Berryhill assistant dean for student affairs, with responsibility for student admissions, counseling of students, and the vitally important function of transferring the students to four-year medical schools for their two clinical years and the MD degree. Berryhill added these duties to those he already had as university physician in charge of the student health service and as the faculty member responsible for the clinical courses in the second-year medical curriculum.[21]

The New Medical and Public Health Building

The modest faculty additions to the medical school and the establishment of the Division of Public Health resulted in further pressure on the space available in

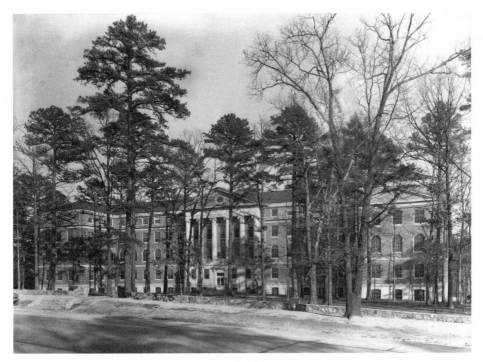

The Medical and Public Health Building (later MacNider Hall) was occupied in 1939.
(NCC)

Caldwell Hall, which the medical school had occupied since 1912. Based on the earlier work of Deans Manning and Mangum, MacNider worked with Graham and the university to obtain a state appropriation for a new building to house the School of Medicine and the new Division of Public Health. Through the influence of Rosenau and the state health officer, Carl Reynolds, MD, a construction grant was obtained from the federal Public Works Administration to supplement the state funds.[22] MacNider wrote to a friend that this new building would be "in the woods across the Pittsboro Road from the new high school [site of the current School of Pharmacy] in such a location that in some years to come this initial laboratory unit will be ready to have added to it a University hospital."[23] The building was occupied in 1939. After MacNider's death in 1951 it was named MacNider Hall by action of the university board of trustees.

The dedication of the new Medical and Public Health Building was held on December 4, 1939, as part of the university's celebration of the sesquicentennial of its chartering in 1789. James King Hall, MD, of Richmond, who had completed the two-year medical course at UNC in 1902, delivered the address. He concluded, "I look upon the New Medical Building with pride and satisfaction and with gratitude," but reminded the students and teachers in the audience that he looked upon them "as the spirit of the medical school. Such as you constitute the basis of the hope of a mad world. May God keep you in strength and in courage."[24]

Berryhill would occupy a small office in this building to the right of the main entrance during his years as acting dean and then as dean of the two-year school, from 1940 until 1952. After the medical library moved to its new quarters in the clinic building in 1952, Berryhill, as dean of the four-year school, had a larger office and a suite of adjacent offices in the old library reading room just across the hall from the original dean's office until his retirement as dean in 1964. Subsequent deans occupied the same suite in MacNider Hall until the dean's offices were moved to the renovated Bondurant Hall in 2006.

This new Medical and Public Health Building was to be the cornerstone for a vast new academic medical center that would evolve over the next decades.

Acting Dean, 1940–1941

MacNider resigned in 1940 after four years as dean to devote his time to his first loves, research and teaching. He particularly wanted to pursue his observations of the influence of aging on the body's reaction to injury—an outgrowth of his work in experimental nephritis. After the atomic bomb was dropped in 1945, it was revealed that MacNider had also consulted secretly with the Manhattan Project during the war because he was one of only a few scientists who had studied the effects of uranium on living tissue. He remained as Kenan Research Professor and chair of pharmacology until 1943, when failing health compelled him to resign as chair. He continued to teach a second-year course on the history of medicine until 1950, when he retired from the university after forty-eight years of faculty service. He died in June 1951. The last class of sophomore students he taught honored him by establishing the MacNider Award, given annually to the second-year medical student "who is selected by his classmates as most nearly possessing the philosophy and various intangible traits of good character which were typified by Dr. 'Billy' MacNider during his forty-eight years as teacher and physician at the University of North Carolina School of Medicine."[25]

Robert House, dean of administration (and later chancellor at UNC–CH), and President Graham asked Berryhill to be acting dean during 1940–1941 while the search for a permanent dean was under way.

Dean of the Two-Year School, 1941–1952

The search committee for MacNider's replacement recommended that Berryhill be appointed to the deanship and that he be charged with planning the school's expansion.

Berryhill later commented that the deanship was one "which he did not wish and which he was ill prepared to discharge." He finally accepted it, he said, because of the influence of former Dean Isaac Manning, Sr., who insisted "this had to be his decision if the future of the school was to [be] made secure by its expansion to a four-year status." He added, "For the next five years, until his death

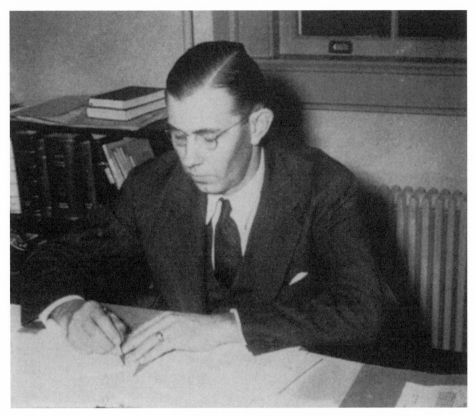

Dr. Berryhill, the new dean of the School of Medicine, *Yackety Yack,* 1942. *(NCC)*

in 1946, Dr. Manning's continued support and wise counsel were invaluable." Berryhill also observed that he was in an unusual position as dean in 1941, when four of the five departmental chairs who reported to him had been his teachers in 1923–1925 and were close friends. He said that "the understanding, patience, and support of these men was most helpful" as he undertook this leadership role in the school.[26]

After Berryhill's appointment as dean was announced in September 1941, the *Charlotte Observer* published a news item headlined, "Mecklenburger Named Dean of UNC Medical School: The Trustees Make the Natural Choice."[27] Those on campus were equally enthusiastic about his appointment, as noted in the 1942 *Yackety Yack:* "Young, capable, and energetic, Dr. Berryhill took office with the applause of faculty and students alike."[28]

The World War II Years, 1941–1945

The surprise Japanese attack on Pearl Harbor on December 7, 1941, just months after Berryhill became dean, plunged the nation and the university into a world war that was to last another four years and make profound changes in American society, education, and medicine.

Preliminary efforts by medical schools to prepare for possible war had been going on for some time. A report was made to the administrative board of the UNC medical school three days before Pearl Harbor concerning the recent meeting of the Association of American Medical Colleges (AAMC):

> To meet the increased demand for physicians due to the war emergency the medical schools last year were asked to increase their entering classes by 10%, if such could be done without lowering the standards . . . The placing of medical schools on a 12 months teaching basis was considered, but more deliberate consideration led to the conclusion that the shortage of physicians is probably more apparent than real, due to reluctance, perhaps, of physicians to enter the Military Service. Since the lowering of the draft age limit from 35 to 28 years many medical seniors and young M.D.'s holding internships who were given a deferred classification to complete their medical training passed the 28 year age and subsequently declined to enter the medical service of the Army and Navy. This did not, of course, create a very favorable impression with the Surgeon Generals of the Army and Navy and there was talk of a refusal to defer medical students; however, a committee from the association went to Washington and conferred with officials and recommended that medical students be given a deferred classification throughout the first two years of their medical training. If at the end of that time they declined to enter the Medical Reserve the Deans of the medical schools would not ask for further deferment. This is the plan in effect at present.[29]

Immediately after Pearl Harbor, however, the AAMC recommended that the four-year medical school course be shortened to three years. At most medical schools the entrance requirements were relaxed, and the students were enrolled in a 9-9-9-9 accelerated curriculum that allowed only a two-week vacation between the four 9-month terms. The traditional contents of the curricula were not watered down or eliminated, but topics of a military nature were added or enhanced in areas such as tropical medicine, infectious diseases, trauma, and shock. Internships were cut from 12 to 9 months, and the duration of most residencies was cut in half.[30]

At UNC the medical curriculum was changed by early January 1942. The two-year course was adjusted to approximately eighteen months, and the schedule was changed so that students could transfer into the accelerated clinical programs at other schools. A new class was admitted in June 1942 and every nine months thereafter until the war was over. Much later Berryhill commented that both faculty and students during the war years "accepted the necessary adjustments, the longer hours, and the added strain in a fine fashion and attempted to make the most of the situation."[31]

The UNC campus soon became a sea of military uniforms as the navy established a preflight school and an officer training program, and the army established Army Specialized Training Programs (ASTP) in medicine, language, and

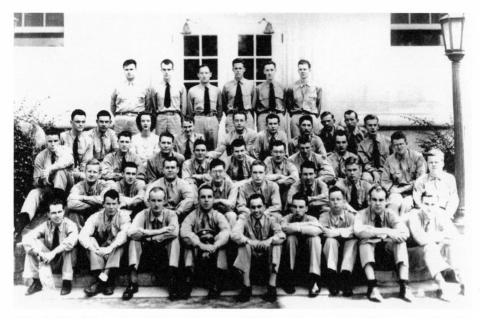

School of Medicine, class of September 1944. All the students are in uniform except for the sole woman, Margaret Swanton, who later became professor of pathology at UNC. *(NCC)*

other areas. Although the UNC prewar civilian enrollment of some 3,600 fell to some 1,400 during the war, the total enrollment increased to some 5,000 at the height of the wartime educational programs. A total of more than 20,000 young men—including a future US president, Gerald Ford—attended the university during the war in various military training programs.[32] Most medical students whose active duty was deferred were enlisted in the service and wore military uniforms to class.[33]

The medical students had the pressure not only of an accelerated curriculum but also of knowing that their military service was postponed while others their age were fighting and dying. One alumnus, a second-year student during the war years, said that his group had been excused from class one morning to go to Watts Hospital in Durham to participate in an autopsy. After it was over the students decided to stay in Durham to eat at the Chinese restaurant and then to cut their 1:30 P.M. class so they could study for an exam the next morning. Berryhill learned of their truancy and called the group to his office the next morning. He told them that "boys were dying overseas and here we were flaking off and his first impulse was to just call up the army and navy and tell them to draft every one of us and just send us off to the war." Later they were somewhat relieved when one of their professors told them that Berryhill was in the midst of a legislative struggle for medical school funding and "if you'd have dropped a pen in front of his door that day you'd have gotten the same response."[34]

Berryhill's report to the administrative board of the medical school at the end of the war demonstrated the effects of the draft and the lowered admissions standards on the medical student body:

The class entering in September [1945] consisted of 46 students and . . . the record to date indicated that it was perhaps the poorest class in the history of the school. Many of the better prepared students who were originally accepted were drafted before the opening of the school year. Of those in the class, many were unprepared and some disinterested, having been sent here by the Army in some cases without previous intent on the part of the student to study medicine.[35]

Berryhill elaborated on the end of the accelerated wartime program in an annual report to Chancellor House for the year ending December 31, 1945:

The Medical School has begun its program of deceleration, which will be completed by the end of the present academic year [1945–1946]. The present second-year class began its work in June and will graduate in March, while the present first-year class began on the regular schedule in September and will finish the school year in June. There will be no summer session [for the first time since the war began] and both first and second-year classes for 1946 will begin at the regular opening of school in September . . .

All Navy students [twenty-four in the two classes at the beginning of the 1945–1946 school year] have been discharged and the [fifteen] Army students will receive their discharges at the end of the present quarter. It is interesting to note that in this connection the mortality rate in the present first-year class has been excessive, both because of academic failures and voluntary withdrawals. As you recall, due to the shortsighted policy of the Selective Service, War and Navy Departments premedical students have not received deferment for over one and one-half-years. Almost one-half of the qualified students accepted for admission in September 1945, were drafted before the end of the war. We were, therefore, forced, as far as civilian students [fifty-five originally in the two classes at the beginning of the 1945–1946 academic year] to scrape the bottom of the barrel. For those students who were in the Army and Navy, and particularly in the Army, the School had little to do with their selection, and many had no real interest in medicine. This experience, which is fairly common throughout the country, merely confirms the opinion of medical educators that selection of students should be by those qualified from experience and not by the "Brass hats" and "top sergeants" in the military organization.

Berryhill went on to say that forty-six students successfully completed the two-year school at Chapel Hill in June of 1945 and had been transferred to MD-granting medical schools. All of the transfers were to out-of-state medical schools and included Jefferson Medical College (nine students); the University of Maryland (eight); Harvard University (seven); the University of Pennsylvania (four); Washington University (three); the Medical College of Virginia (three); the University of Virginia (three); and one or two students to each of seven other schools.[36]

In his annual report to Chancellor House for the year ending in December 1946, Berryhill concluded his lamentations over the accelerated wartime program with these comments:

> The enrollment for the session 1946–47 is lower than in the last few years. This is due to two factors: in the first place, the second year class is the smallest since the '30s because of a very high academic mortality, and second, to the voluntary withdrawal of a considerable proportion of the ASTP trainees sent here by the War Department. When this class was selected in the summer of 1945, the deferments for premedical students had been discontinued and medical schools were forced to make their selection from civilian students who were IV-Fs or women. Many of these were obviously poorly qualified to the study of medicine. All of the Army trainees sent to this school were from other sections of the country. Most of them had no interest in medicine and selected this course of training in preference to going into the Infantry. It is the feeling of the faculty that the profession and the University are well rid of these students.

Berryhill added that the postwar applications for admission were probably the largest in its history: "The encouraging feature is the large number of qualified State residents who are applying for admission." In spite of a large increase of applicants from out of state as well, "the Medical Faculty has taken the position that insofar as possible the enrollment should be largely limited to State Residents . . . [and] that students from counties and sections in North Carolina that are now most deficient in doctors should be given a priority wherever they present adequate qualifications and preparation . . . It is likely that the number of applicants will increase over the next few years and if the Medical School is expanded, the demand for places here will certainly increase."[37]

The accelerated program for medical education in the United States during World War II did result in the graduation of approximately 25,000 doctors, an increase of about 5,000 over the comparable peacetime period. Although this was an impressive output, many medical educators viewed the lowering of standards and the acceleration of medical learning with great alarm. Apparently no other nation adopted such a course during the war. One medical historian observed, "The greatest legacy of World War II for American medical education was in creating a resolve never again to risk compromising standards." When a need for more doctors arose at the outbreak of the Korean War, a joint committee of the AAMC and American Medical Association (AMA) recommended against repeating the accelerated program: "The price of acceleration has proved to be lowered quality of graduates, exhaustion of faculties, and serious curtailment of research . . . The rapid production of half-trained men will make statistical charts look better but will not improve the health of the nation."[38]

The Immediate Postwar Years, 1945–1952

By the fall of 1946 the university campus was crowded with some 6,500 students, including more than 4,000 veterans, and some 500 teaching faculty. Because of the GI Bill (which paid educational expenses for veterans) and the great demand for admission to the university after the war, the trustees set up a priority system, giving preference to former students returning from military service, and among those the highest priority was given to North Carolinians. According to the director of admissions, however, "it is the aim of the university to attempt to admit all qualified students, who can provide their own housing." He added, "The Trustees' policy of providing dormitory space for some current North Carolina High School graduates will be continued. [The new] Alexander Dormitory is this year the home of 150 1946 North Carolina High School graduates. The completion of the new dorms will give relief to the housing shortage." Nonetheless, the university's policy with regard to women students continued, with the Woman's College in Greensboro (now UNC–Greensboro) providing full four-year access for (white) women. Only women students in pharmacy and those who were residents of Chapel Hill were eligible for admission as freshmen at Chapel Hill, but women were eligible to transfer into the junior year at Chapel Hill after two years at the Woman's College or other colleges.[39] A few women students were accepted to the medical school beginning in the 1920s, but it was not until 1972, with the passage of federal Title IX legislation, that women were admitted to all programs on an equal basis with men.

Relationship with Students

Berryhill accepted his new duties as dean with dedication and energy, as attested to by numerous students whose admission to medical school, progress in medical school, and transfer elsewhere were determined by Berryhill's involvement.

Berryhill also remained active as a physician to students and townspeople. His daughter recalls that he always kept his black doctor's bag by their kitchen door and that she and her sister enjoyed playing with the contents.[40] His care was remembered by a student who had completed his undergraduate coursework early in order to graduate in December 1942 and volunteer for the US Army Air Force. He was married in November and had to move from UNC's Old East dormitory to a residence in town. Both he and his new bride came down with the flu, and their landlord insisted on calling Dr. Berryhill to see them. The former student remembers sixty years later that the dean of the School of Medicine made a house call on a student in town.[41]

Berryhill's informality and personal approach to medical students was underscored by a member of the class who entered the school in the fall of 1940, when Berryhill became acting dean. Berryhill knew everyone in the school by their first names, and there was a very close student-faculty relationship. When his class graduated from the two-year school it was 1942, and the war had begun. They hated to leave Chapel Hill, but they knew that "Uncle Sam needed us as MD's" for the war effort. Just before their graduation ceremony, "'Peaches' Dunlap, Dr. Berryhill's Girl Friday, said I needed to drop by her office to complete my records." What she needed was the student's application for admission to medical school—something that Berryhill had apparently considered superfluous because the student and his classmates had visited the medical school across from the arboretum since their undergraduate years and had known many of the UNC medical students and faculty before applying for admission.[42]

Another student was asked by Norma Berryhill to stand by the dean "to prompt him with the names of my classmates at a lawn party at the Berryhill home." Recognizing the problem of the dean's knowing all their names—even in those days of much smaller classes than today—the student agreed. His services, however, were not needed: "To my surprise, I did not have to come up with even one reminder: he was quite able to greet each of us with our name and a warm smile."[43]

One student said that he first met Dr. Berryhill when he was applying in 1940 for admission to medical school before completing his AB degree:

Dr. Berryhill was kind but firm. He found my credentials quite adequate, but he felt it necessary to remind me that being Jewish, I might encounter difficulties in transferring from Chapel Hill to a good four year school for completion of my clinical training two years hence. Completion of a fourth year of college, he believed, would obviate the problem. (In that era racial and religious prejudice, both overt and covert, was known to exist among medical school admissions committees.) He left the decision to me, and I gratefully accepted his advice. This encounter with Dr. Berryhill, painful though it was, first evoked my admiration for him. The willingness to discuss a sensitive issue openly, candidly, and with great kindness was to me an early revelation of his greatness and the beginning of an enduring friendship.[44]

Another student approached Dean Berryhill after the war for advice about entering medical school. The student had majored in commerce before his military service and didn't have the required science courses for medical school. When he talked with Berryhill he was married, with two children and a job. Berryhill's reply to the student's question about going to medical school was, "I think it's a damn fool idea." The young man didn't take the dean's advice, but instead took the required science courses, was accepted to medical school, and graduated. His record was so good he was asked to stay on and teach. One day while he was still a resident, Berryhill asked him, "How on earth did you do it?" The young physician replied with a grin, "You made me so damned mad I had to."[45]

Norma Berryhill was an equal partner with Berryhill with regard to the students' welfare. One former UNC medical student said that he was an undergraduate freshman at Chapel Hill when his father, a physician and personal friend of the Berryhills', was killed in an automobile accident while on his way to a meeting in Raleigh. "Instead of calling me on the phone, my family called Norma Berryhill and she came to my dorm and found me and told me in the most kind and gentle way about the accident. She told me to pack my clothes and that *she* was taking me home." He concluded, "There are not many friends as dear as that and I shall love her and treasure her friendship as I did . . . Dr. Berryhill's all of my life."[46]

An Evaluation of the Dean

In July 1951 James B. Bullitt, MD, professor emeritus of pathology, received a letter from B. S. Guyton, MD, in Oxford, Mississippi, concerning the search by Bullitt's alma mater, the University of Mississippi, for someone to be the director of the Medical Affairs Division at the new academic medical center to be built in Jackson for the university. He elaborated, "We are wondering if Berryhill might be available, and if he might be a good man for this position. He has not been approached, and will not be if we get an unfavorable reply from you." He added, "A committee [from Mississippi] will be up there in about ten or eleven days, looking over the new set-up which you have." Bullitt's frank and concise reply provides an insight into Berryhill's performance as student, faculty member, and dean. He began by saying, "If you could secure Berryhill for the position in Mississippi, you would be most fortunate. I doubt, however, if he would consider the offer." (He didn't.) Bullitt went on:

> He was a student under me twenty-five years ago, at which time he was at the top of an unusually good class. He completed his medical education at Harvard and had service in a Boston hospital and also in Cleveland. He returned here in 1933 as University Physician and as a member of our medical faculty. He proved to be both an excellent teacher and a fine administrator. He became Assistant Dean some twelve or thirteen years ago and for the past seven or eight years has been Dean. He has been a real wheel horse in the very difficult task of securing support for and finally building our new hospital, which will make possible our full four-year medical school. No man has all the qualities that are desirable for this type of administrative job, but Berryhill has an unusually large number of them. He knows medicine well. He is a good judge of men. He is an extremely hard worker. He has nothing of the "orator" but makes a clear plain statement on any proposition; to me this is far more effective than florid speech. He has strong opinions of his own which he does not change easily, but he listens with an open mind to any opinions that are opposed to his. There are times when he may not be as tactful or diplomatic as might be desirable. When this is the case, it is

because his own straightforward mind forbids any roundabout methods. He can always be counted upon to carry out to the best of his ability anything that he promises to do.[47]

Coexisting Challenges

While Berryhill was dealing with the challenges of wartime and postwar medical education as the dean of the two-year school, he was simultaneously planning the expansion of the medical school and the building of a university hospital at Chapel Hill.

PART III

A University Medical Center for the People
of North Carolina, 1941–1964

*It is bad enough that a man should be
ignorant, for this cuts him off from the
commerce of men's minds. It is perhaps
worse that a man should be poor, for
this condemns him to a life of stint and
scheming, and there is no time for dreams
and no respite for weariness. But what
surely is worse is that a man should be
unwell, for this prevents his doing anything
much about either his poverty or his
ignorance.*

— G. H. T. Kinball, quoted in E. H.
Beardsley, *A History of Neglect*, 1987

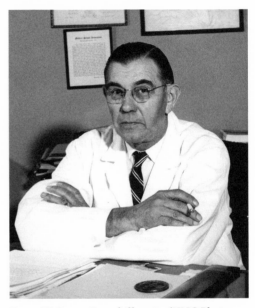

Dean W. Reece Berryhill, 1963. (*UNC Photo Lab, NCC*)

*When Aycock became Governor he
supplanted the old slogan, "We are too poor
to educate," by substituting, "We are too poor not to educate," and all succeeding
Governors and the people have gone forward in that spirit . . . When [Governor]
Morrison said North Carolina must get out of the mud and issue bonds to build good
roads, there were those who said, "The State is too poor." But the people said, "We are
too poor not to have good roads." . . . And now there are some jeremiads [sic] who are
saying, "We are too poor for the State to give hospitalization to those who need it and
to establish a State four-year medical college." But these present day men with eyes in
the back of their heads are in a minority. All wise leaders and the people say, "We are
too poor not to have the health policy which has been approved by all forward-looking
organizations in the State" . . . Schools—Roads—Health. This is the trinity that will
give North Carolina primacy.*

— *Raleigh News and Observer*, August 24, 1946

Chapter 6

The Poe Commission, the Sanger Report, and the Good Health Movement

Medical, university, and political leaders in North Carolina attempted for almost half a century to marshal public and political support to establish a university hospital and a four-year, MD-granting medical school at the University of North Carolina. Three separate attempts during the first four decades of the twentieth century each failed. Berryhill was either uninvolved or a bystander in these unsuccessful attempts. He then was the catalyst for, and leader of, the fourth and successful effort in the 1940s and 1950s.

By the end of World War II in 1945, the state was the site of two relatively new but very promising privately supported four-year medical schools: the Duke University School of Medicine in Durham and the Bowman Gray School of Medicine of Wake Forest College in Winston-Salem. Many of the students attending these schools were from out of state. In the early 1940s approximately 75 percent of the Duke medical school class was from out of state, and the state board of medical examiners annually licensed an average of only about fifteen Duke MD graduates to practice in North Carolina. Approximately twenty MD graduates of the two-year Wake Forest medical school were licensed annually from 1939 to 1943. This figure was expected to at least double once the Bowman Gray school began to award MD degrees in 1943.[1]

In 1945 the state university system had only a two-year basic science medical school at the University of North Carolina at Chapel Hill. Almost all of the approximately forty students in each class were from North Carolina. Most had to go out of state to complete their clinical training and obtain their MD degrees. Although some Duke and Bowman Gray graduates stayed in North Carolina and many UNC students returned to North Carolina after earning their MD degree elsewhere, the ratio of doctors to general population was almost the lowest in the United States. To reach a desirable physician-to-population ratio of 1 to 1,000 by 1960, it was predicted that North Carolina would need an additional 75 licensed physicians per year entering practice. This was calculated to require from 87 to 132 additional entering North Carolina medical students per year.[2]

The extremely high rejection rate of North Carolina young men for service in the armed forces in World War II helped provide the impetus for finally obtaining public and political support for an academic medical center for the people of the state. The political will for such an innovative program was enhanced by the public's positive attitude toward medicine because of wartime successes in trauma care, treatment of infectious diseases with antibiotics, and many other areas of medicine and surgery. The fiscal means for converting this public support into bricks, mortar, and people were provided by the state's post–World War II budget surpluses and by the passage in 1946 (and funding in 1947) of the federal Hill-Burton Act to help states finance hospital and health center construction by providing federal funds to match state and local funding.[3] The state's urgent health care needs were publicized in the mid-1940s throughout the state by the Good Health Movement, an exceptional campaign that enlisted the support of local and national entertainers, elected officials, physicians, public health officials, ministers, and the public.

This chapter explores the developments over the first half of the twentieth century that ultimately led to the decision in 1947 to build a teaching hospital and to expand the medical school at Chapel Hill. These decisions in turn led to the opening of North Carolina Memorial Hospital in Chapel Hill in September 1952 and to the first MD graduates at UNC–CH in 1954.

THE FIRST EFFORT TO EXPAND THE MEDICAL SCHOOL, 1902–1910

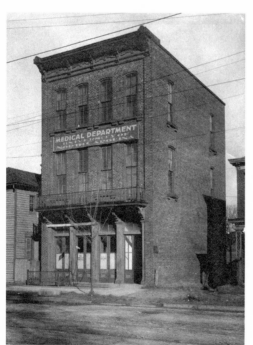

The UNC medical department at Raleigh, 1902–1910. (*Health Sciences Library, UNC at Chapel Hill*)

Reece Berryhill was still a youngster in Steele Creek at the time of the university's first, temporary MD-granting program in the first decade of the new twentieth century. He first learned about it while a medical student at Chapel Hill in the 1920s, and his future mentor was an MD graduate of this medical school.[4]

A Medical Department was established by the UNC trustees in Raleigh in 1902. It had its own building and a respected Raleigh surgeon, Hubert A. Royster, MD, as dean. The primary reason for its establishment was the desire to increase the number of practicing physicians in North Carolina. Although the two-year basic sciences school at Chapel Hill was relatively inexpensive for students, they had to transfer to much more expensive northern schools for the last two clinical years and the MD degree, which excluded many potential medical students. The expenses at the Raleigh school were low because instruction was provided by practicing physicians, who welcomed the supplementation of their incomes from tuition payments. Furthermore, two hospitals, a public dispensary, and several state institutions provided patients and clinical facilities, so that it was not necessary for the state to make major capital expenditures. Finally, the successive deans at Chapel Hill had a continuing concern about the time when the four-year, MD-granting schools would no longer accept transfers to their third-year classes from Chapel Hill and other two-year schools.

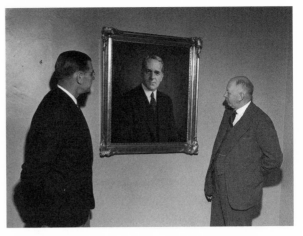

Dean Berryhill and Chancellor House view a 1953 portrait of Dr. Hubert A. Royster, dean of the medical department at Raleigh from 1902 to 1910. *(UNC Photo Lab, NCC)*

The Medical Department at Raleigh provided two years of clinical experience for those students completing the two-year basic science curriculum at the Chapel Hill campus. During its eight years, seventy-nine physicians graduated from the school with an MD degree, and sixty-six became practicing physicians in North Carolina. Among the graduates were two outstanding medical leaders who had a major impact on medicine in North Carolina and well beyond its borders. William de B. MacNider, recognized internationally for his research in kidney disease and in gerontology, was a faculty member at UNC for almost half a century, served as dean of the medical school, and was Kenan Professor of Pharmacology. John A. Ferrell, MD, served as a distinguished member of the

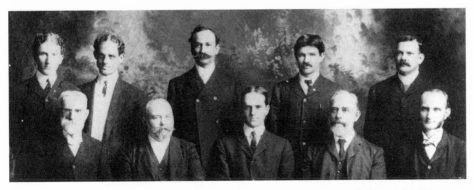

The faculty of the medical department in Raleigh in 1904. *Front row, left to right:* Drs. Wisconsin Illinois Royster, Richard Henry Lewis, Hubert A. Royster (dean), August Washington Knox, and Kemp Plummer Battle, Jr. *Back row, left to right:* Drs. William de Berniere MacNider, Henry McKee Tucker, Andrew Watson Goodwin, Robert Sherwood McGeachy, and James William McGee, Jr. *(NCC)*

Poe, Sanger, and the Good Health Movement   127

International Health Board of the Rockefeller Foundation, president of the John and Mary R. Markle Foundation, and later as director of the North Carolina Medical Care Commission.

In February 1909 Abraham Flexner, an educator studying medical schools in the United States and Canada for the Carnegie Foundation for the Advancement of Teaching, inspected the two-year school at Chapel Hill as well as the Medical Department in Raleigh.[5] Henry Pritchett, president of the Carnegie Foundation, informed UNC President Francis Venable that the "clinical department . . . at Raleigh is . . . perhaps the very worst department of its kind to be found in the United States." Probably because this was one of the first schools Flexner visited, the UNC Medical Department at Raleigh was one of only a few schools cited as bad examples in Flexner's 1940 autobiography: "The State University of North Carolina gave the first two years of its medical course at Chapel Hill, while the two clinical years were given at Raleigh. The medical-school building at Raleigh was filthy and absolutely without equipment. I employed a photographer who took photographs of every room in the building. When I returned to New York, Dr. Pritchett sent these photographs to the president of the university with a letter saying that they would be reproduced in facsimile in the forthcoming report. The president, who had probably never visited the medical school, was horrified."

Pritchett suggested to UNC President Venable that the annual appropriation of $750 for the Raleigh branch could much better be spent in upgrading the medical teaching laboratories at Chapel Hill. Simultaneously the American Medical Association's Council on Medical Education (CME) notified Venable that the council would no longer place the Raleigh branch on their "acceptable list" of medical schools. The CME stated that they would continue to list the Chapel Hill basic science school if the Raleigh school were closed.

In the face of these threats, President Venable met with the university board of trustees on February 9, 1910. Venable recommended that the Raleigh department "either be properly equipped or discontinued at the end of the current session." Because the estimated $3,000 needed to upgrade the facilities was not available, the trustees elected to discontinue the Raleigh school at the end of the academic year, and Venable notified the faculty members at Raleigh, the AMA CME, and the Carnegie Foundation.[6] The CME continued to list the Chapel Hill school on their acceptable list.

The Flexner Report, published later in 1910, did not list the Raleigh department, as Pritchett had promised if it were closed. The report on the Chapel Hill school was generally favorable, with the exception of the "inferior" anatomy facilities (which were housed in a wooden building at the edge of the campus). The school was complimented for "work [that] is intelligently planned and conducted on modern lines." Flexner emphasized that the medical school was "an organic part of the university," a condition he and other leading medical educators of the day were forcefully advocating. He documented that the resources of the medical school included $12,000 annually in the university budget and fees of $6,500.[7] (See Appendix D.)

In Venable's letter of February 10, 1910, concerning the trustees' decision to discontinue the Raleigh department, he added: "If the State does not provide for the further equipment of the Medical Department at Chapel Hill within the next few years, it also will have to be discontinued." The national criticisms of the medical school and this warning worked, for the state appropriated $50,000 to build the first building on the Chapel Hill campus specifically designed for the medical school. This building of some 28,000 square feet was named Caldwell Hall in honor of the university's first president, Joseph Caldwell, a mathematics professor and Princeton-educated Presbyterian minister who was the son of a physician. It was opened in 1912 with dedicatory exercises that included state and national medical leaders. This building (with renovations in the 1930s to open the previously unfinished third floor) continued to house the medical school (and later the Division of Public Health) until MacNider Hall, the first building at the site of the future hospital and academic medical center, was occupied in 1939.

Following the Flexner Report in 1910, the North Carolina Medical College, founded at Davidson College in 1886 and located in Charlotte since 1907, merged with the Medical College of Virginia and moved to Richmond in 1914. Leonard Medical School at Shaw University in Raleigh had operated since 1882 to educate much-needed black physicians and pharmacists but was forced to close in 1914 for lack of funds to meet current standards.[8] Thus, by World War I the state was left with the only the two basic science medical schools, at Chapel Hill and Wake Forest, the latter founded in 1902 on the campus of the Baptist-supported Wake Forest College in Wake County. The state became totally dependent on other states with MD-granting medical schools to furnish practicing physicians for a growing population.

THE SECOND EFFORT TO EXPAND THE MEDICAL SCHOOL, 1921–1923

Berryhill had just received his undergraduate degree from UNC and was teaching school in Charlotte when the second effort to expand the university's medical school came, in the 1920s.[9] The university had a new president, Harry Woodburn Chase, a polished and energetic New Englander. During Chase's tenure (1919–1930) the campus was the site of a building boom: it gained new classroom and laboratory buildings, new dormitories, Kenan Stadium, and the magnificent Wilson Library. In addition, Chase began the process of recruiting outstanding faculty that would be continued by his successor, Frank Porter Graham. These efforts would lay the foundation for the university's growing recognition as a regional and then a national institution.

Chase was equally devoted to enhancing the standing of the university's professional schools. His efforts to convert the law school from "a coaching school for bar examinations" to "a real professional law school in the modern sense" were successful: the admission requirements were increased, the required course was increased to three years, a new permanent home was completed in Manning Hall, a new dean and faculty were recruited, and full accreditation was achieved.

Chase's attempt to develop the medical school into a four-year, MD-granting medical school with a teaching hospital ultimately failed, but he started with the same determination and drive that he exhibited in his successful transformation of the law school. Chase's motivation for expanding the medical school was similar to that which resulted in the formation of the Medical Department in Raleigh in 1902—the need for more physicians in the state and the perceived fear of increasing difficulty in ensuring places in MD-granting schools for those students who completed the first two years at Chapel Hill.

President Chase took these concerns to the executive committee of the university board of trustees on December 9, 1921. At the next meeting of the executive committee, on January 7, 1922, President Chase, Medical School Dean Isaac Manning, and Dr. Richard H. Lewis (a member of the board) were appointed as a committee to study the issue of an expanded medical school and to report back to the trustees. Their preliminary conclusions were presented to the executive committee on March 23, 1922, and a final written report was presented to the board on June 1, 1922. The committee noted that the physician-to-population ratio in North Carolina was 1 to 1,600, while nationally it was 1 to 720; only two states had a ratio worse than North Carolina's. The number of hospital beds in relation to the population was about half that for the nation, and only four North Carolina hospitals provided internships. These statistics, along with the desire to provide an inexpensive education for North Carolinians wanting to become physicians, led the committee to conclude that the state should provide a four-year medical school and teaching hospital for its citizens. The committee recognized the problem of building a teaching hospital in a small community but cited the success of the Mayo Clinic and of the Universities of Iowa, Michigan, and Virginia in having hospitals in relatively small towns. They suggested that not having a divided school (basic science years on the university campus and clinical years elsewhere) was a further argument for locating the teaching hospital and expanded school at Chapel Hill.

The trustees agreed that this matter needed further study, so Governor Cameron Morrison appointed a new committee composed of President Chase, Dean Manning, MacNider, and four members of the board of trustees: Senator J. L. DeLaney of Charlotte, W. N. Everett of Rockingham, R. P. Grier of Statesville, and Representative Edgar W. Pharr. During the summer and fall of 1922 this committee studied the situation in depth. Their activities included meeting with leaders of the North Carolina Medical Society as well as trips to Chicago, New York, and Baltimore to consult with national leaders in medicine and medical education. Most of the advice from the national leaders was that the university should proceed with building a teaching hospital and expanding the school at Chapel Hill, although concerns were naturally expressed about the availability of patients in Chapel Hill. Only President Pritchett of the Carnegie Foundation leaned toward a divided school to obtain the necessary patients, but he felt that the clinical facilities should be as close to the campus as possible.

As the study continued, other communities became interested in having the hospital and clinical portion of the medical school located in their city. Charlotte was particularly vocal in this regard, having recently lost its medical school. Other cities in the state also joined in the scramble for this presumed plum to be dispensed by the legislature.

During this debate the director of the state board of health, G. M. Cooper, MD, wrote MacNider in October 1922 to express his personal opinion about "the 'free for all' now going on among the profession pertaining to the location of the university Medical School."[10] Cooper suggested that in considering this issue the "door to the past should be completely closed, because medical training and the conditions governing medical practice are now undergoing more epochal changes than at any time in the past three hundred years." Because of the Good Roads Program then in progress in the state, he stated, an ambulance would soon be able to transport a patient from Raleigh or Greensboro to Chapel Hill "much quicker and easier than it was done from the suburbs of Baltimore when Hopkins was first opened some thirty years ago." He added that he had no doubt that "ten year[s] from now an airplane ambulance [will be able to] make the trip to and from Wilmington, Charlotte, or Asheville bringing a patient in three or four hours with more safety than an auto bus now carries children to consolidated schools." He also argued that a hospital and teaching hospital in a smaller town was more likely to train physicians for practice in "small villages and country places" and to inspire them to consider medicine as "a profession of service to humanity and not a commercial enterprise." He concluded by citing the success of the Mayos in situating their clinic and hospitals in a small Minnesota community and of Leonard Tufts in building his resort hotel in the village of Pinehurst.

When the committee met at the governor's mansion in Raleigh on December 19, 1922, to prepare for their presentation to the full board of trustees the next day, they received a surprise proposal by President William Preston Few of Durham's Methodist-supported Trinity College. Few stated that he had assurance from an anonymous donor of $8 million to build a first-class medical school and teaching hospital in Durham that would be operated by an independent board as a joint enterprise of the University of North Carolina and Trinity College (along with Davidson and Wake Forest, should they desire to be included). He felt that North Carolina should have one good school rather than two that might be mediocre, but that if the state could not accept this offer Trinity would carry the plan forward itself.[11]

The next day at the trustees' meeting, President Chase presented the Few proposal for discussion rather than the committee's prepared report. The proposal engendered a heated debate among the members that soon spread throughout the state.

A news report the next day in the *Raleigh News and Observer* summarized the trustees' immediate reaction:

> Simple as is the proposal in theory, inquiring members of the board developed a labyrinth of ramifications, the implacable opposition of the Baptist denomination to any coalition [of the state and a denominational college], the constitutionality of any such combination, the means and machinery of control, whether it would be a University school, or a Trinity school, what voice would the State have in its management if it were located off the University grounds—the suggestions were endless.[12]

In an accompanying editorial entitled "Matter for Careful Consideration," the *News and Observer* added:

> The consensus of opinion now seems to be that the participation of the State in a denominational enterprise is impractical and unwise. But more careful inquiry in the light of the urgent need for a first class medical college and of the many calls for public funds for other purposes possibly will lead to different conclusions. It is a matter not to be disposed of in haste but worthy of the most careful study and reflection.

President Chase, speaking for the committee, made a statement to the press on December 21 declaring, "Any plan which may be devised must be acceptable to the Trustees of the institutions concerned, to the national authorities in medical education, and it must not violate the constitutional provision guaranteeing the separation of church and state."[13]

Over the next several months the debate raged. The Baptist denomination expressed unyielding opposition to this church-state endeavor. At the same time delegations from Charlotte, Durham, Greensboro, and Raleigh made proposals to the trustees regarding financial commitments for the establishment of the expanded medical school in their communities. During the spring the state's budget commission turned down a proposal by the board of trustees for the funding of the expanded medical school. The 1923 General Assembly also made extensive reductions in the university's budget requests for both existing programs and improvements.

In view of these developments, on June 12, 1923, the university board of trustees passed President Chase's resolution that the matter of an expanded medical school be deferred for two years until the next General Assembly. In fact, it would be another decade before the expansion would be seriously considered again.

Berryhill years later analyzed this second failure to provide a state teaching hospital and MD-granting medical school for the citizens of North Carolina:

It is difficult to determine precisely what influence Dr. Few's proposal had on the outcome. Dr. Manning said, however, "at any rate, it seems clear that his proposal succeeded in contributing to the confusion and ultimate failure of the plan." If, as he stated, Dr. Few had long been interested in establishing a medical school at Trinity College, one wonders why this interest had not been communicated to university officials or trustees during the twelve months it was public knowledge that the university through a special committee was studying and planning for the expansion of the university's two-year medical school.

Possibly the lack of agreement on the location for an expanded school was of some importance in the outcome. The most important factor, however, was undoubtedly the fear on the part of President Chase and important members of the board of trustees that funds requested for construction and operation of an expanded medical school and university hospital would jeopardize the university's request for legislative appropriations for other urgently needed buildings and developments.[14]

An insight into Few's action is provided in a biographical sketch published with Few's *Papers and Addresses* in 1951. Few had had a medical school for Durham in mind for some time. When it appeared that UNC might build one, he urgently wrote B. N. Duke in early December 1922 (shortly before his December 19 public proposal):

I wish you and your Brother would give just a few moment's [sic] thought to the Medical School matter about which I have spoken to you both. I consider it practically certain that if we do not get it, it will still be put in Durham, built partly by the Rockefeller money, and controlled by the University of North Carolina. If there is to be a medical school in Durham, Trinity ought to have its hand on it. With one of the most important departments in Durham and a hard-surface road making Chapel Hill almost a suburb of Durham the time might come when we might have to struggle for educational leadership in our own town. While there can be no rivalry in good works, we ought to look out for the causes we have on our hearts. I expect Trinity to become one of the great institutions of America. It may take years . . . [but] we must do our best to keep the road open . . . Whatever is done must be done within the next few weeks. And this seems to me to be a matter of so great importance that I could never forgive myself if I had to feel through the years that I had left any stone unturned.[15]

In December 1924 the founding of Duke University was announced, and the charter of Trinity College was subsequently amended to accommodate the

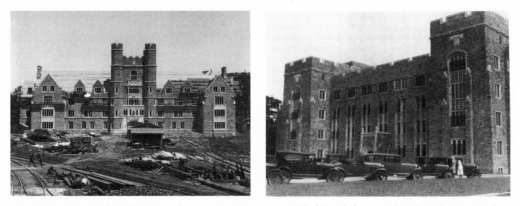

The Duke School of Medicine under construction in 1928 *(left)* and the completed Duke Hospital in 1930 *(right)*. (Gifford, *The Evolution of a Medical Center,* 1972; Duke University Press)

name change. Wilburt C. Davison, MD, a pediatrician at Johns Hopkins, was appointed the first dean of the Duke medical school on the basis of the recommendation to President Few by the Johns Hopkins medical dean, William Henry Welch, MD. The Duke Endowment allocated $4 million for the medical center, and not too long afterward construction began on the hospital and medical school. Duke Hospital opened in 1930, and the first medical students (who had transferred from other medical schools into the third-year class) graduated with MDs from Duke University in 1932. Thus, after a hiatus of a decade and a half, North Carolina now had an MD-granting medical school—in Durham, supported by private funds, without a state appropriation.[16]

THE THREAT TO THE EXISTENCE OF
THE TWO-YEAR SCHOOLS IN THE 1930S

In 1929 Acting Dean Charles S. Mangum reported to the medical school's administrative board on the recent meeting of the AAMC in New York City:

A great deal of stress was laid upon the fact that large numbers of students are applying for admission to Medical Schools only to be rejected, in some instances, by as many as from thirty to forty different schools. Last year, less than 50% of the students who applied finally gained admittance into a Medical School. A significant fact reported was that a great many of these rejected applicants are going to Europe for their medical education. In the English schools alone, there are approximately 1,000 medical students whose names appear upon the lists of those rejected in this country. In France, there are between 250 and 300, and in Germany 25. Many of these men, after receiving their degrees abroad, are returning to America to practice medicine. It is admitted that we are badly in need of more properly equipped schools to meet the demand for medical education and, of course, a large percentage of the rejections were for lack of sufficient scholastic preparation, but the majority were rejected because of "personality" and "undesirability." Running beneath the whole discussion was an unvoiced realization of the fact that there exists, in the American schools, a wide-spread discrimination against Jews and applicants from the "foreign element." One had the courage to say so in very plain language. The others only hinted at it. The influx of the "foreign element" into the large Medical Schools is to our advantage in the transfer of our students. One Dean told me that he needed our students to dilute his foreign population and another that he welcomed our transfers because we sent him "blue-eyed men."

. . . Of the ten two-year Medical Schools now in operation, eight were represented at this meeting. We held a conference and organized, within the larger Association, an Association of Two-Year Medical Schools. This group is to meet each year and talk over the problems of the two-year schools . . .

The general impression I received at this meeting of the Association of American Medical Colleges was encouraging. The two-year schools are accepted as American Medical Colleges on equal basis of respect and credit with the others. The need of a few such schools is generally recognized and it is admitted that the students transferred from them should improve the personality and the scholarship of the classes they enter.[17]

In the early 1930s the effects of the worldwide economic depression were being felt throughout the nation. People lacked money to buy many of the items and services they needed, and surpluses were developing. In response, the government told farmers to reduce supply by destroying cattle and plowing under every third row of cotton. Many physicians could not collect enough fees to support themselves, and some were turning to other work. The AMA began to explore ways to reduce the perceived oversupply of physicians.[18]

Mangum's optimistic outlook on the future of two-year medical schools was shattered in September 1935 with the announcement that after July 1, 1938, the AMA Council on Medical Education and Hospitals would no longer include two-year schools on their list of approved institutions.[19] The two-year schools had always been at a disadvantage because of difficulties they experienced in recruiting and retaining the most able faculty and because they feared that their graduates might not be accepted into the third-year class of the MD-granting schools. The AMA council's decision had the effect of limiting the number of the nation's physicians through the accreditation process and could have doomed the two-year schools.

Thurman D. Kitchin, MD (Cert. Med., UNC 1906; MD, Jefferson 1908), dean of the Wake Forest College of Medicine from 1919 to 1936 and president of Wake Forest College from 1930 to 1950, was outspoken in an interview with the *Raleigh News and Observer* about the intent of the proposed AMA action, which would have closed both the Wake Forest and UNC two-year medical schools. An editorial in the paper on October 1, 1935, entitled "Plowing Up Doctors," said that "the time has come to change an old injunction, 'Physician, heal thyself . . . 'to 'Physician, diagnose thyself.' For if, as Dr. Kitchin says, organized physicians are deliberately undertaking to create a scarcity profitable to themselves in the practice of medicine, the practitioners of an ancient, an honorable, a learned profession ought to realize that they are not immune to the disease of rapaciousness which is the plague of our times." The editorial concluded, "Plowing up cotton was an emergency measure justified only by the crisis of the depression. But plowing up doctors, not merely for the present but for the whole future in which men who might now be educated . . . would be plowing up humanity in order that profits might be reaped."[20]

MacNider and President Graham were furious when they learned of the AMA council's proposed action and immediately organized a campaign to reverse it. As a first step, they both attended the meeting of the AAMC in Toronto in October 1935. Although Graham could not participate in the floor debate, he worked tirelessly behind the scenes on a resolution in favor of the two-year schools. The dean of the University of Pennsylvania School of Medicine provided support with his statement that UNC had furnished almost one-third of the graduating students from his school; some of these had become leading physicians in Philadelphia, but most had returned to their native North Carolina to practice. His motion that the two-year schools be judged on their merits, rather than arbitrarily rejected, was passed unanimously.

Graham carried the battle further in November at the meeting in Washington of the National Association of State Universities. Five of the two-year schools were represented, but he was the only person there who had attended the Toronto meeting. A resolution supporting the two-year schools was passed unanimously with the instruction that it should be presented to the next meeting of the AMA council.

Graham, MacNider, and the president of the University of Utah presented convincing arguments for the existence of the two-year schools at the meeting of the AMA council in Chicago in December. At the conclusion of the discussion the council overturned its previous action and agreed to judge each school on its individual merits. After the meeting the council's chair, Stanford President Ray Lyman Wilbur, told Graham, "You gentlemen have won your reconsideration, but my advice to you is that you get your house in order and prepare the way for the expansion of your school into a four-year medical program."[21]

Although Berryhill was not an active participant in the fight to preserve the accreditation of UNC and the other two-year medical schools, he was acutely aware of the struggle through his frequent contacts with Graham and MacNider during this time. When he became dean, this lurking threat provided one more motivation for his drive to achieve a four-year medical school for the university and the people of North Carolina.

The increased demand for physicians during World War II required the full support of the two-year medical schools and made their threatened closure a moot point. In the years after the war, however, all ten of the two-year schools in operation during the 1930s converted to four-year schools. Some new postwar schools (including East Carolina University medical school in North Carolina) started as basic science schools and then evolved into four-year schools, but today there are no separately accredited two-year medical schools.[22]

The Third Effort to Expand the Medical School, 1937–1938

As he was during the accreditation crisis in the mid-1930s, Berryhill was the university physician and a medical school faculty member when the third effort to expand the medical school at Chapel Hill failed. As assistant dean to MacNider, however, he was much more informed about the issues, even though he still did not actively participate in the fight.

Berryhill wrote in the centennial history of the medical school that an attempt was made in the early 1930s by a loyal and prominent medical school alumnus to revive the UNC Medical Department in Raleigh to serve both the two-year school at Chapel Hill and the one at Wake Forest. "This movement," he added, "although conceived with the best interest and motivation, did not gain much support."

The General Assembly of 1937, recognizing the threat to the two-year schools and concerned about the supply of physicians in the state, called upon the governor to establish a commission to study the issue and report to the 1939 General Assembly. Governor Clyde R. Hoey appointed a Commission on Medical Education composed of physicians and members of the legislature. It was chaired by a 1915 graduate of the two-year medical school, T. W. M. Long, MD, and included two other UNC medical school graduates, William Coppridge, MD, and B. J. Lawrence, MD, as well as Dean MacNider of the UNC medical school and Dean C. C. Carpenter of the Wake Forest medical school. Long and the two other commission members, O. M. Mull and J. W. Garrett, were also leaders in the General Assembly. A committee of the state medical society worked closely with the commission.[23]

The Hoey Commission, as it came to be known, thoroughly explored the various issues and alternatives. They sent questionnaires to deans throughout the country asking about medical school and hospital costs, hospital location and control, and number of students and faculty. Answers were tabulated and distributed to the members. Individuals on the commission also visited other academic medical centers. The commission tentatively finished its work in early November 1938 with a majority report calling for a four-year, MD-granting medical school as an expansion of the two-year school as well as the construction of a 300-bed teaching hospital at Chapel Hill. It urged that the "institution should be established as soon as practicable."

The commission met a few days later to review its recommendations with the medical society committee before making its report to the governor and the 1939 General Assembly. Mull, an attorney from Shelby, surprised the commission with the announcement that private money was available for the expansion and endowment of the medical school if it were built in a city of the state other than Chapel Hill. Mull asked that the commission amend its previous report to remove any reference to the location of the proposed school so that this offer could be considered.

Mull's proposal was vigorously opposed by Dean MacNider, who stated it was better to have no school at all if it were not located on the university campus in Chapel Hill. MacNider convincingly argued—based on his thirty-five years of experience with medical education—that the only way for the four-year school to succeed was to put it on the university campus and give it its own teaching hospital. Following the discussion the Mull amendment to the commission's report striking out any references to the location of the recommended medical school was defeated, with four votes against, two votes for, and one absent. Mull then submitted a minority report that concurred "in the report of the Commission in that there is a need for a Medical School, owned and operated by the State," but reiterated his view that the location of the medical school should not be specified: "I do not think the location of the Medical School at Chapel Hill is of sufficient importance to make it necessary to refuse a large donation which was conditioned upon building the School elsewhere." (At the time it was generally agreed that it would take from $5 million to $10 million to build a new medical school and teaching hospital, and Mull was under the impression that the proposed donation from the Bowman Gray estate amounted to over $5 million. Later Wake Forest medical school Dean Coy Carpenter said that he, Mull, and Wake Forest President Kitchin were shocked when they learned it was only about $600,000.)[24]

MacNider, in a letter to Mull, complimented him on his interest in the medical school but elaborated his position concerning the importance of the location of the expanded school:

The greatest danger, and the danger which has killed so many schools and which has completely changed the point of view of medical educators about medical education, is that it is just a matter of time, if the school is not on the University campus and an integral part of it, before influences other than those of a University order insert themselves into the various departments, attempt to run the departments in an improper manner and lead to disintegration.[25]

Mull replied to MacNider's letter graciously but insisted that the state should accept the proposed donation:

I appreciate your letter . . . as well as your willingness to fight for a position you conscientiously believe to be right. I certainly concede sincerity of purpose and ask the same for myself. I understand that you are definitely of the opinion that a School of Medicine operated by the State at any other place than Chapel Hill would be a failure because it would not have the use of certain necessary facilities which can only be furnished by such a school as the University. I therefore understand that your position is that you prefer for the State to have no [four-year] Medical School unless it is located at the University for the reason that you do not want the State to own and operate a failure, rather than a personal wish to have new school located at your old home base. You can afford to fight for such a position and I admire you for doing so.

Yet I am equally convinced that the location of a Medical College is not limited to the campus of some University. Being of that opinion I can not eliminate good business judgment from my decision that the State should accept large donations for establishing and maintaining a Medical School although the donors required same to be located at some other city within the State. Your splendid presentation of your opinion on the subject convinced the majority of our committee and I congratulate you. I am convinced that the course followed by our committee makes it impractical to establish the desired school at this time, yet the future will afford many other opportunities and the day may come in our lifetime when the State will be both able and willing to make your ambition and dream come true by erecting a great Medical School at Chapel Hill.[26]

MacNider did live to see the day when such a teaching hospital and expanded medical school were located in Chapel Hill, although he died a year before the hospital opened.

The resulting confusion and subsequent developments following the Bowman Gray proposal by Mull ended the work of the Hoey Commission, as had the proposal by President Few from Trinity a decade earlier.[27]

The proposed gift was never officially presented to the university trustees, and in August 1939 it was announced that the Bowman Gray Foundation was going to fund the expansion of the two-year medical school at the Baptist-supported Wake Forest College into a four-year school located in Winston-Salem, with North Carolina Baptist Hospital as its teaching hospital. The expanded school moved in 1941 and was named the Bowman Gray School of Medicine of Wake Forest College. The first MD class graduated in 1943. The entire Wake Forest College moved from Wake County to a new campus at the edge of Winston-Salem in 1956 and became Wake Forest University in 1967. The medical school was renamed the Wake Forest University School of Medicine in 1997.[28]

Berryhill and colleagues commented on this third failure to establish a full medical school for the university:

Among many alumni of the university and of the School of Medicine as well as among friends of the institution and the general public, the university was

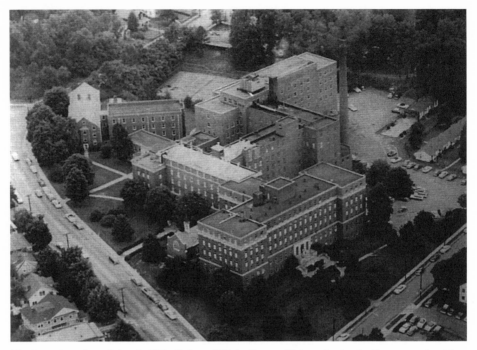

The Bowman Gray School of Medicine of Wake Forest University in the foreground, with the expanded Baptist Hospital in the background, 1954. (Garrison, *Wake Forest University: One Hundred Years of Medicine*, 2002; courtesy of Wake Forest University Health Sciences)

severely criticized for not accepting "the offer from the Gray family." It was felt that this probably was the end of any possible hope for the expansion of the two-year medical school. . . .

This development continued to plague the university for some years. In retrospect it was most unfortunate that the majority of the members of the Hoey Commission were unwilling . . . to explore to the fullest the information he [Mr. Mull] had presented, whatever might have been the final decision with respect to the wisdom of acceptance . . . It was even more unfortunate that the university leadership did not make an effort to follow up or explore in detail and weigh carefully the possibilities of whatever proposal the Gray family wished to make . . . Even if a thorough study might have led eventually to the university's inability to accept the proposal, its position would have been much stronger after making such a study.[29]

Although the process was undoubtedly flawed, the university's decision not to accept monies that might have severely compromised its academic and public service mission was in keeping with the advice of UNC President Francis P. Venable in his 1900 University Day address:

The founders of this State in their sturdy independence and far-seeing wisdom recognized the importance of such an institution, and so, while the struggle for freedom was still upon them, provided for the establishment of this University—the chief safeguard of their children against the loss of those liberties for which they fought. And should some one come and offer to endow this institution with many millions and remove it from the control of the State, it would be a sale of the birth-right of those children, a betrayal of the trust of the fathers. The citizens of this State cannot afford to have this University narrowed down to the political platform of any one part, to the creed of a single sect, to the economic belief of any individual philanthropist. Parties, churches, philanthropists, all can centre their efforts here and unite in the making of a great people, a grand Commonwealth, but the people must control.

Success at Last: The Fourth Effort to Expand the Medical School, 1941–1952

Berryhill Appointed Dean

When MacNider resigned in 1940 after four years as dean to return to his research and teaching, Chancellor House and President Graham asked Berryhill to take the position of acting dean. He served in this capacity during the 1940–1941 academic year.

A search committee for MacNider's successor as dean was appointed: Drs. Robert E. Coker, professor of zoology (chair); Ralph Bost, professor of chemistry; W. Critz George, professor of histology; and Grant L. Donnelly, professor of pharmacology. The committee studied the situation of the two-year schools of medicine and concluded that they were not viable in the long run. They then recommended that Acting Dean Berryhill be appointed dean of the medical school and charged with planning for the expansion of the school to a four-year program.

Berryhill initially declined the appointment. But once he was assured that the university was committed to expansion of the school when funds became available, he accepted the deanship in 1941 for a five-year term. Berryhill was convinced to accept a second five-year term beginning in 1946 as the planning for the expanded school intensified. After the initial funding for the school and the hospital at Chapel Hill were obtained, he submitted his resignation, but President Graham refused to accept it. Thus he continued his service as dean for thirteen years during the most critical time for the establishment of the academic medical center in Chapel Hill, until his resignation in 1964.[30]

In a report to President Graham in December 1940 after Berryhill had assumed the position as acting dean for 1940–1941, he reconfirmed the medical school's commitment to educating "well qualified . . . medical students, largely from this state, in the hope that they will return to this section to practice their profession. This function of the school of course is seriously curtailed and handicapped because our work is limited to the first two years. *We should never give*

*up hoping, planning and working to bring into actual being here on this campus
a University hospital, and the establishment of a four-year school"* (emphasis
added).[31]

In his annual report to Graham for 1940–1941, Berryhill began in earnest his
unwavering campaign for an academic medical center for the citizens of North
Carolina:

> In spite of the national emergency we should not lose sight of our ultimate
> goal of establishing a four-year school, and we ought to be continually think-
> ing and planning so that we will be in a position to take advantage of any
> private endowment or support from the national government when the ap-
> propriate time arrives for this further development. It is inevitable that we
> take this step if this school if to survive, and what is more important, if the
> State and University are to fulfill their obligations to the people of the State
> in the way of both training practicing physicians, public health physicians,
> and nurses and at the same time provide adequate medical care for the entire
> population.[32]

In 1942, in his second report as dean, Berryhill recognized the reality of wartime conditions but did not lose sight of the goal:

> During the nine years I have been connected with the Medical School, but
> particularly during the last two years when that connection has been that of
> the administrative officer of the School, it has become more and more appar-
> ent that in order to survive this School must develop into a four-year school.
> Under the present emergency and with the great shortage of doctors, it seems
> fairly clear that the two-year schools will be encouraged to continue, and it
> certainly would be most unwise to take definite steps now to expand into a
> four-year school before the end of the war.
>
> This does not mean that we should sit by and wait hopefully for something
> to happen. We ought to be planning now for the development of the School
> in the post-war era, and we ought to have certain fairly definite approaches
> to the problem worked out so that we may be able to take advantage of both
> State and Federal support and private support.[33]

In keeping with this view, in early 1943 Dean Berryhill began discussions
about the expansion of the school and its financing with a group composed of
medical faculty members (James Bullitt, MD, and Russell Holman, MD, and
two former deans, Isaac Manning, MD, and William de B. MacNider, MD); a
faculty member in public health (Herman G. Baity, PhD); a faculty member
from the biological sciences (Robert E. Coker, PhD); and university administrators (Chancellor Robert B. House and Controller William D. Carmichael). Simultaneously, continuing discussions were held with William Coppridge, MD, a

1916 graduate of the UNC two-year medical program. Coppridge predicted that federal funds would become available to support the planned expansion and had conveyed this possibility to President Graham on several occasions. In the summer and autumn Dean Berryhill continued discussions with Chancellor House, Controller Carmichael, and the members of the medical school's Alumni Visiting Committee (Donnell Cobb, MD, Cert. Med., UNC 1919; Roy McKnight, MD, Cert. Med., UNC 1918; and Coppridge).

The Committee of Physicians and the Board of Trustees

At Berryhill's request, in the fall of 1943 President Graham convened a meeting in Chapel Hill to discuss the soundness of the medical school expansion proposal. Included were medical alumni Drs. Coppridge, Cobb, McKnight, Karl Pace, and Foy Roberson (also a member of the UNC board of trustees); Paul P. McCain, MD, superintendent of the State Tuberculosis Sanatorium; state medical society president James W. Vernon, MD; former state medical society presidents F. Webb Griffith, MD, and Hubert Haywood, MD; and two representatives of the state medical society, Street Brewer, MD, and Grady Dickson, MD.[34]

These medical advisors unanimously recommended to President Graham that the university lead a statewide effort to plan and seek funding for the expansion of the medical school and for the construction or renovation of medical care facilities in medically underserved areas of the state. President Graham wanted to present this plan to Governor Broughton and, if he supported it, to the UNC board of trustees meeting at the end of January 1944. He asked five physicians who were present or past presidents of the state medical society (Drs. Cobb, Haywood, McCain, Vernon, and Paul F. Whitaker) to prepare such a proposal with the help of Drs. Coppridge and Hamilton McKay. Graham asked Dr. McCain to chair the committee and asked Dean Berryhill to serve as the university's representative and as secretary for the committee.

The Committee of Physicians met in Raleigh with Governor Melville Broughton in January 1944 to present their approach to addressing the critical health care needs of the people of North Carolina. The committee's report (see Appendix E) began with an assessment:

> One of the most important problems facing the State and the medical profession is that of providing opportunities for more adequate medical care in the post-war period for all groups of citizens. Some provision must be made for the low-income group to have adequate medical care at fees they can afford to pay and for the indigent to receive both hospital and ambulatory medical services.
>
> In any attempt to solve this problem we are immediately faced with critical shortages of general hospital facilities and trained medical personnel of all types. In 1941 North Carolina, the 11th largest state and the 5th most rapidly growing, stood in 42nd place, tied with South Carolina, in the number of

general hospital beds per thousand population and in a comparable position in the number of doctors. In addition, we have always had in this State too few trained medical personnel, nurses, dietitians, doctors of Public Health, sanitary engineers, sanitarians, medical technicians, and health educators.

The committee clearly recognized the magnitude of what they were being asked to deal with: "[That] the problem is too large and complex for any one group of individuals or institutions to satisfactorily and adequately solve seems obvious. It is a responsibility and obligation and an opportunity of the entire community, that is, the State."

The committee suggested two major steps for dealing with these problems. First, the "building of a large well-equipped general hospital, initially 500 to 700 beds, in a more or less centrally located place in the State" to provide "a diagnostic and treatment center" for both ambulatory and hospitalized indigent patients and to "train needed medical personnel of all types—doctors of medicine, doctors of public health, nurses . . . and perhaps dentists." In addition, it should provide postgraduate education for practicing physicians and serve as a "central laboratory for research in medicine and public health." In view of the controversy that would soon arise in regard to the location of the new hospital, it is of interest that the committee unequivocally stated:

Such a general hospital for the State would logically be placed adjoining the present buildings of the Schools of Medicine and Public Health and the Navy Hospital on the Campus of the University at Chapel Hill. The present two-year Medical School, now adequately housed in a new building representing an outlay of approximately $500,000, should be expanded into a four-year School of Medicine and the clinical teachers of the Medical School should serve as the professional medical staff of the hospital . . . Past experience has shown that the best progress in Medicine is attained through the maintenance of the closest possible physical and spiritual relationship between patient, "student" (teacher, student, investigator), library, and laboratory, including the science laboratories of Chemistry, Physics, and Biology, best afforded by universities. Thus, the hospital should be integrated with the Schools of Medicine and Public Health and other facilities at the State University and would undoubtedly work in close cooperation with the State Health Department and with the other State hospitals and agencies devoted to medical care and the improvement of the general health of the State.

The committee's second major recommendation concerned the statewide need for adequate health care facilities:

Obviously, one hospital could not care for all the indigent in the State who need medical attention . . . smaller hospitals, well equipped for diagnostic work and treatment, should be set up in different sections of the State in which there are now no hospital facilities. In certain sections existing hospitals might be enlarged. The professional direction of those additional hospital facilities should be in the hand of the medical profession in those communities and sections of the State. A well coordinated plan could be worked out between the smaller hospitals and the larger central unit whereby the latter could supply professional consultation when requested, or obscure cases in the former presenting problems in diagnosis or treatment could be sent to the central hospital for study.

The building of small hospitals in areas where no such institutions exist and the enlargement of some of the present hospitals would not only provide vitally needed medical facilities but would tend to attract young graduates of Medicine and all other types of trained medical personnel to those areas to begin the practice of their profession. This would help greatly to improve the maldistribution of medical personnel in the State.

The committee concluded that such a plan "might eventually provide an opportunity for adequate medical services for the citizens who have not been able to afford [them] . . . [and] might well serve as a model for other states and for the nation as a whole in improving the health and the general usefulness of our people."

Governor Broughton accepted the committee's proposal. As chairman of the board of trustees of the Consolidated University of North Carolina, he presented the recommendations to the full meeting of the board in Chapel Hill on January 31, 1944, with the comment that:

There is great concern on the part of all members of the medical profession . . . over the prospect of what is broadly termed "socialized medicine" . . . While such [a] prospect is naturally viewed with apprehension, it is at the same time fully recognized by the profession that certain broad and deep trends in the field of social welfare as affecting medical service cannot and should not be resisted. These conditions spring from a deep-seated feeling that good health and adequate medical attention should be the right and privilege of every man, woman, and child regardless of race, condition, or financial circumstances . . .

It accordingly would seem wise under a suitable basis of cooperation between the Federal Government, the respective state governments, local governments, and various foundations and funds, to make provision for adequate medical care and service to those of our citizenship who by reason of unemployment or low income are unable to provide this service for themselves . . .

The [North Carolina Medical] Society is not only favorable to such general plan, but would be glad to join in the sponsorship of any move that may be made in this direction.

It is believed that the University of North Carolina, which already has a standard two-year medical school and has recently had its medical facilities substantially enlarged in connection with the Navy program, should join in sponsoring such [a] proposal. In fact, it is felt by officials of the Medical Society and by many who have given consideration to this matter that the University should have an active part in any plan that is proposed . . .

The ultimate purpose of this program should be that no person in North Carolina shall lack adequate hospital care or medical treatment by reason of poverty or low income.[35]

Following the governor's presentation of the physicians' recommendations, "Mr. Walter Murphy moved that the trustees go on record as unanimously and enthusiastically approving the Governor's recommendations and report; and that a Commission be appointed by him to make a comprehensive study of the whole subject and submit recommendations to the next General Assembly." The motion was seconded and unanimously approved.[36]

The North Carolina Hospital and Medical Care Commission, 1944–1945

Governor Broughton wasted no time in selecting Clarence Poe of Raleigh, the respected editor of the *Progressive Farmer*, as the chairman of the new North Carolina Hospital and Medical Care Commission.[37] The sixty-three-year-old Poe was an ideal choice to lead the commission. Although neither a physician nor an elected office holder, he had waged a campaign for more than forty years against poverty, ignorance, and illness through the pages of the *Progressive Farmer*, which he had purchased at age eighteen and which had grown to a circulation throughout the South of well over one million. His personal struggle with illness began when he was just nine days old, when he developed whooping cough. The story was retold many times through the years about how his "mother continued working with untiring fingers to expel the choking phlegm from my little throat and help my heart overcome the constantly recurring spasms of coughing that each time left me gasping for breath." In rural Chatham County, where he was raised, childhood illnesses devastated whole families: "Joe Elkins had four children; all died of diphtheria. Hath Gilmore lost four boys in two weeks from diphtheria. A man named Malone lost seven grown children the same fall from typhoid fever." The cemeteries of his childhood thus had a disproportionate number of "short graves" of children as compared with today's cemeteries. Poe had been active in the early 1900s in promoting the Rockefeller-supported program to rid the South of hookworm, "the physical and mental anemia that was sapping thousands in the South." Following his service as head of the North Carolina Hospital and Medical Care Commission in the mid-1940s, he was asked by President Truman to serve on the Committee on Health Needs of the Nation from 1951 to 1952. Based on his long campaign for better health, he championed in this report the principle that "our democracy will never be complete until every person, rich or poor, high or low, urban or rural, white or black, has an equal right to adequate hospital and medical care whenever and wherever he makes the same grim battle against ever-menacing Death which sooner or later we must all make."[38]

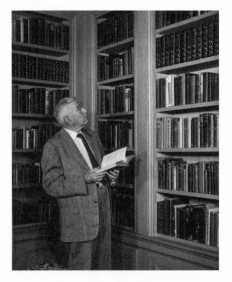

Clarence Poe of Raleigh, chair of the North Carolina Hospital and Medical Care Commission. *(Authors)*

Sixty citizens from around the state representing a broad spectrum of medical professionals and other citizens were appointed to the new commission. Carl V. Reynolds, MD, the state health officer, was appointed as secretary. The organizational meeting of the commission was held in Raleigh on February 28, 1944, at which time seven subcommittees were formed:

1. Hospital and Medical Care for Our Rural Population
2. Hospital and Medical Care for Industrial and Urban Populations
3. Special Needs for Our Negro Population
4. Four-Year Medical School for the University and Hospital Facilities
5. Mental Hygiene and Hospitalization
6. Statistical Studies
7. Hospital and Medical Care Plans in Other States

Dean Berryhill, along with Deans Coy C. Carpenter of the Bowman Gray medical school and W. C. Davison of the Duke University medical school, were members of the subcommittee on the four-year medical school for the university. P. P. McCain chaired this committee of eleven persons, and Josephus Daniels served as vice chair.[39] At the end of months of deliberation and visits to other medical centers, McCain and Daniels asked Berryhill to write the formal report for the committee.[40] The subcommittee's report reiterated the findings of the other subcommittees that a severe shortage of all types of medical personnel existed in the state.

As part of its study, the subcommittee on the four-year medical school visited the medical schools at the Universities of Iowa, Michigan, and Virginia as well as the Medical College of Virginia. The officials of these schools all advised the visitors that the expanded medical school should be located on the campus at Chapel Hill because of the many advantages offered by close association with the parent university. They recognized that Chapel Hill's small size might make it hard for the area to furnish enough clinical material for teaching in some fields but suggested that affiliations with hospital obstetrical and other services in larger cities could address this problem.

The medical school subcommittee recommended that the existing two-year medical school at Chapel Hill be expanded to a four-year, MD-granting school; that a teaching hospital of 600 beds be built at Chapel Hill; that a dental school and a nursing school be established at Chapel Hill; and that the existing pharmacy school be expanded. They also recommended that dental and medical education for Negro students be provided on a regional basis with other states.

The seven subcommittees labored for eight months to develop a comprehensive survey of the health status and needs of North Carolinians. The commission approved a preliminary report on October 11, 1944, after presentations to Governor Broughton. Chairman Poe later observed:

> While resolutely determined to discover and uncover all the facts about North Carolina hospital and medical care conditions, the highlight of all our activities was not the discovery about the shockingly high 57% rejection rate of North Carolina boys in the American armies but rather the far more astonishing discovery that among draftees who had grown up in North Carolina orphanages and who had had not-too-expensive hospital and medical care plus sound but not-expensive nutrition, the rejection rate had been only 3%!

To respond to this and other identified health needs in the state, the report called for "More Hospitals, More Doctors and More Insurance" for the people of North Carolina. As part of this statewide effort the commission gave "its unqualified endorsement to the proposal that the present two-year medical school at the University of North Carolina be expanded into a standard four-year medical school with a central hospital of 600 beds." It was their opinion that "North Carolina students trained in North Carolina will likely remain in North Carolina to follow their chosen profession." The preliminary report concluded with a plea that all "work together to make real a new ideal of democracy": "The equal right of every person born on earth to needed medical and hospital care whenever and wherever he battles against Disease and Death."

The commission's written report (see Appendix G) was later described by a participant in the debates at the time as "a remarkably accurate inventory of the State's woefully inadequate hospital facilities, the increasing shortage of physicians, dentists, and nurses, especially in rural areas, the extraordinary high percentage of North Carolina draftees rejected in two wars because of physical and mental defects, and the inadequate educational and training facilities for supplying the necessary trained personnel for the task ahead. So thoroughly and accurately was the work of the Poe Commission done that no one was able to refute either its findings of fact or its conclusions."[41]

The new governor, R. Gregg Cherry, had not been actively involved in the early discussions about the proposed statewide health program. Shortly after his inauguration in January 1945, a group had a long evening meeting with the governor at the mansion in Raleigh to discuss the commission's major recommendations for state and federally funded hospital and clinic construction throughout the state and for the expanded medical school and teaching hospital at Chapel Hill. Those present included several medical society and political leaders, UNC President Graham, and Dean Berryhill. Paul Whitaker and Berryhill were so zealous in educating the new governor about the need for the entire program that one participant commented afterward, "Doctors Berryhill and Whitaker did not seem to realize that they could not talk to the Governor of North Carolina like he was a medical student." The governor finally told Graham that he was reluctant for the state to finance hospital and clinic construction, but he could support the expansion of the medical school and the building of the teaching hospital if the other recommendations were dropped. Graham made it clear, however, that he and those present were committed to the entire program:

> Governor, I am pledged to support the entire program recommended. I believe that there is a great need for it and that the people of our state will support it. You have the opportunity to go down in history as the Health Governor of North Carolina as Governor Aycock did in education and as Governor Morrison did in building good roads. This, in my opinion, is the third great epic movement in North Carolina. There is more of God in it than any program with which I have ever been connected. Naturally, as president of the University of North Carolina, I would like to see its medical school expanded. It is sorely needed but all of the program is needed, and I must say to you, Sir, that I am pledged to support the program in its entirety, and this I will do.[42]

The commission's recommendations were then presented to a joint session of the 1945 General Assembly on February 10, 1945. The members of the General Assembly had been provided in advance a clothbound book entitled *To the Good Health of North Carolina* containing the Poe Report and additional pamphlets and statements. Poe began his presentation with the exclamation that this was "a program of great hope, of almost infinite promise, and yet of great practicability!"[43] On this critical occasion, according to Graham, Governor Cherry "threw his personal, political and official weight in support of the program" when he introduced the presentation with a challenge to the members of the General Assembly (see Appendix H):[44] "You have the responsibility and privilege of making another decisive decision in the history of our state. I ask you to believe with me that better schools, better roads, and better health constitute the main high roads for advancement of North Carolina. I have confidence that you, in this hour of destiny, will make the decision embracing a program for the future happiness and welfare of North Carolina."[45] In view of the fact that the war was still raging, the governor did not ask for appropriations for buildings, but did request funding for a new permanent Medical Care Commission to carry on the work of the ad hoc Poe Commission. He reminded the legislators:

The voices of the sick, the suffering, and even the dying cry out to us at this time for help. These voices which we hear, voices too long unheard, come to us across the plains and hills of every part of our state. It is my belief that we should answer their calls and minister to their needs by laying the foundation of a balanced and humane program for more adequate medical care for the people of this commonwealth.[46]

The presentation of the commission's recommendations began a vigorous public debate that lasted two years and had repercussions for long afterward, as Berryhill later observed: "The lines were quickly drawn, and there began a battle which raged throughout the state with considerable fervor—sometimes with ferocity. Its effects were evident for some years following the action of the 1945 and 1947 General Assemblies, which finally passed legislation which implemented essentially all of the recommendations of the Medical Care Commission."

Although the report was positively received in general, some people expressed concerns regarding the size of the long-term financial commitment the state would have to make in order to implement the entire program. Wealthy citizens were especially concerned about what this could add to their taxes. One financial leader in the state was quoted as saying, "North Carolina [which already had two private medical schools] needs a medical school like I need three legs."[47] An editorial in the *Raleigh News and Observer* answered those "jeremiads [*sic*]" with "eyes in the back of their heads" who say "we are too poor for the State to give hospitalization to those who need it and to establish a State four-year medical college" with the counterpoint that "we are too poor not to have the health policy which has been approved by all forward-looking organizations in the State."[48]

Specific concerns included the fear by some physicians and civic leaders that the state's oversight of the local hospital and health care facilities' construction would be a step toward "socialized medicine." Proponents of the commission's recommendations made clear that the proposed new state medical care commission would leave the professional and financial control of local facilities in the hands of their own boards of trustees.[49]

Some in the state's larger cities, while supporting the expansion of the medical school, felt that the teaching hospital and clinical years of the expanded school should be located in their city, not in the small village of Chapel Hill. On the other hand, as one editorialist pointed out, no city in North Carolina at the time was large enough to provide all of the patients needed for a complete medical education. The fact that medical students would have to go elsewhere for part of their clinical experience was thus not unique for a teaching hospital located in Chapel Hill. This is still true fifty years later, when more than one-third of the medical students at any one time are receiving their clinical training at sites outside of Chapel Hill in order to provide a diversity of educational experiences for a much larger student body.

Some of the bitterest and most persistent opposition to the recommendations that a teaching hospital be built in Chapel Hill and that the UNC medical school be expanded came from some officials and alumni in the state's two existing private medical schools.[50] (Similarly, several decades later, initial opposition to a proposed state medical school at East Carolina University in Greenville came from some UNC alumni and officials.) The main argument in both situations was that any new state appropriations should support the expansion and enhancement of the existing schools rather than being put toward establishing a new school. Whitaker later observed that there "was highly vocal and powerful opposition to the medical school facet of the program, much of it centered in the Duke Endowment. Dr. W. S. Rankin, secretary of the Duke Endowment, and Dean Wilburt C. Davison of the Duke University medical school opposed the program vigorously but at the same time openly and cleanly . . . but once the expansion was decided upon they offered their wisdom and experience to make it a success."[51] Berryhill said that Rankin visited him some time after the medical school issue had been resolved to express his regret that he had been obligated to oppose the school. He added that Rankin's "efforts and advice were of considerable assistance" for the next decade or more. Rankin was especially helpful in making it possible for the annual Duke Endowment indigent-care grant to the North Carolina Memorial Hospital to be set aside in a fund that could be used for special hospital needs not covered by the state appropriations.[52] Whitaker said that President Thurmond Kitchin of Wake Forest College also opposed the medical school expansion behind the scenes, with most of the active opposition coming from several Wake Forest alumni who were practicing in the state. He added that most of the faculty members at the two private medical schools were not opposed to the expansion, although there were a few detractors in each school.[53]

As a result of strong and courageous leadership in the legislature, a compromise act was enacted on March 21, 1945. It adopted most of the major recommendations of the Poe Commission (with some added conditions):

1. A permanent North Carolina Medical Care Commission, reporting to the legislature and the governor, was established and funded to assume the leadership for coordinating the planning and implementation of the statewide plan for improved health care for North Carolinians.

2. The legislature authorized the trustees of the university to expand the medical school to a four-year school and construct a teaching hospital but appropriated no funding, with the intention that this was to be requested from the 1947 session. An amendment to this section required that the North Carolina Medical Care Commission assemble a group of out-of-state experts to study the best location for the expanded school and hospital as well as the need for an expanded school.

3. A sum of $50,000 was appropriated for the next biennium for loans to medical students who would practice in rural areas.

The North Carolina Medical Care Commission and the Sanger Report

The Medical Care Commission came into being in July 1945, replacing the ad hoc Hospital and Medical Care Commission appointed by Governor Broughton in February 1944. The new commission had twenty members appointed by the governor. The state health officer and the state commissioner of public welfare served as ex officio members. Many of those appointed to the commission had served on the earlier Poe Commission. James H. Clark of Elizabethtown was elected chair,[54] and Clarence Poe was elected vice chair (see Appendix H). The state appropriation also provided for an executive secretary and other support staff. Later additions to the staff included field representatives to conduct hospital surveys, hospital administrators, and hospital architects and engineers, who were to be involved in approving construction projects partially funded by the state through the commission.

Although the 1945 legislature did not appropriate funds for hospital construction throughout the state, they did instruct the commission to do a county-by-county survey of the state "to determine the need for some kind of state aid for construction and enlargement of local hospitals to insure adequate hospital facilities for all sections of the state." The act further authorized the commission to establish and administer a statewide plan to use the proposed federal funding for construction of hospitals and other health care facilities. North Carolina was thus well prepared to make good and prompt use of the federal funds that did become available through the Hill-Burton Act in 1947.[55]

One North Carolina layman, who had been a member of the UNC board of trustees and an active supporter of the medical school expansion, observed two decades later, "The creation of the Medical Care Commission in the area of good health takes equal rank in importance with the creation of the State Highway Commission in the area of good roads."[56]

The Sanger Report

One of the first acts of the new commission was to engage outside consultants as required by the legislative act. Officially known as the National Committee for the Medical School Survey, its report came to be known as the "Sanger Report" after its chairman, William T. Sanger, PhD, president of the Medical College of Virginia in Richmond. The committee of seven members spent more than six months reviewing the work done by the Hospital and Medical Care (Poe) Commission, interviewing various state leaders, and surveying various proposed sites for the new teaching hospital and the expanded medical school.

A total of eight North Carolina towns and cities—Asheville, Charlotte, Elizabeth City, Gastonia, Greensboro, Raleigh, Salisbury, and Wilson—petitioned the National Committee for consideration as the location of the proposed teaching hospital and expanded medical school instead of Chapel Hill.[57] Some, such as Greensboro, prepared bound volumes of letters, maps, and other documents supporting their superiority as the site for the state's new medical center.[58]

An editorial in the *Durham Morning Herald* in March 1946 was entitled "Chapel Hill Has Competition for Medical School" but concluded:

> Ever since the expansion was first intimated, *The Herald* has contended that Chapel Hill is the proper site for the hospital and school. There the coordinated institution would have the advantage of accumulated facilities of the University; it would be located in a strategic medical center of the State; it would be easily accessible to all parts of the State; and it would enjoy a nonpartisan administration that some fear might be serious [*sic*] if its location becomes a political football.
>
> ... Until [the committee's] report is made public there is little basic justification for having a lot more to say about it. But we keep right on hoping, sincerely and unselfishly, that the location will be Chapel Hill.[59]

During the spring of 1946 the national committee did visit and inspect possible sites for the new teaching hospital in Charlotte, Greensboro, and Raleigh. It also visited the Chapel Hill campus and held discussions with University officials.

Five of the seven members of the committee filed a majority report on July 1, 1946, agreeing with the recommendations of the Poe Commission that the medical school be expanded and a teaching hospital built in Chapel Hill (see Appendix I). The committee added two provisions that were to guide Berryhill and future deans in the years to come:

> That such a school of medicine and associated services of the medical center, responsive to the will of the people, be integrated effectively and continuously with a State-wide network of hospitals and health centers in so far as these volunteer to cooperate; merely to expand the two-year medical school at Chapel Hill in order to graduate a greater number of physicians is not regarded as sufficient justification for such expansion ...
>
> That the University of North Carolina develop a philosophy of medical education, research, and medical care which will make it a service facility for the whole State.[60]

Two members of the survey committee (one formerly with the Duke Endowment and the other a staff physician from the American Medical Association, an organization that had recently been charged in federal courts with restraint of trade as a result of its efforts to control the supply of new physicians in the United States) filed a minority report strongly disagreeing with the majority opinion that an expanded medical school was needed and that it should be on the university campus in Chapel Hill (see Appendix J): "There is no evidence to support the conclusion that another school as such would add a single physician to the number now practicing in the State." (In fact, in 2000—almost fifty years after the expanded school opened—some 3,500 physicians who graduated from the UNC medical school and/or had their residency training at Chapel Hill or in the affiliated AHEC hospitals were in the practice of medicine in North Carolina.[61] This figure does not include those who were no longer in practice owing to their retirement or death, nor does it include the thousands of allied health professionals, dentists, nurses, pharmacists, PhD biomedical scientists, or public health physicians educated at the UNC medical center during the past half century.) Furthermore, they questioned the need for more physicians: "The nation's existing medical schools, including the two in North Carolina, will provide [the state] with all the physicians, dentists, nurses, public health officers and other health personnel it needs."[62]

Paul Whitaker, chairman of the Committee on Medical School Expansion of the Medical Care Commission, had this to say about the minority report:

> The minority report has completely disregarded the exhaustive studies submitted by the Poe Commission which show clearly the shortage of not only doctors, but trained personnel in public health fields, in sanitary engineering, in nursing, in hospital administration, in medical technology, in dietetics, and in all other personnel ancillary to medical and hospital service. The conception of the expanded medical school as set forth by these two gentlemen is to graduate more doctors, period.
>
> The complete lack of comprehension and imagination which characterizes this minority report is no more strikingly illustrated than in the sentence, "The comprehensive educational and service program recommended in this [the majority] report has not been attempted in all its details anywhere in the world." The implication is that since that is true it should not be attempted. The standpat attitude of the American Medical Association on all progressive issues regarding medical care is a matter of history. The same attitude prevailed toward hospital insurance and prepaid medical care insurance when these measures were first proposed.[63]

Although some newspapers lamented the fact that their city was not recommended as the site of the new state medical center, most accepted and supported the majority recommendation of the Sanger Report about the location of the teaching hospital in Chapel Hill. The *Durham Sun,* in an editorial entitled "Where It Belongs," observed:

> The medical school and hospital belong in Chapel Hill because there the liberal arts school of the Greater University is established. Apart from the facts that Chapel Hill provides a beautiful setting with ample room for growth and expansion, that it is centrally located for North Carolinians, that it is next door to the great medical center at Duke University and to the Veterans

Hospital soon to be erected, *it will complement the present university in Chapel Hill and the university will complement it.*[64] (Emphasis in original.)

The *Wilson Times* editorialized:

Since Chapel Hill is the center of learning for the commonwealth of North Carolina, it seems most fitting that to the other aggregation of facilities for the dispensation of knowledge, we should also add facilities for the care and treatment of the body as well as the mind . . . One of the nice things about the enterprise is that it makes the University a complete entity for the instruction and care of our people, and will give those aspiring to be adept in the . . . care of human mind and body that sort of care and training that will complete the facilities that our State is so proud of and boasts about, that makes North Carolina a great and complete state in every line or calling.[65]

The *Asheville Citizen* chastised the *Charlotte Observer* for its "vehement" eruption in opposition to the Sanger Report, which the *Observer* called "virtually an absurdity."[66] The *Citizen* correctly predicted that the controversy over the expansion of the medical school would not end with the national committee's report.[67]

The North Carolina Medical Care Commission held a meeting in Raleigh on August 7, 1946, to discuss a report from a subcommittee chaired by Whitaker recommending that the commission accept the majority report of the Sanger Committee. They also heard a statement from five past presidents of the state medical society endorsing the national committee's majority report. Following a long and heated discussion by proponents and opponents, the commission approved the majority Sanger Report by a vote of thirteen (several with qualifications) to four. The commission added a recommendation that the expansion of the medical school at Chapel Hill "be timed in relation to the program of construction and expansion of the hospitals and health centers throughout the State to effect the coordinated advancement of the total State-wide health-service project of North Carolina."[68] The commission then forwarded to Governor Cherry and the 1947 General Assembly their recommendations, along with a budget request for $5.29 million to establish the new medical center at Chapel Hill.

THE NORTH CAROLINA GOOD HEALTH ASSOCIATION

As the findings and recommendations of the Poe Commission, the Sanger Report, and the North Carolina Medical Care Commission worked their way through the various steps toward receiving final legislative approval and appropriations for the ambitious program to better the health of all North Carolinians, many concerned state leaders recognized the need for a broad campaign to inform the public of the state's needs and to influence the actions of the 1947 General

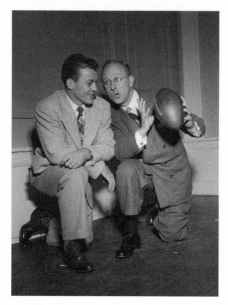

Bandleader Kay Kyser (with football) enlisting the support of UNC football legend Charlie "Choo-Choo" Justice for the Good Health campaign. *(NCC)*

Assembly. The campaign would draw parallels to the state's Good Schools Program, begun in the early 1900s, and the Good Roads Program, begun in the 1920s.

Some 200 of the state's leaders, representing many groups, met in Thomasville on March 14, 1946, at the invitation of I. G. Greer, superintendent of the Baptist Orphanage in Thomasville, to organize the North Carolina Good Health Association to provide publicity for a broad-based good health program for all North Carolinians. Greer was elected president, and regional chairmen were appointed for the west, piedmont, northeast, and southeast. Within a short time more than 1,500 citizens representing a wide range of individuals and organizations in the state had signed the association's charter, which had been adopted unanimously at the first meeting.

Although some progress was made in its first few months, the Good Health campaign took off when Kay Kyser, a native of Rocky Mount and UNC alumnus who was a nationally known bandleader and star of radio and film, got involved. In presentations to the Good Health Association and others, Kyser made an "impassioned appeal" to "build a bonfire at the grass roots. We must merchandise health to the people, and we must employ the same technique of a large manufacturer in marketing a new product." He pointed out that "the smart industrialist knows it's smart business to keep his workers healthy. So does the farmer. Our State is too poor to stay unhealthy."[69]

Kyser enlisted his colleagues in the entertainment industry to help with the Good Health campaign. Notable was a song entitled "It's All Up to You (to Make North Carolina No. 1 in Good Health)." The legendary team of Sammy Cahn and Jule Styne (who had written "I'll Walk Alone," "Let It Snow," and many other popular songs of the day) composed the words and music. Twenty thousand copies of the sheet music were distributed free throughout the state, and a recording featuring the Kay Kyser Orchestra with vocals by the young singing stars Frank Sinatra and Dinah Shore filled the state's airwaves. The Columbia Recording Corporation provided 10,000 free records, which were distributed by North Carolina's forty-eight radio stations to their listeners. The catchy words made it clear to the listeners that "it's all up to you" to "preach the Good Health view" so that "we will be the state where the weak grow strong and the strong grow great." According to the *Raleigh News and Observer* in February 1947, the song "was sung by hundreds of thousands of teen and pre-teen age voices last week during Good Health Week in the public schools. 'It's All Up to You' today

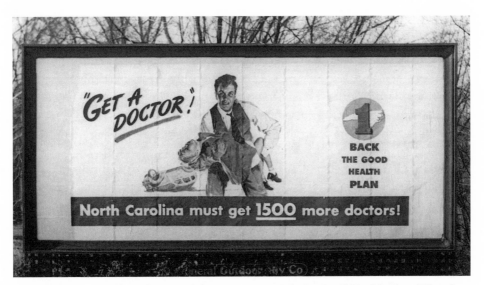

One of numerous billboards around the state supporting the Good Health Plan. (*Chapel Hill Herald*)

is basking in state favor second only to the nutty novelty smash, 'Open the Door, Richard.'"[70]

The results of this Good Health campaign were vividly described in Frank Porter Graham's dedicatory address at the medical center in Chapel Hill in 1953:

> The people's movement rolled on in gathering power from the mountains to the sea. Petitions by the people from all parts of the state, mass meetings of people, the uprisings of communities, columns of news and editorials of support east and west, signboards along all the highways told in facts and figures the needs of the people for doctors, nurses and hospitals here and now.[71]

THE HILL-BURTON ACT

An essential part of fulfilling the dream of the Good Health Program for North Carolina was the parallel development on the national scene of a program for federal funding of construction and renovation of hospitals and other health care facilities. This legislation, called "The Hospital Survey and Construction Act," was enacted on August 13, 1946. It is generally known as the Hill-Burton Act after its co-sponsors, Senator Lister Hill (D-Alabama) and Senator Harold Burton (R-Ohio). The success of North Carolina's Good Health Program hinged on the passage of the federal program, and North Carolinians played a significant role in its successful enactment and eventual funding in 1947.

UNC President Graham took a gamble in 1947 by agreeing that the state's funding of the comprehensive health plan be contingent upon the federal government's payment of at least one-third of the cost of the construction. This was based on his knowledge of the Hill-Burton Act, the funding of which was working its way through Congress at the time. Josephus Daniels, however, had warned him of the dangers to this bill in the House. As it turned out, both the federal and the state plans came close to being shot down over the question of the formula for the federal matching funds, which originally was to be one federal dollar for every local and state dollar.

Graham, who as chairman of the President's National Advisory Committee on Social Security had come to know Lister Hill, said that Hill called one evening and asked him to fly to Washington to help mediate a dispute between two North Carolina representatives that could have killed funding for the Hill-Burton Bill (which had already been passed by the Senate). Graham arrived the next day, was briefed by Hill, and met with each of the congressmen. A compromise acceptable to both the Senate and House was eventually devised: the federal government's share of the construction costs was to be one-third, and the local and state governments' share would be two-thirds. Shortly afterward Hill sent Graham a letter thanking him for his efforts to save the hospital construction bill.[72] Graham later observed that Representative Bayard Clark of Fayetteville, through his strong support of the bill in committee and on the floor of the House, helped achieve "a decisive victory" that saved both "the Hill-Burton Bill and the North Carolina Medical Care and Hospital Program."[73]

POLITICAL DEBATE AND DECISIONS

Governor R. Gregg Cherry, in a Christmas radio message to the people of North Carolina on December 25, 1946, set the stage for the crucial political decisions about health care that were soon to be made by the 1947 General Assembly:

> Our state, as you know, is devoting much attention to this whole question of better health. The North Carolina State Medical Care Commission, after months of careful study, has formulated a Good Health Plan. The plan will be presented to the General Assembly, which convenes next month. We need not wait until then, however, to say that North Carolina will be a better state because of the unselfish time and energy expended by members of the State Medical Care Commission in formulating the Good Health Plan and because of the efforts and work of the Good Health Association in acquainting the people with that plan. I do not believe there is another state in the union which today is more health conscious than North Carolina . . . History shows that once the people of North Carolina know the facts in connection with any state-wide problem, action is bound to follow . . . And so, on this Christmas Day, 1946, all of us can rejoice that we in North Carolina have, in a measure at least, humbly caught the spirit of the Great Healer, Jesus Christ, who said, "I have come that ye might have life and have it more abundantly."[74]

Berryhill later observed that "no one who was present in the packed and overflowing chamber of House of Representatives on February 13, 1947, will ever forget the drama which took place" in this public hearing before the Joint Appropriations Committee concerning the funding of the North Carolina Good Health Plan. A large group of prominent citizens from around the state appeared to support the request for a total of $48 million—less than half of it from state appropriations—to be spent during the next five years to improve the health of North Carolinians. Those speaking in opposition to some or all of the program included, among others, Rankin of the Duke Endowment and a member of the North Carolina Medical Care Commission.[75]

A member of the UNC board of trustees, who spoke in support of the program, later put the hearing in perspective:

> By this time opposition to a permanent Medical Care Commission, with authority comparable to that of the Highway Commission with respect to roads and highways, and to a three-way financing plan by state, local authorities, and the federal aid, for a system of local hospitals and health centers, had all but disappeared, leaving only the amount of the appropriation under serious debate. But this was not true of the proposed expansion of the Medical School, the construction of a training hospital, and dental and nursing schools. There were prominent and well-meaning citizens who argued that there were other and less expensive ways to produce more physicians, dentists, and nurses; that the original cost was staggering, from ten to fifteen million dollars, and the operating cost would constitute a permanent drain upon the future revenue of the State to the detriment of other essential public services. Although not vociferous, there were those in academic circles who felt that the future financial support of our orthodox education programs in the public school and institutions of higher education would be endangered.[76]

During the vigorous debate, one proponent expressed the citizenry's admiration and appreciation of the state for the work of the Duke Endowment, but added, "No individual and no organization had—or should have—the power to tell the state of North Carolina what it should or should not do for the education or medical care of its citizens."[77] In response to an opponent's statement that the AMA had said no more doctors were needed, he said he wasn't aware of this study but that he did know the AMA had just been convicted in federal court for being a monopoly. He said all you had to do was just ask the people of the state whether there were enough doctors; they would tell you there weren't.

The proponents' arguments won the day. On March 18, 1947, the Joint Appropriations Committee approved without further debate the appropriations for expansion of the medical school and construction of a teaching hospital at Chapel Hill. Governor Cherry's belated support of the full program and Graham's willingness to make state appropriations contingent on federal funding were both thought to have been critical in winning the legislature's final approval.[78] Once the funding for the federal Hill-Burton Act was passed by Congress later in 1947, the recommendations of the 1945 Poe Commission could finally begin to be implemented.

THE MOSES CONE HOSPITAL PROPOSAL

On June 8, 1947, Bertha Lindau Cone died at Blowing Rock, making available the endowment she had established in 1911 for a hospital to be built in Greensboro as a memorial to her husband, Moses H. Cone. By this time the endowment was estimated to be worth $15 million, with a significant annual income. Shortly thereafter, at the request of the Moses Cone trustees, Governor Cherry appointed a committee of university trustees to work with a committee of Moses Cone trustees "for the purpose of exploring all possible methods of cooperation between the Cone Hospital and the University Medical School."

Although Dean Berryhill and most faculty members would have much preferred that the expanded school and teaching hospital be located in Chapel Hill—especially once this issue had finally been resolved by the action of the legislature—they were also well aware of the unique nature of this offer and of the continuing negative feedback that the university had received from turning down "the offer from the Gray family" in the late 1930s to support the expanded medical school and teaching hospital if it were built in Winston-Salem. The Moses Cone proposal was different: the Cone Endowment was very much larger, and a branch of the Consolidated University existed in Greensboro. Because the legislature might be reluctant to appropriate operating funds for the new medical school if the university were again perceived as having arbitrarily turned down a generous offer of private monies, Berryhill was very sensitive to the need for a through study of the Cone proposal. As a result, he made a point of recording the Moses Cone negotiations in detail in his annual report for 1947.[79]

After some delay, the university and the Cone committees had their first joint meeting in August 1947 at the O. Henry Hotel in Greensboro. Neither side had a definite proposal or any advance information. Toward the end of the day, UNC Controller William Carmichael, Jr., and Dean Berryhill were invited to join the discussions. To them, "it was obvious that much ill will had been engendered and the university trustees were attempting to have the Cone trustees to agree that nothing feasible could be worked out, which the latter group was loathe [sic] to do. A public announcement was made, however, that it did not seem feasible to work out a merger of the two institutions." The newspapers immediately responded with criticism of the university for turning down a $15 million endowment and a hospital.

When a proposed merger of the two hospitals was rejected after only one meeting, Carmichael and Berryhill were surprised and concerned that history was repeating itself. They went to Governor Cherry and to a representative from the Cone trustees to request a continuation of the discussions. Later in August the governor called a meeting saying that "he felt the situation had not been sufficiently studied. " He elaborated "that this was of great importance because if the idea got around the University was turning down endowment[s], it would be hard to get adequate maintenance funds in the legislature, that rumor still persisted that the University might have had the Gray-Reynolds money, and finally that if a merger could be worked and the State funds could be joined with the endowment income, he could visualize the greatest medical institution in the South."

The governor then appointed a subcommittee of the university trustees to work with the Cone trustees, make a thorough study of a possible merger, and report their findings to him and the full board of trustees. He asked the state's attorney general and Dean Berryhill to serve as advisory members of the trustees' subcommittee.

The university subcommittee worked for several months, meeting with the Moses Cone committee and with the executive director of the Moses Cone Foundation. The Moses Cone trustees prepared a specific offer that included deeding twenty-five acres of land (out of the sixty-seven acres granted to the Moses Cone Hospital by Bertha Cone's trust) to the university for a university hospital of no fewer than 300 beds that would be adjacent to a similarly sized hospital on the Cone property, and making available $100,000 annually for ten years from the Cone Endowment to support the operation of the joint hospitals along with an additional allocation based on the number of indigent patients from Guilford County admitted to the joint 600-bed hospital. Furthermore, the university would be financially responsible for the operation of the joint hospitals; a joint board would operate both hospitals; the university would appoint the teaching staff, with the joint board appointing the attending physicians from the local community; and the joint hospital would be called the Moses H. Cone Memorial Hospital, in keeping with Bertha Cone's bequest. At the end of ten years, either institution could give notice and the agreement would be terminated two years later; each hospital would then operate independently.

This proposal was discussed by the representatives from the Moses Cone trustees and by the executive committee of the university trustees in a meeting in the governor's office on December 10, 1947. They reached the "unanimous conclusion that the purposes and objectives of the two institutions could not be reconciled [by a merger] . . . and issued a joint statement to that effect."[80] According to one participant, who was both a university and a Moses Cone trustee, "The conclusion reached was both honorable and amicable and received wide publicity throughout the State."[81]

Berryhill was pleased that the issue had been thoroughly explored and that both sides (and the public) realized that Bertha Cone's mandate for a hospital to serve the people of Guilford County and the state's commitment to a teaching hospital to serve all the people of North Carolina were irreconcilable in a joint-operated facility. On the one hand, violation of the Cone trust "could result in forfeiture of the entire trust in favor of certain other beneficiaries" outside North Carolina. On the other hand, because the university would have ultimate financial responsibility for both hospitals (with the aid to be given by the Cone Foundation), the legislature would undoubtedly have difficulty supporting a hospital that could be perceived as primarily benefiting only 1 of the state's 100 counties.[82]

Berryhill's experience with this proposed merger is reflected in a 1950 presentation at a national conference on medical education where he forcefully advocated locating a medical school on a university campus. He cited the experience in North Carolina, where the university could not "secure that control of any hospital in the larger cities which [the university trustees] deemed essential to assure a sound teaching program. Many existing hospitals offered their facilities to the university 'as far as practicable,' but this did not seem a sufficient guarantee in perpetuity of a workable arrangement." He noted that "University standards are more easily maintained and the medical school enjoys more freedom from 'pressure groups'—medical and other—when it remains physically a part of the parent institution." He quoted a prominent medical educator who had addressed this issue in a 1945 report about the proposed University of Missouri medical school: "I know of no medical school in a large city which, within my memory, has not had at least one serious quarrel between the university and the powerful and privileged professional leaders in the city. Unless your university medical leaders are resigned to offering teaching positions in return for support and collaboration of clinicians with few other claims to attention, they may [as] well prepare themselves for a decade of pressures and political maneuvers. Usually if appointment[s] are made quid pro quo and at a distance from the university the character of the school depends on forces only slightly under its control."[83] (See Appendix K.)

Berryhill did conclude his report of the Moses Cone–UNC discussions with the prediction that "this end of negotiations we hope does not preclude close professional cooperation in the future between the two hospitals and an arrangement which would aid in both undergraduate and graduate training between the Cone and University hospitals." He was able to make this prediction come true almost two decades later when he became director of the Division of Education and Research in Community Medical Care after his retirement as dean.

AN OVERVIEW OF 1947

Berryhill's annual report as dean to Chancellor House captured the excitement of the events of 1947 as well as the tremendous challenges he, the medical school, and the university faced in achieving the ambitious goals they had proposed for the coming years:

> The year just ended has been perhaps the most significant in the fifty-seven years of the School's history. At long last the State appropriated funds for the establishment of a 400-bed teaching hospital, authorized the University Trustees to expand into a four-year school, and this apparently secured the future development of the institution. This is the first step in the realization of the hopes and dreams of the medical faculty and alumni over the last fifty years.
>
> At the same time it immediately brings the University face to face with many tremendous and serious problems for the next decade. This venture into complete professional education in medicine to be successful and to accomplish the ends desired in the State must be carefully planned and adequately financed.[84]

With the location of the expanded medical school and the teaching hospital finally assured and the funding for their construction appropriated, Berryhill could now focus his attention on organizational issues, planning and construction, and recruitment of those who would lead and staff the medical school clinical services and the new teaching hospital.

CHAPTER 7

Building and Recruiting

The years from the legislative decisions of 1947 to when the first MDs graduated from the School of Medicine in 1954 were "among the most exciting, important and productive years in terms of tangible activities and results in the history of the School; it was also among the most trying and, in a measure, frustrating periods for many reasons," according to Berryhill writing in the late 1970s.[1] During these years he and his colleagues were responsible for planning and constructing the teaching hospital and the expanded medical school facilities as well as for the recruitment of those who would lead and staff the university's clinical endeavor. Marshaling the funds and having the administrative flexibility necessary to accomplish these goals would prove to be a constant struggle.

ORGANIZATIONAL EVOLUTION

Board of Trustees

Although University President Frank P. Graham had the ultimate responsibility for working with the university's board of trustees, Dean Berryhill worked closely with the trustees in the late 1940s and early 1950s during the legislative approval process and during the planning, construction, and recruitment phases of the medical school expansion.

Recognizing the developing momentum toward expanding the medical school and building a university hospital, President Graham in 1944 set up a four-member medical committee of university trustees chaired by Lennox P. McLendon, Sr., a UNC alumnus and an attorney from Greensboro.[2] This committee, with some changes in name and composition, provided a liaison during the next few years between the trustees and those advancing the plan for the expansion. Members of this committee were also active in representing the trustees in the negotiations in 1947 over the proposed merger of the university teaching hospital with the Moses Cone Memorial Hospital in Greensboro.

The Medical Committee (which later became the Health Affairs Committee) of the trustees was expanded by Governor Cherry in 1948 to help coordinate the planning of the new hospital and expanded school. The committee, which was chaired by McLendon until 1955 (and thereafter by Victor S. Bryant and then George Watts Hill, Sr., both of Durham), was split in 1948 into two subcommittees, one to deal with buildings, chaired by Collier Cobb, Jr., of Chapel Hill, and one to deal with policies and personnel, chaired by Bryant.[3] All of the committee members were later commended for their hard work, but Cobb was singled out for his "extraordinarily effective work as Chairman of the building committee which finally supervised the expenditure of approximately ten million dollars."[4]

Division of Health Affairs

In his first annual report to President Graham in 1940, Acting Dean Berryhill noted that the Division of Public Health (formed in 1936) had become the School of Public Health. He stated that "there is still close cooperation and coordination between the School of Medicine and the School of Public Health" and that "this of course should be still further encouraged and increased."[5]

In 1942 a Division of Medical Sciences, approved by President Graham and Chancellor House, was established in the university, with an advisory board chaired by the dean of the medical school and composed of three representatives each from the Schools of Medicine and Public Health, one from the University Health Service, and one from the Orange County Health Department.[6] (The School of Pharmacy, which then still occupied a building on the main campus some distance from the medical and public health schools and the future medical center, was not represented.) The goal was to coordinate the teaching and research activities of the various units and to assist in future planning for the Division and its components. However, Berryhill, in his annual report to Graham in December 1943, expressed frustration over the difficulty he was having "in accomplishing the purposes which you and Dean House had in mind in the organization of the Division of Medical Sciences" owing to the fact that the representatives of the School of Public Health (with the exception of Professor Baity) "resented the formation of this advisory board and of the Division" and had "no disposition . . . to discuss with other medical representatives of the University problems that concern the organization as a whole." He added, "This is most regrettable in the light of our opportunities here in the state and in the Southeast and particularly in relation to what we hope one day to accomplish."[7] Berryhill later reported, "After a few frustrating years the Division of Medical Sciences as an organization was dissolved."

The origins of the Division of Health Affairs and the reasons behind its successes and failures have been debated in medical school circles for some time. According to Berryhill's account written in the late 1970s:

> Despite written statements by an uninformed few, and the general impression of many within and without the university, the much discussed Division . . . was not initiated by the report of the National Committee on the Medical

School (the Sanger Report) of 1946 nor by the university administration of that period. President Graham, Chancellor House, and Controller Carmichael were initially lukewarm—if not actually opposed—to the proposal for forming such an administrative structure in the university. In retrospect it can be seen that their reasoning and judgment were sound . . . The idea and early formation of this organization [were] urged by the dean of the medical school [Berryhill] for the following reasons. After the 1949 General Assembly had created a School of Dentistry, the problems of planning the hospital structure, recruiting clinical faculty, and administering the two-year school—together with understandable pressures from the nursing and dental groups for immediate action in selecting deans for these schools—became too arduous for one person. At that period there were no funds available for the employment of assistant or associate deans in the medical school who could have assumed some of the responsibilities.

Berryhill cited as models similar administrative structures that had been set up at other well-known medical centers at that time but added that several were later abandoned. He stated that the deans of the Schools of Public Health and Pharmacy could accept such an arrangement, but "senior members of the medical school faculty were strongly opposed because they feared such an administrative structure would handicap the development of the school. Later these fears were proven to be well founded."[8]

John B. Graham, MD, a 1940 graduate of the two-year school and later professor of pathology and an associate dean, wrote in 1984 about Berryhill and the Division: "The position [of administrator of the Division] was offered first to Dr. Berryhill. After consideration, he declined, arguing that organizing the medical school properly was as much as he could handle, besides he knew nothing about the methods and standards of the other disciplines." Graham said he had to share some of the blame in this regard: he and Berryhill discussed his pending decision on a trip to an AAMC meeting in Colorado in 1949, but "I was not experienced enough at age 31 to advise him wisely." Graham believed in retrospect that Berryhill's decision "was probably a mistake. [Berryhill's] two major contributions—the successful political campaign and the recruitment of the clinical chairmen—had been largely completed by 1950, and as time has shown, the job of Administrator of Health Affairs is largely ceremonial." (In fact, because of funding delays the recruitment of the clinical chairs did not begin until 1951 and were not completed until the summer of 1952.) Graham continued, "He could probably have melded this position with the deanship and managed both, thereby avoiding the troubles to which his declination was to lead." Graham supported this assertion by citing the fact that "Christopher Fordham held both positions successfully 3 decades later when the demands of administration were much greater."[9] (Since that time the span of responsibility of the dean of the medical school has continued to expand, so that by 1998 the dean of the UNC medical school also served as vice chancellor for medical affairs and CEO of the UNC Health Care System. See Appendix M.)

In the spring of 1949 the university administration and the trustees approved the recommendation of a committee chaired by Berryhill that a Division of Medical Sciences and Services be formed to "effectively administer and correlate the work of the Schools of Medicine, Public Health, Dentistry, Nursing, and Pharmacy and the Hospital Division and to integrate their educational and research and service activities with the health needs and progress of the State."[10] The committee recommended that the full-time director of the Division have the title of vice chancellor, which would have been the only such position on the campus at that time. The first permanent director of the Division later stated that he reluctantly agreed to the change of title to administrator because the university leaders "wanted to avoid taking a step which would lead to a proliferation of Vice Chancellors in the University."[11] The five deans of the health sciences schools and the hospital director would be co-equals reporting to the administrator.

The new Division came into being in the spring of 1949 with Dean Edward G. McGavran of the School of Public Health as the acting administrator. Henry Toole Clark, Jr., MD, assumed the duties as the first administrator of the Division on June 1, 1950. A native of Scotland Neck, North Carolina, Clark was an undergraduate at UNC in the class of 1937 and completed two years of medical school at UNC in 1939. He received the MD from the University of Rochester in 1944 after a three-year interruption as he recuperated at the Trudeau Sanatorium from tuberculosis he had contacted from an indigent patient when he was a third-year student. He then took a year in pathology at Rochester under George Whipple, MD, the Nobel laureate and medical school dean, who advised him to consider a career in "administrative medicine," presumably for health reasons. Following an internship in medicine at Duke in 1945–1946, he was the assistant director of Strong Memorial Hospital, the teaching hospital of the University of Rochester, from 1946 to 1948. Before returning to Chapel Hill he was the director of the Vanderbilt University Hospital from 1948 to 1950.[12]

Clark served in this position until July 1965, when a new chancellor, Paul Sharp, reorganized the chancellor's office and eliminated Clark's position and the dean of the faculty, replacing them by a single vice chancellor for the university. During 1965–1966, Clark was on a sabbatical leave from the university, serving as an advisor to the director of the National Institutes of Health (NIH) on the implementation of the proposed Regional Medical Programs legislation and then as a consultant to help plan a large central university hospital for the University of Leiden in the Netherlands. Clark left UNC the end of September of 1966 to take a position as director of the Connecticut Regional Medical Program and to become a faculty member at both the Yale and University of Connecticut medical schools.[13] Chancellor Sharp was soon replaced by Chancellor Carlyle Sitterson, who established a new position as vice chancellor for health sciences

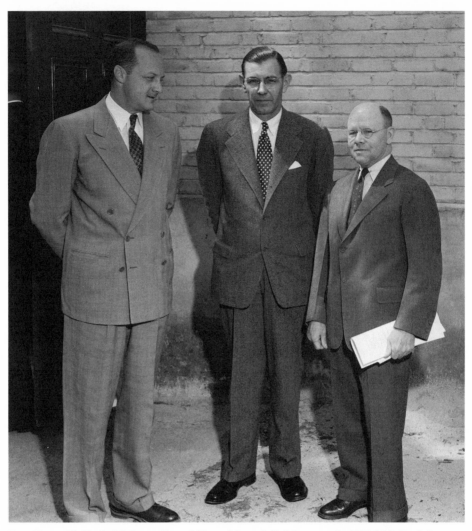

Drs. Henry T. Clark, W. Reece Berryhill, and Joseph T. Wearn at the UNC Medical Center dedication ceremonies, 1953. Wearn, dean of the Western Reserve University School of Medicine, delivered the opening address. *(UNC Photo Lab, NCC)*

and in 1966 appointed Arden Miller, MD, to fill it. Miller, a former dean of the University of Kansas School of Medicine and a pediatrician with an appointment in the Department of Maternal and Child Health at the UNC School of Public Health, served until 1970.[14]

Clark much later recalled in an oral history interview that he was first asked to come to Chapel Hill in 1949 to consider becoming the director of North Carolina Memorial Hospital after Berryhill had received some strong recommendations about Clark's work with the Vanderbilt Hospital. He recalled that Dean Berryhill and his wife "were very cordial hosts for Blanche and me during that visit. I declined an invitation to take that position because I felt I had an obligation to Vanderbilt to solve some of their major hospital problems before moving on." He added that Berryhill "was a prime advocate for the creation of the Division of Health Affairs at UNC. I think he [then] actively supported the choice of me as its Administrator in the absence of other promising candidates."[15]

Although Clark had had relatively few interactions with Berryhill when he was a medical student at UNC in 1937–1939, he stated that "my relationship [as Administrator of the Division] with Reece [Berryhill] was somewhat strained from the start. Reece was seventeen years older than I and I had the feeling that he approached our beginning relationship as one of professor to student." Not long after he arrived at UNC, in the summer of 1950, Clark had a conversation in Chancellor House's office about an issue with Berryhill. He said that House then "reflected on the process of [Clark's] selection as Administrator of the Division . . . saying that Reece had first been asked to take the job and he [House] had actually, at one critical point, telephoned Reece at 6:00 AM one morning to urge him to do so with the admonition that Reece would never be satisfied with anyone who was placed over him."[16]

Clark much later commented on Berryhill's "commanding personality, strong qualities of leadership and strong personal convictions, mostly along quite conservative lines. He was an indefatigable worker. . . . He put a high value on loyalty and rewarded those who supported his views. . . . His central mission in life was to establish an outstanding School of Medicine. . . . I was soon to learn that his models were Harvard and Western Reserve, where he had trained, rather than the brave new world of the Sanger report. Reece was also an astute politician with an extensive 'Old Boy' network of physicians and lay leaders around North Carolina."[17]

In the same interview, Clark said he soon realized "that there was also a serious 'down side' to Reece. He was obsessed by his conviction of the primacy of medicine as an academic discipline and was openly disdainful of the other Health Affairs schools as lesser sciences. This produced strained personal and professional relationships in the University 'family.'" Clark was also distressed that Berryhill would go outside regular university channels to accomplish his goals. While "this made him a hero to his inner circle of Medical School supporters," Clark saw it as "an affront to me and the Chancellor and President, and I was dismayed that the top administration made so little effort to discourage this type of activity."[18] Others who knew him, though, saw Berryhill as a clear-sighted leader who would not let academic politics get in the way of fulfilling his vision.

After Clark and the deans for the new Schools of Dentistry (John C. Brauer, DDS) and Nursing (Elizabeth L. Kemble, RN, PhD) had been appointed, the nonmedical deans successfully mounted an effort to remove "Medical" from the Division's name and rename it the Division of Health Affairs, according to Berryhill. Clark recalled years later that "Billy Carmichael [the university comptroller] was persuasive in advocating 'Division of Health Affairs,' saying 'Health Affairs' had a positive, happy ring, like 'Love Affairs,' and that it was a broad term which covered Public Health, Nursing, Dentistry, and Pharmacy in addition to Medicine."[19]

Berryhill later lamented, "From that time, 1950, the battle was joined." The medical school, which contributed to the teaching of students in the other schools and which had the largest budget, faculty, and research grants, was "in fact a minority member of this coalition" in a situation where the other four deans, the hospital director, and the Division administrator could easily outvote the dean of the medical school.[20]

In the first annual report in 1950 for the Division, Clark described it "as a fiscal unit of the University [functioning] administratively from the Deans and the [Hospital] Director of the six units through the Administrator to the Chancellor." He listed a number of reasons for the creation of the Division: the advantage of having "one overall administrative organization" for the closely related health sciences programs and the hospital; the savings in having a central faculty to teach subjects that are needed in several schools (for example, the anatomy and pathology courses for dental and nursing students were to be taught by medical school faculty members rather than duplicating these departments in the other health science schools); the physical closeness of the buildings; the development of teamwork among future members of community health care teams through their "living and working and playing together"; and the "great stimulus to research which will come from the fact that all branches of the health sciences are represented in a concentrated area." He observed, "There are few complete medical centers in the world of the type envisioned for the University of North Carolina."

Clark extolled the benefits of the Division to the people of North Carolina:

1. "The foremost contribution . . . will be the training of men and women in all of the primary fields of health services and in many additional specialized fields to be our community health leaders."

2. " . . . An expanded program of post-graduate instruction to keep our graduates abreast of current advances . . . through refresher courses [at Chapel Hill] . . . and in the various counties of the state through extension courses."

3. A gradual increase in consultative services to the people of the state along the lines of the "consultation services rendered to county health departments . . . by men in our School of Public Health." In the future "many of the new hospitals being constructed in North Carolina will get help in the form of interns and residents rotating from the University Hospital, part-time services of . . . [various medical specialists] and the consultation services of a trained hospital administrator and his assistants."

4. "Individuals with medical or dental problems which are too difficult to be handled at the community level will have ready access to the best of treatment facilities at the University."

5. "In a broad sense the Division . . . will take the lead in teaching the people of our State what to expect and what to demand of a good health program. This will be done by means of a positive general public relations program . . . and by laying stress in our University training programs on the future civic responsibilities of our trainees. The latter is sadly neglected in many health training centers today. In this educational process emphasis will be placed on prevention as well as cure."[21]

In his annual report for 1950–1951, dated June 12, 1951, Berryhill was not so sanguine about the benefits of the Division—especially in regard to the medical school. He began:

Admittedly, it may be unfair to pass judgment on the administration of the Division of Health Affairs after eighteen months of operation; nevertheless, the patterns that are being set and the policies and procedures that are evolving are so disturbing that this could not be an honest chronicling of the events of the year without regretfully calling your attention to certain factors that seriously disturb the medical faculty and administration. Furthermore, these developments have disturbed representatives of the Council on Medical Education and Hospitals of the American Medical Association and of the Association of American Medical Colleges.

Berryhill said this situation was also affecting recruitment and cited the fact that one outstanding prospect for the chair of medicine turned down an offer because of "the potential danger to the School of Medicine in the administration of the Division." He admitted:

The Administration of the Medical School [that is, Berryhill] was primarily responsible for providing the impetus for the creation of the Division. The value of such an administrative organization had it followed the plan originally visualized seemed clear. It was an attempt to coordinate the teaching, research, and service activities of a group of professional schools with somewhat related interests, and those of the University Hospital which is primarily linked with the School of Medicine . . . It was hoped, too, that a full-time administrative officer of wide educational experience and vision could aid the heads of the several units involved in expediting solutions for some of their problems [while] it was intended that the several schools should have a great deal of freedom and autonomy within the University framework . . . and enjoy some budgetary discretion once the annual funds for a particular

School had been determined . . . The attainment of these hoped for objectives . . . [now] seems improbable. The position of the Medical School in the Division is particularly vulnerable and insecure. This unit will represent the largest instructional and research budget and staff, upon the adequacy and competency, even eminence, of which depends the quality of medical care and teaching the institution offers and therefore the extent of its services to the State and its national reputation. And yet in determining policies vital to its own development it has on the Division Board just one vote out of eight—the same as the smallest unit.[22]

In the annual report for 1953–1954, Berryhill reiterated that the "most serious and most important" of the many problems facing the School of Medicine was the "local organization—or specifically . . . the relation of the Medical School to the Hospital and the position of the Medical School in the Division of Health Affairs." He reminded the chancellor that this issue had been noted in previous annual reports, as well as "more recently in the form of a resolution from the Executive Committee of the Medical Faculty" and in the report of the AMA/AAMC accreditation survey of the school in the fall of 1953. Berryhill argued that "the State through its General Assembly considered education and teaching as a primary objective of the hospital—not only by locating it on the university campus but by specifically designating it a 'teaching' hospital." He thus reasoned that the hospital's "wards and outpatient clinics should be looked upon as the teaching and research laboratories of the clinical departments and bear the same relationship to the School of Medicine as do the laboratories and classrooms of the basic science departments located in this [the Medical School] building."[23]

In his annual report for 1954–1955, Berryhill became philosophical about the organizational dilemmas faced by the School of Medicine. He cited the material needs for further development but said: "The greatest priority is not of a material but of a morale [sic] and spiritual nature, which—ironically enough—seems hardest to come by. Never was the Biblical statement that 'man does not live by bread alone' more true or more apropos than in this situation." He stated that "the best faculty has been selected" and "they have built wisely and soundly . . . The School has the potential to move forward. Perhaps better than at any time in the last fifty years the faculty is working as a unit . . . " He concluded, "The University and the people of the State have imposed great responsibilities upon us. If these are to be discharged, initiative should be encouraged, and that degree of authority and freedom of action commensurate with the responsibilities permitted."[24]

John Graham said that in the early days of the expanded school the administrative structure of the Division led to many frustrations among the young and eager medical school clinical faculty members, "who were very interested in advancing their careers through teaching and research. The new organizational structures forced them into frustrating and wasteful inefficiencies." They found

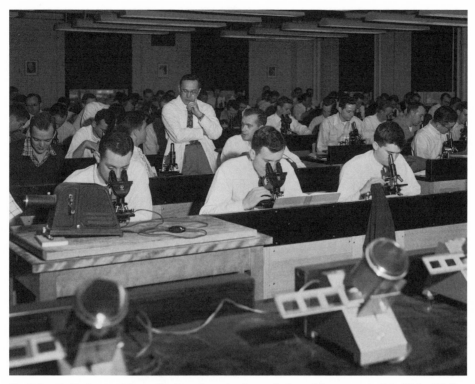

Dr. John B. Graham with medical students in the pathology laboratory in MacNider Hall, 1954. *(UNC Photo Lab, NCC)*

that they had to turn to Berryhill for some issues and to the hospital administrator for others, "and the boundaries of responsibility between the two were very hazy." According to Graham, "the conflicting goals and the strong personalities involved led" to what he called the faculty "Revolt of 1956" over the issues of Berryhill's leadership as dean, the administrative structure of the hospital, and the standing of the medical school in the Division of Health Affairs. The medical faculty in two mass meetings in March 1956 affirmed their confidence in Berryhill's leadership, called for the administrative placement of the hospital under the medical school, and expressed their concern over the Division of Health Affairs. In spite of the opposition of the Division administrator and the other health affairs deans, the university administration placed the hospital under Berryhill's direction. The reorganization of the Division to provide the School of Medicine itself with more independence and influence would have to wait.[25]

Thanks to the decision to place the operation of the hospital under the School of Medicine, Berryhill's annual report for 1955–1956 concluded in a much more optimistic mood:

This tangible evidence of confidence by the University Administration and the Trustees in the Medical Faculty has first of all vastly improved the morale and while such a change will not resolve all the major organizational

Building and Recruiting 173

problems with which the development of the School of Medicine has been plagued, it is believed to be a step in the right direction. . . . The Medical Faculty . . . is well aware of the tremendously increased responsibilities. They are prepared and indeed determined to carry out these responsibilities to the best of their abilities and judgment in response to the confidence that has been placed in them.[26]

In January 1956 the Trustees' Health Affairs Committee asked William B. Aycock, professor of law (and later chancellor of the university from 1957 to 1964), to do a study of the Division of Health Affairs and to "prepare an administrative code for the Division." The widespread frustration with the structure and function of the Division was reflected in trustee Victor Bryant's letter to Aycock after he had accepted the assignment: "I want to thank you for agreeing to undertake to help the Health Affairs Committee from the Board of Trustees. Heaven knows we need it."[27]

Aycock did a thorough study of the pertinent laws, the minutes of the trustees, the University Code, and various committee minutes and documents in the Division of Health Affairs. In a preliminary report to the Division's Advisory Committee in February, Aycock indicated that the proposed code would not deal with "internal affairs of the units in the Division," but would cover "matters affecting the entire Division . . . as an operating unit, and with interrelationships among the units." In the active discussion that followed, "Professor Aycock reasserted that only existing material would be codified—what is, not what should be," although he indicated that recommendations might be made for clarification of policy in "ill-defined areas." After widespread consultation with all those involved, Aycock submitted a report and a proposed code to Chancellor House. In June House wrote Aycock to say, "Your project of writing the Code for the Division of Health Affairs was, from my point of view, an outstanding success and I am most grateful to you for it." Berryhill sent Aycock a handwritten note: "Your forceful, knowledgeable . . . scholarly statement on the Medical School in the University was magnificent! You stimulated the interest and helped the morale of alumni, faculty, and students. For all of us—and for myself especially, I want to thank you most sincerely for your interest and your leadership."[28]

With revisions through the years to reflect changes in the practice plans and the statutory creation of the UNC Health Care System in November 1998, the Health Affairs Code has been used from the mid-1950s to the present as a guide to the operation of this complex area of the university.[29]

The concerns about the administrative structure of the university's hospital and health sciences schools were also noted in the reports of the Liaison Committee on Medical Education (LCME) on their accreditation visits to the new medical school in the 1950s and early 1960s. A survey of the two-year school was made in 1950 and "a favorable report" issued. The school was resurveyed in October of 1953, the first semester that all four medical classes were enrolled.

According to the ensuing report, "The survey team was favorably impressed by the efficient way in which the expansion to a full four year curriculum had been carried out," but the team did comment on several problems that needed attention. One concerned the observation that "there is an undercurrent of dissatisfaction in many segments of the medical school faculty, with certain aspects of the medical school administration" having "to do with the interrelationships between the dean and the director of the Division of Health Affairs." The 1953 survey recommended that the "Teaching Hospital be placed under the control of the Dean of the Medical School," and this was done in 1956.

The 1963 LCME report noted that the hospital director now reported to the dean of the medical school, as the 1953 survey had recommended. The report observed that the full-time administrator of the Division of Health Affairs, Henry T. Clark, MD, was "assisted by an Advisory Board composed of the Deans of the various professional schools concerned, the Director of the North Carolina Memorial Hospital and the Chief of Staff of the hospital. All major decisions in any school including appointments and promotions are brought before this Board for information and approval." The survey team raised questions about "the desirability of the present administrative function of the Advisory Board of the Division of Health Affairs, under which the purely internal affairs of the School of Medicine must be approved by the Deans of the other professional schools. It would seem that this [is] potentially an awkward arrangement which conceivably could cause difficulties in the future."[30]

Berryhill wrote later that the difficulties with the administrative structure of the Division were "an important factor" in his resignation as dean in 1963, which took effect on August 31, 1964. Yet, he added, "even then there were no efforts to review the structure during the year 1963–1964." This hampered the search for a new dean "because all those sought for the position were wary of the existing structure . . . Finally in 1965, *after* the new dean [I. Taylor] had been selected, Chancellor Paul F. Sharp and President William Friday agreed to certain modifications of the previous administrative structure: (1) a name change to the Division of Health Sciences; (2) abolishment of the Advisory Board of the Division to permit more freedom and independence for the individual schools, and (3) a change in title from administrator to vice chancellor for health sciences."[31]

While Dean Berryhill and many medical school faculty members continued to be frustrated during this time with having to deal with the Division and its administrative structure, the faculty and deans in the other schools viewed this administrative structure as a means of leveling the playing field for the smaller health sciences schools and programs in relation to the vast medical school–hospital complex. One of the first faculty members (now retired) of the dental school gave voice to this view when he was overheard to exclaim: "Henry Clark was our hero!"

Berryhill was so single-mindedly committed to the establishment of a first-class medical school and hospital that he could be blind to the needs of the other areas and became angry when resources went to them while he could still see major medical school and hospital needs going unmet. For instance, in his 1950–1951 annual report, Berryhill noted, "It is ironical that the [Medical] School which is fundamental to the success of the whole Division—indeed the unit to which the State Legislature and the University gave first priority—should now be the one most severely and dangerously handicapped by the encroachment of important but definitely ancillary units. Funds are being spent to extend the periphery, so to speak, while the core and the heart of the undertaking is being crippled."[32] For his uncompromising dedication to the task at hand, Berryhill is widely recognized as the founding father of the expanded medical school and of the UNC hospitals at Chapel Hill.

The organizational turmoil and reorganizations in the health sciences arena were not unique to Chapel Hill. Most academic medical centers in the nation have faced or are now facing similar problems owing to the multiple and overlapping missions and responsibilities of the various health sciences schools within ever-expanding and complex universities.

The Five Health Sciences Schools

Today the UNC hospitals and all five health sciences schools are on the university campus adjacent to each other in modern and expanding physical facilities, and they continue to develop in terms of faculty, students, clinical services, and research. Much of the unique value of this complex comes from the many formal and informal interactions between the various components of the medical center and with other university departments, schools, and programs. All five of the schools are highly ranked among their peers around the nation. They and the university have reciprocally enhanced one another's fine reputations.

The School of Medicine, the first of the health sciences schools, first opened from 1879 to 1885 and has been in continuous operation since 1890. After being located in one building on the main campus from 1912 to 1939 and another one from 1939 to 1952 on the medical campus, the School of Medicine in the early 2000s now occupies almost 2 million square feet of space in some 21 major buildings, while the UNC Hospitals occupy another 2 million square feet of space. As of 2005-06, 642 medical students were enrolled in four classes. In addition, there were 746 graduate students, 384 post-doctoral research fellows, and some 400 allied health sciences students. At end of 2005-06, the full-time faculty were 232 in the basic sciences departments and 959 in the clinical sciences departments, plus 75 in the allied health sciences department. The School of Medicine budget (excluding AHEC and the UNC Hospitals) for 2005–2006 amounted to $694 million, with 11% ($79 million) from state appropriations, 42% ($289 million) from grants, and 34% ($233 million) from clinical income.[33]

The School of Pharmacy, established at UNC in 1897, was the second health sciences school on the UNC campus and is one of the oldest in the nation. It was housed in various university buildings for a quarter of a century and then from 1925 to 1959 on the main campus in Howell Hall, which was named for Edward V. Howell, the first dean. In 1959 the school moved to the medical campus on the west side of South Columbia Street at the site of the former Chapel Hill High School, where it occupied Beard Hall, named for John Grover Beard, the dean from 1930 to 1946.[34] A major addition, Banks D. Kerr Hall, was completed in 2002 and more than doubled the school's space, to 166,000 square feet. Afterward Beard Hall underwent a major renovation. Construction started in 2005 on a Genetic Medicine Building, which will provide research space for both the medical and pharmacy schools.

As of 2005, the pharmacy school was one of only three in North Carolina and the state's only public pharmacy school. After offering the BS degree in pharmacy from 1925 to 1996, in 1996 the sole degree in pharmacy became the doctorate (PharmD). This professional degree requires a two-year pre-pharmacy course followed by a four-year program in the School of Pharmacy. The school also offers a graduate curriculum leading to the doctor of philosophy (PhD) degree in pharmaceutical sciences. The number of students in the School of Pharmacy has grown from 17 in 1897 to 468 in 1996 and 511 in 2005. In 2005 the pharmacy school had sixty full-time faculty members and an operating budget of almost $54.35 million (19 percent of which came from state funds); that same year it received $7 million in research grant support.[35]

Public health came into being at UNC in 1936 as a division in the medical school and shared space with the medical school in Caldwell Hall on the main campus.[36] When established in 1939, the UNC School of Public Health was the fourth school of public health established in the nation and the first school of public health within a state university. When MacNider Hall was opened in 1939, the School of Public Health occupied the ground floor. The space reverted to the medical school when the new School of Public Health building was completed in 1962. This building, now known as Rosenau Hall after the founding dean of the school, Milton J. Rosenau, MD, incorporated as a wing a small venereal disease research laboratory built with US Public Health Service funding in 1949.[37] Since then two major additions and renovations have more than tripled the original space available for the School of Public Health to a total of 373,000 square feet. Today it is the only such school in North Carolina and one of thirty-seven accredited public health schools in the nation. It awarded its first graduate degrees in 1940 and today awards doctoral, master's, and undergraduate degrees as well as certificates to students who take courses on campus or via the Internet as distance learners. In 1939 the public health school "consisted of five full-time faculty members, four departments and twenty-four students" and "by 1950 had grown to forty full-time faculty members, eleven departments, and one hundred forty-five full-time students who were working towards a wide variety of public health degrees."[38] In 2005 it had 213 full-time faculty and 1,648 students (including degree, certificate and distance education program students). The operating budget for fiscal year 2004–2005 was $98 million, of which 21 percent was from state funds and $68 million was from research and training grants.[39]

The 1949 General Assembly approved construction and operational funding for a new dental school, which admitted first-year students in 1950. Until the two wings of MacNider Hall were completed in 1952 and 1953 and the first dental school building was completed in 1953, the dental faculty members were housed in Miller Hall, and the student classrooms and laboratories were in two temporary Quonset huts located beside MacNider Hall.[40] The first class of thirty-four students graduated with the DDS degree in 1954. Since then other buildings and renovations have provided a dental research center and new facilities for clinical practice, research, and teaching, with a total of some 315,000 square feet by 2005.

Today the School of Dentistry remains the only one in North Carolina and is one of 56 accredited schools in the nation. In 2005 it had a total of 120 full-time faculty and 520 students in a four-year program leading to the DDS degree, in MS and PhD programs, and in allied dental health programs (dental hygiene and dental assisting). Its budget for fiscal year 2004–2005 was $46 million, of which 25 percent was from state funds and $10.2 million was from research and training grants.[41]

The School of Nursing, which opened in 1952, was the first degree-granting (BS) program in North Carolina at a time when most nursing education was in hospital-based schools with no university connection. The first class of seventeen nursing students entered in the fall of 1952 and occupied the new nursing school building and the student nurse quarters adjacent to the new hospital. The nursing school moved to its current quarters in Carrington Hall in 1969. A major addition to the nursing school was completed in 2005, giving it some 139,000 square feet of space.

In 2005 the UNC School of Nursing was one of three nursing schools in North Carolina at an academic medical center. There are some twenty other North Carolina nursing schools in community colleges and community hospitals and at other branches of the University of North Carolina. The UNC school now offers a full range of degrees, from the BS to the MS and PhD in nursing and degree programs for nurse practitioners. In 2005 there were 106 full-time faculty and 560 students. The operating budget for fiscal year 2004–2005 was $17.7 million, of which 44 percent was from state funds and $9.3 million was from research and training grants.[42]

UNC–CH does not have a separate school of allied health sciences, but rather a Department of Allied Health Sciences in the School of Medicine, established in 1970 to consolidate the various allied health programs that had previously been administered by North Carolina Memorial Hospital. Beginning with 105 students in 1971, the department by 2005 had some 400 students and 75 faculty members. It offers academic programs ranging from entry-level professional certificates to advanced professional doctorates and research PhDs in seven allied health disciplines.[43] Since 2006 the department has been housed in the newly enlarged and renovated Bondurant Hall.

The Medical Library

Caldwell Hall had a medical library room in 1912 when the medical school occupied this first building specifically designed for the school. Dean Isaac Manning and Louis Round Wilson, the university librarian, were said to have personally moved the medical school's collection of books and journals into the new library. For many years the dean's secretary apparently managed the library. By 1936 the medical library was listed as a departmental library under the aegis of the university library, and its first official librarian was a medical student who provided part-time care for the library while a full-time student. In 1937 the medical library became a member of the Medical Library Association, and the first Medical Library Committee was appointed, chaired by W. Critz George. When the medical school moved to its new building in 1939, the library was on the first floor (where the dean's office was located from 1952 to 2006) and the stacks directly below, with access by the winding stairway. For the first time the medical library had a professional librarian, a graduate of Columbia University's School of Library Science.

In his annual report for 1951, Dean Berryhill commented, "While the Library is theoretically at least a Division of Health Affairs project, actually in financial support, in the work that has gone into its planning and development, and in its use by faculty and students, it is primarily still the Library for Medicine and Public Health. The physical facilities for the new library [in the Clinic wing of the Hospital] were never planned nor intended for a Division library and cannot now be transformed for that purpose." He praised "the tireless and enthusiastic efforts of Professor W. C. George, long the able Chairman of the Library Committee, to build up our book and journal collection for Medicine and Public Health, and also for Nursing and Dentistry. He has literally scoured the larger medical libraries of the East, South and Midwest and with comparatively little cost to the University secured thousands of volumes through gifts and exchanges. In addition he has carefully and wisely spent some $50,000 for volumes that are necessary for the clinical years of medicine and the departments in the allied schools." He added that these accomplishments were "all the more noteworthy when one realizes that Dr. George has been practically unaided and in addition has carried his usual teaching load . . . The schools involved and the University owes [sic] him a deep debt of gratitude for this essential service."[44]

In 1952 the library ceased being a branch library of the university library and with its move into the new library in the clinic wing of the new hospital buildings became the Division of Health Affairs Library. During the 1950s the library collection was greatly expanded and reclassified using the National Library of Medicine system.

The library had grown to 1,863 journal subscriptions and 109,030 volumes by 1968, when the name was changed to the Health Sciences Library to reflect its broader mission. In 1970 the library moved to its current location, its own building in the courtyard of MacNider Hall. During the next decade all the library collections and reading rooms of the five health sciences schools were consolidated into the Health Sciences Library. In 1982 the library building was doubled in size with the addition of three floors. Another major renovation completed in 2004 accommodated the library's increased use of electronic services for users on site and around the state. It also provided expanded space for the exceptional History of Health Sciences collections, part of the library's heritage. By 2004 the library employed sixty-five full-time librarians and staff, and the collection included 317,261 volumes and more than 3,500 journal subscriptions. The library now also has subscriptions to more than 2,000 electronic journals that are available locally as well as to students and other health care professionals statewide through the NC AHEC Digital Library.[45]

Hospital Naming and Organization

The idea of making the teaching hospital of the university a living memorial to those North Carolinians who served in World War I was first promulgated in June 1922 by the unanimous action of the university board of trustees as part of the recommendation that the medical school be expanded to four years. Josephus Daniels elaborated in a letter to the *Raleigh News and Observer* published the next week:

> That would be indeed a living memorial, worthy of the noble youths who made the supreme sacrifice and the commonwealth which was enriched by their nobility. It would be a memorial, too, that would carry benefaction to the people in every county in the State, alleviate suffering, save lives, and be a fresh proof that North Carolina is regarding the health and life of its people as its greatest possession. A living memorial: That is what the brave youths would feel was the fittest honor that a grateful State could pay them.[46]

Although the four-year medical school did not materialize at UNC in the 1920s, the concept of making the university's hospital a memorial to North Carolina's war dead persisted.

As the planning and construction of the new university hospital at Chapel Hill proceeded, the university board of trustees approved the name: North Carolina Memorial Hospital. Their action was affirmed by a resolution of the 1951 General Assembly.[47] The resolution specified that the hospital would be a memorial to those who gave their lives in all the nation's wars, not just World War I. A plaque was installed in the main entrance of the hospital in 1952 and relocated in later years whenever the hospital entrance moved:[48]

The North Carolina Memorial Hospital
To serve as a continuing memorial to those North Carolinians
who have given their lives, and who may hereafter give their lives,
as members of the Armed Forces, in protecting the freedom and
common welfare of their fellow citizens.

Robert R. Cadmus, MD, was recruited by Henry Clark in 1950 as the first director of NC Memorial Hospital. A native of New Jersey, Cadmus was an MD graduate of Columbia University and had a residency in surgery at Columbia-Presbyterian Medical Center. He served as a flight surgeon in the air force during World War II, rising to the rank of lieutenant colonel. After the war and prior to coming to Chapel Hill, he served as director of the Vanderbilt Clinic at Columbia-Presbyterian Hospital in New York City and then as assistant director of University Hospitals of Cleveland (where Berryhill had worked in the early 1930s).[49]

Cadmus served in a part-time consulting capacity from May 1950 until he began his full-time position on September 2, 1950—two years to the day before the hospital opened its doors to patients.[50] He served as the hospital director until 1962, when he was succeeded by E. B. Crawford, who, after joining the hospital in 1952, had risen to the rank of associate director. Cadmus then served as professor and first chair of the UNC Department of Hospital Administration from 1962 until he resigned in 1966 to assume the presidency of the New Jersey College of Medicine and Dentistry.[51]

Cadmus and his assistant, Rachel Long, who was hired as the hospital's first employee in 1950, had temporary offices in Miller Hall. The navy had built this small building adjacent to the Carolina Inn in 1942 as a dormitory for those in the various naval training programs at UNC during World War II. In 1950 the building was brick-veneered and converted to temporary offices for the hospital director, the administrator of the Division of Health Affairs, and the deans of the dental and nursing schools until construction was completed on the various new buildings on the medical campus.[52] For almost a year and a half Cadmus and Long were the only hospital staff. They then recruited the hospital department heads and the first director of nursing, who in turn began recruiting their staffs.[53]

When Cadmus returned in 1977 to speak at the twenty-fifth-anniversary celebration of the opening of the North Carolina Memorial Hospital, he reminded the audience, "This hospital is not your hospital. You, as was I, are but transient care-takers. It belongs to the people of North Carolina, as your stationery says [Operated for and by the People of North Carolina].[54] Patients come here not to offer their bodies for education and research, but to find health, comfort and compassion. The fact that we learn and conduct research is both a planned and a fortuitous opportunity, but in return, there must be giving; there must be caring; and there must be loving."[55]

The hospital director initially reported to the administrator of the Division of Health Affairs. Berryhill related that "the problems of administering the hospital became so overwhelmingly frustrating that the faculty of the school, with the support of a majority of the Trustees' Committee on Health Affairs . . . recommended to the chancellor and the president that the hospital be made a division of the medical school with its director responsible to the dean of the School of Medicine for hospital policies and operation. This was approved by the chancellor and the president of the university to become effective September 1, 1956, despite strong opposition of the division administrator and the deans of the other schools within the Division of Health Affairs."[56] With this change the hospital director became a department head in the School of Medicine and reported to the dean.[57]

Hospital Medical Staff Organization

When the hospital opened in 1952, its active medical staff consisted of physicians and dentists who were privileged to attend patients in the hospital, who were licensed to practice medicine or dentistry in North Carolina, and who were full-time faculty members in the School of Medicine or Dentistry. Only active medical staff members could admit patients or vote on matters related to medical practices and policies in the hospital. Over the years the rules have been changed to permit physicians in the community who have part-time faculty appointments to admit patients on the teaching services, to serve as attending physicians, and to bill for their professional services.

The chairs of the clinical departments in the medical school served as the chiefs of the corresponding clinical services in the hospital. The governing body of the medical staff was the medical board, which included the chiefs of the then eight clinical departments (medicine, obstetrics and gynecology, pathology, pediatrics, preventive medicine, psychiatry, radiology, and surgery), the director of the nursing service, the hospital director, the deans of the Schools of Medicine and Nursing, and the director of the student health service. Four other representatives of the preclinical and clinical departments were elected annually to serve one-year terms on the board. The administrator of the Division of Health Affairs served as a nonvoting member. A smaller executive committee met more frequently and had the power to act of behalf of the board, but its actions were subject to the board's review. Additional clinical chairs were added to the medical board over the years as new clinical departments were established in the School of Medicine. In later years a member of the medical faculty was appointed chief of staff and served as the operational chief of the medical staff. Still later the chief of staff also served as executive associate dean for clinical services in the School of Medicine.

The Women's Auxiliary

In the spring of 1952, while hospital construction was being completed and hospital and medical staff were being recruited, an enthusiastic group of some 190

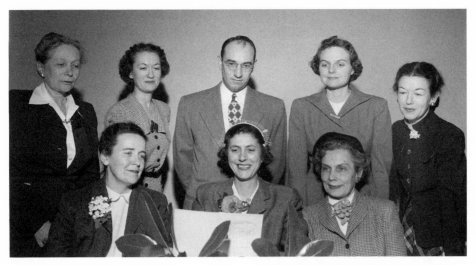

Dr. Robert R. Cadmus at the organizational meeting for the North Carolina Memorial Hospital Women's Auxiliary, 1952. Seated at lower left is Norma Berryhill. At lower right is Viola Jacobs, the hospital's first director of volunteer services. *(UNC Photo Lab, NCC)*

local women met at the Institute of Pharmacy building to organize a Women's Auxiliary to serve the hospital and its patients. Norma Berryhill played an active role in the organizational efforts, which received the full support of Robert Cadmus and of Mrs. M. L. (Viola) Jacobs, who served as the hospital's director of volunteer services from 1952 to 1967.

In recognition of the increasing numbers of male volunteers, "Women" was dropped from the auxiliary's name in 1967, and in 1981 the auxiliary changed its name to the NCMH Volunteer Association. In 1972 the faculty of the UNC School of Medicine presented its Distinguished Service Award to the hospital auxiliary and volunteer services for their meritorious service to medicine.

In its first half century thousands of volunteers have supported patients and their families through some two million hours of service. In addition the volunteer association has generated millions of dollars from its gift shops and other fund-raising activities to provide special care and equipment for patients and families as well as scholarships for those entering a health care career.[58]

FUNDING

State Appropriations

Although he continually struggled to acquire the state appropriations necessary to complete and operate the academic medical center at Chapel Hill, Berryhill was sensitive to the impact these developments might have on the university in general. In his 1947–1948 annual report he strongly advocated that "a sizable endowment" be secured; that the hospital's operating expenses be separated from the university's educational budget because "the cost of medical care is a community responsibility—and not the function of the educational institution to provide"; and that "the remainder of the University [be protected] from the drain that medical education—the costliest of all professional training—may make on the total institutional budget." He felt so strongly about these concerns that he concluded: "Unless these essentials can be provided and an outstanding School of Medicine assured, we should unhesitatingly abandon at once the expansion program."[59] In Berryhill's 1948–1949 annual report he did note that the legislature, which had approved the construction appropriations for the hospital and expanded medical school, had also appropriated "approximately $1,000,000 for maintenance of the Medical School for the next biennium, and, very important, the separation of the Medical School budget from that of the general University."[60]

Although the 1947 General Assembly had authorized the expansion of the medical school and the building of the teaching hospital at Chapel Hill, it was not until 1949 that the General Assembly made the funds available. In the interim, some of the funds previously allocated from the federal Hill-Burton program for the university hospital and other state-supported institutions had been reallocated by the Medical Care Commission for construction of community hospitals across the state. Berryhill later commented, "The Medical Care Commission's decision . . . to assign first priority on the Hill-Burton funds to the community hospitals, while temporarily disheartening to the university and the other state institutions involved, was wise and in the long run the best decision that could possibly have been made so far as the state institutions were concerned. Thereafter no one could accuse the university of having received federal funds for construction which might otherwise have gone to improve community hospital facilities in the state."[61]

The 1949 General Assembly did act upon the Medical Care Commission's recommendation to restore to the university $1.5 million in construction funds to replace those Hill-Burton funds that had been diverted to the community hospitals. This made a total of $5.29 million available for the construction of the hospital and clinic building, the School of Nursing building, and quarters for house staff and student nurses. Additional funds were specifically appropriated for a tuberculosis sanatorium to be constructed on the university campus adjacent to the teaching hospital. Two other developments, however, still left the university short of funds needed for the total hospital project. One was the realization that the funds appropriated for construction of the hospital were not going to be adequate to provide what was needed for patient care, teaching, and research in the teaching hospital. Another was the appropriation of $1 million for construction of the dental school. Although Berryhill and others supported this development after the hospital was built, the appropriation further compromised the funds allocated for the hospital, and it was estimated that an additional $2 million would be required. Because of other university needs and political considerations, a supplemental appropriation was not aggressively pursued. Berryhill stated, "In retrospect, the decision to move rapidly in letting the contract [for the hospital] and not to request supplementary appropriations from the 1949 General Assembly—while based on the trustees' genuine concern and that of other interested persons . . . —proved to be a serious error." Senator Clarence Stone, the chairman of the Advisory Budget Commission and a strong supporter of the medical school expansion, "later blasted Dean Berryhill for failure to communicate with him, indicating that this commission would undoubtedly have approved the supplementary request." But by that time it was too late to get the additional funding, and alternate plans had been made.[62]

The area that suffered most from this funding shortfall was the obstetrics and gynecology service, which would have had the entire eighth floor in the new hospital if the funding had been adequate. Edward Hedgpeth, the director of the student health service, generously offered a floor of the student infirmary (the 1942 navy hospital, which to this day still has the navy emblem in the lobby floor). It was remodeled, and funds were found to add a fifth floor. A visiting neonatologist from Washington, DC, in the early 1950s expressed dismay that the smallest and the most vulnerable of patients—the newborns and their mothers—were given these secondhand accommodations. Charles H. Hendricks, MD, the third chair of obstetrics and gynecology (1968–1980), accepted his appointment with the understanding that "the labor and delivery facilities were outmoded as a site for clinical practice and completely inadequate for an obstetric teaching service" and that their replacement would be given high priority by Dean Taylor. He added, "Despite the Dean's good will, however, the actual construction of adequate new facilities became a tedious, frustrating, years-long struggle." The "temporary" 4M and 5M floors—with renovation for a large modern delivery suite in 1973 and the move of the gynecology patients to the fourth floor in the main hospital—were utilized until the Robert A. Ross Labor and Delivery Suite in the new Patient Support Tower building was dedicated in June 1981 by Governor James Hunt. The governor pointed out that the new unit "was a model of state-of-the-art thinking in the delivery of medical services" but also recognized that the department and patients "had waited many years for the fulfillment of the dream." The space for obstetrics was doubled, and the hospital "became a more viable and credible referral center for critically ill newborns and women with complicated pregnancies." During the next year the service delivered almost 1,600 babies, and 500 sick or premature babies were cared for in the hospital's special-care nurseries. With these facilities the hospital "became the preeminent state regional referral center for sick newborns and women with complicated pregnancies."[63] Twenty-one years later, in 2002, the North Carolina Children's and Women's Hospitals opened with complete inpatient and outpatient care for women and children, the only facility in the state to offer these services in one location.

Through the efforts of state representative John W. Umstead of Chapel Hill and of the State Hospitals Board of Control, the 1951 General Assembly made an additional appropriation of $1 million for an addition to Memorial Hospital for psychiatry, known as the South Wing. The unit was created in order to train more professionals for the mental hospitals in the state and to help improve the mental health of North Carolinians.[64]

Clinical Income and the Private Patient Service

As late as 1944 Berryhill lamented the fact the medical faculty's salary scale, though better than it had been, was "still not up to the level of the salary scale in the Schools of Law and Public Health." He stressed the importance of this issue "not only in keeping promising members of the faculty but also in enabling us to secure other worth-while teachers and investigators as vacancies develop in the present staff and as the School expands."[65]

Although maintaining salary levels competitive with peer institutions around the country would be a challenge for Berryhill and all subsequent medical deans, the internal salary discrepancy between the medical school and some other professional schools within the university soon disappeared as the clinical activities of the medical faculty began to generate significant clinical income and as research grants provided further support for salaries. In the following decades, faculty members elsewhere in the university would look with envy at the salaries of their colleagues in the medical school. A journalist who interviewed UNC liberal arts faculty members in 1958 about salary discrepancies between them and the medical school faculty quoted an English professor as justifying the doctors' higher salaries: "Doctors can go into private practice at any time. They are free to leave. Academic men must go to another academic institution." Another professor remarked, "For their own salvation we have to work them over occasionally to keep them from getting uppity." A history professor added, "There won't be any trouble about the doctors getting more money as long as they don't start acting like they're worth it."[66]

The concept of private practice for medical school faculty was well established around the country by the 1950s and was already operating at the medical schools of both Duke (in the Private Diagnostic Clinic or PDC) and Wake Forest. Abraham Flexner in the early part of the twentieth century had advocated a "strict" full-time plan for academic clinical physicians, who would be paid a straight salary by the university and who could not engage in private practice. This never took hold, and what evolved in most medical schools was what is called "geographic full-time." Physicians on the clinical services could see and bill for their services to private patients in the academic medical center, but the resulting income would go to the faculty practice plan. The professor would receive a medical school salary that might include funding from various sources, including state appropriations, research grants, and the faculty practice plan.[67]

For the dental school, this was a new concept, and a vocal group in the North Carolina Dental Society made a bitter and eventually unsuccessful attempt to have it rejected. In a presentation at the 1954 annual meeting of the dental society, Chancellor House responded with a strong argument for the importance of private practice for clinical faculty:

Whatever your opinion may be about this question of intramural [private dental] practice, there are not any two opinions about this: you say, and we say, that we want an excellent School of Dentistry. Let us not talk about dentistry for a second. Let us talk about university education. We want an excellent university. I want to tell you that competent men and women who teach and who do research and who guide young men into their liberal and their professional educations are hard to find. Without this principle of some practice in their profession, we could not have a single member of our faculty in any competent department of the University, whether it is dentistry, medicine, journalism, or the teaching of English. Every college professor has some margin of time which he uses for consultation. The professor of literature will write a book. The engineer will be a consultant. The journalist will write a column in the newspaper; sometimes he will run a paper.

There are economic reasons for this [including having competitive salaries for recruitment] . . . However, there is a deeper and more fundamental education reason for that. Years ago, the great satirist, Bernard Shaw, threw this challenge to the teaching profession. He said, 'those who know how, do it. Those who can, do it. Those who cannot do it, teach."

This business of keeping your hand in play in the profession, in the art of dentistry, we might say, is absolutely essential, in the first place, so that the teacher may have confidence in himself. He has to have it. Education is made of two things: theory and information on the one hand and practice on the other. If the teacher does not have access to practice himself, then he will not have confidence that he really knows what he is teaching.

Just as the teachers have to do this private practice to keep their hands in and to keep their confidence, they also need it so that their students may have confidence in them. There is nothing more successful in teaching how to do a thing than to say, "I use this in [my] private practice."[68]

In the end, the dental faculty practice plan was successfully implemented. It was said to be one of the first of its type in a US dental school.[69]

Dean Berryhill reported in his annual report for 1950–1951 that "the method of remuneration of the clinical staff has been approved by the University Administration and the Board of Trustees; namely, a [base] salary from the University and in addition an income from private patients up to the level of the University salary. The departmental income above that ceiling is to be placed in a special trust fund account to be used on the recommendation of the Department head with the approval of the University Administration for the development and strengthening of departmental teaching and research."[70]

An important and lasting part of the 1956 Health Affairs Code prepared by Aycock was the codification of the concept, then still new at the University of

North Carolina, of clinical income contributing to faculty salary for medical and dental faculty members. At the time of the original 1956 Code, the clinical faculty members were able to double their base university salary, subject to a ceiling for each faculty level. The university base salaries in 1956 for clinical medical faculty members (and the ceilings for total compensation) were: department head, $12,100–13,750 ($25,000); professor, $11,000–12,100 ($23,500); associate professor, $7,975–10,450 ($21,000); and assistant professor, $5,575–7,700 ($16,000).

One of a series of articles on the new UNC Division of Health Affairs in the *Charlotte Observer* in 1958 reviewed the status of the medical school salaries. It commented on the concept of supplementing the base pay for clinical faculty and pointed out that this was common throughout the nation, although the UNC system put a ceiling on such earnings, while some medical schools, such as Duke, had none. The average salary for UNC faculty outside the medical school was cited at $6,752, while the overall average base pay for all medical school faculty was $8,231. Eighty-nine physician faculty members were able to supplement their base salaries with clinical income; their average salary was $13,848. The maximum salary (base plus clinical income) a physician faculty member could earn was $27,500 a year, and five of the eight chairs of medical school departments had earned the maximum the previous year. The clinical salary supplements were funded with about $500,000 from the $850,000 the Private Patient Service (PPS) had earned in 1957–1958. The balance of the $850,000 earnings covered $100,000 rent for hospital space utilized by the Private Patient Clinic; $70,000 for medical school improvements (the Medical School Trust Fund [MSTF] account); and the costs of nurses, other staff, and administrative expenses.[71]

Another important and lasting feature of the code was the initial codification of the use and accounting of clinical incomes for the support of the clinical faculty, the operation of the clinical departments, and the dean's use in support of various medical school endeavors. The MSTF, which the dean could use with few restrictions for "salary supplementations, research activities, and other Medical School projects," initially came from any surplus at the end of the year after the clinical departments had covered their expenses. In later years, the trust fund has been funded by a percentage deduction applied to the departments' net clinical earning after the deduction of certain basic expenses such as liability insurance premiums. Over the years this fund came to be known colloquially (and on occasion, bitterly) as the "Dean's Tax."

All of the clinical income and the associated clinical departmental expenses and faculty benefits were handled through the PPS from 1952 to 1978. During its first year of operation in 1952–1953, the total PPS income for all the clinical departments was $250,000 before any deductions for expenses. During the 1970s, through the efforts of Dean Fordham, the General Assembly recognized the UNC Physicians and Associates Trust Fund statutorily. In return for the resulting fiscal flexibility, the UNC–CH chancellor approves the budget and clinical fringe benefits annually.[72]

Private Funding

Dean Berryhill took advantage of every appropriate opportunity to stress the importance of supplementing state appropriations with private gifts and other funds. In his annual report to Chancellor House for 1943–1944, he said, "I should like once again to call your attention to the absolute necessity of obtaining a substantial endowment to supplement State funds for the maintenance of the School and proposed hospital. I believe it would be impossible to have an outstanding institution on State appropriations alone—subject to the whims of succeeding governors and legislatures."[73] His concern was appropriate, for sixty years later the state support—while still an essential and vital component of the funding—supplied only some 12 percent of the total annual budget for the entire UNC medical center at Chapel Hill.[74]

Following the 1947 and 1949 state appropriations that assured the building of the hospital and expanded medical school in Chapel Hill, meetings were held to consider establishing a mechanism for raising private funds to support the school and hospital. These meetings included Berryhill, University Comptroller Billy Carmichael, and friends and alumni of the school. In his annual report for 1949–1950, Berryhill could exclaim, "At long last the Medical Foundation [of North Carolina, Inc.], whose broad charter and purposes provide aid to medi-

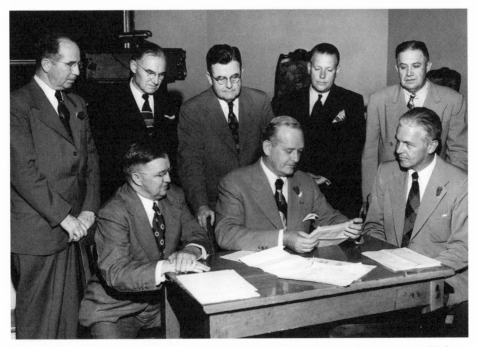

Meeting of officers of the Medical Foundation of North Carolina, early 1950s. Seated left to right are Collier Cobb, Jr., Lennox P. McLendon, and George Watts Hill. Standing left to right are Drs. H. O. Lineberger, Harry L. Brockmann, William M. Coppridge, Paul Whitaker, and Shahane R. Taylor. *(UNC Photo Lab, NCC)*

cal and dental education and research and to worthwhile health projects within the State, has been launched." The foundation was chartered on May 28, 1949, with more than 450 prominent North Carolinians as sponsors, a board of directors, and Lennox P. McLendon, Sr., as president. In 1949 contributions of almost $12,000, largely from the family of John Sprunt Hill of Durham, were received, most of which were used for organizational purposes. C. Sylvester Green, a former president of Coker College who was editor of the *Durham Herald,* became the first full-time executive director for the foundation on January 1, 1950. The foundation's initial goal was to have a permanent endowment of $25 million, with $100,000 available annually to support the schools. During the first full year of operation, more than $100,000 in expendable funds was made available, and progress was made on an endowment. Not long after the establishment of the medical foundation, the dental and nursing schools established their own foundations, while the medical foundation continued to support the medical school and hospital and contributed to the support of the Health Sciences Library.[75]

At a celebration of the tenth anniversary of the school's expansion, a university trustee who had been the first president of the medical foundation recalled the foundation's role in supporting Berryhill's early efforts to recruit an outstanding clinical faculty:

> If you can imagine being Dean of a medical school for almost four years without any way of knowing when it could begin and without any money to employ personnel, hard to get under favorable conditions and all but impossible to get without the certainly of employment contracts, then you can have some appreciation of his difficulties. A man less devoted to an ideal for a great medical school or less determined to do his part, and then some, would have given up in despair. I recall a meeting of the Medical Foundation when it was unanimously decided to clean out the treasury, so to speak, so that Dean Berryhill could have approximately fifty thousand dollars to secure a few key people for the faculty of the Medical School and the staff of the hospital. Knowing the individuals involved I would say that providing this money, at that critical time, added a few years to the Dean's life and fully justified the existence of the Foundation.[76]

In his remarks at the same celebration, Berryhill confirmed that the foundation's support for salary supplements was critical in recruiting clinical faculty in 1951–1954.[77]

A photograph of one of the early meetings of the medical foundation officers in the early 1950s includes Governor Kerr Scott. In comments to the group, Scott advocated that physicians throughout the state voluntarily tax themselves to support the activities of the university's medical school, much as farmers had taxed themselves to support agricultural extension services. Although this plan was never implemented, in recent years contributions by medical alumni to the annual Loyalty Fund drive by the medical foundation have grown at a fast pace. By 2003 almost 40 percent of UNC medical graduates were contributing some $750,000 annually to support their medical school.[78]

Since its origin in 1949, the medical foundation has provided an ever-increasing annual contribution from gifts and endowment income to support the activities of the school and hospitals.[79] More recently, the W. Reece Berryhill Society was formed to recognize those donors to the medical foundation "who, like the society's namesake, choose to leave a lasting legacy to this institution though a bequest, trust or other planned giving arrangement."

Planning and Construction

Hospital and Ambulatory Care Facility Construction

A medical student in the late 1930s who returned after the war to join the faculty in 1946 described "Medical Hill" or "Pill Hill" (Chapel Hillians' nicknames for the medical campus) as "heavily forested in pines and oaks." The only exceptions were the "new Medical Building" (MacNider Hall) and Wilson Hall (home of the Department of Zoology), both built in 1939 on the east side of South Columbia Street, and the navy hospital, built in 1942 east of and parallel to the medical building. On the west side of Columbia Street was the site of the Chapel Hill High School, now the site of the Schools of Pharmacy and Public Health. "The area behind the university buildings sloped eastward toward Kenan Stadium [built in 1927], and a number of small streams converged in the forested glade. In 1950 the glade was quaintly referred to by old timers as 'The Meeting of the Waters.' The rainwater draining from this area entered a large culvert which carried it from 'The Meeting of the Waters' to its final destination in Morgan's Creek" after passing through a large culvert running under the center of the Kenan Stadium football field. Today, the "Meeting of the Waters" is paved over as the Bell Tower Parking Lot.[80]

The $1 million for planning appropriated by the 1947 legislature was released by the governor in 1948 for use in planning and making architectural drawings for the new buildings.[81] The firm of Schmidt, Garden and Erickson of Chicago was engaged to do the hospital architectural plans in association with a local firm, Northrup and O'Brien of Winston-Salem. The Chicago firm had had extensive experience in planning and supervising construction of university hospitals, including those for Chicago, Minnesota, Northwestern, Pennsylvania, and Wisconsin, as well as hospitals at the Texas Medical Center in Houston. A member of the firm was employed to do a long-range site plan that provided suggested locations for a future TB hospital, a psychiatric unit, a handicapped children's unit, a cancer institute, and a chronic disease hospital. Ray E. Brown, director of the University of Chicago Hospital, was employed as a consultant for the planning. Because the state appropriation did not cover payment for the architect doing the long-range site plan or Brown's consulting services, several

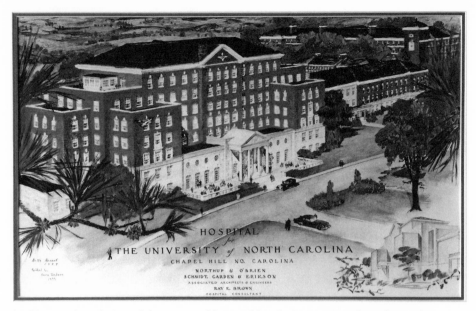

Architectural rendering of the proposed hospital for the University of North Carolina, 1949. *(UNC Hospitals)*

members of the trustees' medical committee raised from private sources the estimated $12,000 needed to cover their fees.[82]

Dean Berryhill ideally wanted to have the chiefs of the five major clinical departments (medicine, surgery, obstetrics, pediatrics, and psychiatry), the hospital director, and the dean of the nursing school on board as soon as possible to help with the planning and design of new hospital, but funding delays made this impossible. As a consequence, the burden of planning the hospital fell on Berryhill, a few other faculty members, the consultant (Ray Brown), and the architects. By the time the new hospital director and clinical chairs were on board, the major decisions about the design and the building had been set, although minor modifications were possible.

As hard as it may be to believe today, during the planning phase for the hospital the small dean's office and the facilities in the medical school building had no readily available table or desk big enough to accommodate the plans for the hospital and other buildings. Catherine Berryhill remembers many occasions when her father, architects, and others pored over massive sets of blueprints at home on their large dining room table, which she has today in her home.

Soon after Henry Clark arrived in Chapel Hill in the summer of 1950 as the Division administrator, he realized that Berryhill had had to focus "heavily during the previous two years on working with architects in planning the main hospital and then serving as the primary 'owner-representative' in discussing many spot construction issues with the builders after the contracts were let in the early fall of 1949. Reece was happy to turn over that latter responsibility to me and, through me, to Bob Cadmus, with whom I talked frequently by telephone."[83]

The *Raleigh News and Observer* reported in July 1949 that the "plans for the proposed seven-story, 400 bed teaching hospital at the University of North Carolina . . . have been completed and are ready for distribution to contractors . . . Bids will be received at Gerrard Hall in Chapel Hill on September 2 at 2 P.M." According to the October 20, 1949, *Greensboro Daily News,* the J. A. Jones Construction Company of Charlotte was the low bidder and was awarded the general contract for $2,626,000. The total cost of the building, including the subcontracts and the architects' fees, was $3,947,150. The seven-story Colonial-Georgian brick building would have administrative functions on the first floor, operating and treatment rooms on the second floor, and inpatient rooms on the third through the seventh floors. Excavation and site preparation for the hospital was started on October 20, 1949. A four-story outpatient clinic building would connect the new hospital with the infirmary (the old navy hospital) and the existing School of Medicine building.[84]

The construction of the classroom building for the School of Nursing and of the quarters for interns and for student nurses, begun shortly after the hospital construction started, was completed in 1952. The School of Nursing building (Medical School Wing A) was vacated in 1969 when Carrington Hall was completed, and the space was used temporarily for various hospital functions before being demolished during the construction of the Patient Support Tower.[85]

The 1949 General Assembly also appropriated funds for construction of a 100-bed tuberculosis sanatorium to be operated by the state sanatorium system as an educational and research hospital in conjunction with the university and North Carolina Memorial Hospital. It was completed in 1953 and was named for Lee Gravely of Rocky Mount, longtime chairman of the State Board of Tuberculosis Hospitals. It was used as a tuberculosis sanatorium until it became part of North Carolina Memorial Hospital in 1975. Since then it has housed various clinical services, including the employee health service, a small inpatient rehabilitation unit, outpatient oncology services, and the radiology oncology department. Gravely is scheduled for demolition after construction of the North Carolina Cancer Hospital is completed about 2009.

The psychiatric wing of the hospital, funded by a special appropriation in 1951, was occupied in 1954. This addition, known as South Wing, provided seventy-five beds for inpatients, outpatient clinics, offices, and research space for the psychiatry department.[86] It housed the psychiatry department until the new North Carolina Neurosciences Hospital was occupied in 1996. South Wing was then demolished to make room for construction of the North Carolina Women's and Children's Hospitals.

The ceremony for the laying of the cornerstone of the university hospital was held on Wednesday afternoon, April 18, 1951, with more than 1,000 people attending, according to the account in the *Greensboro Daily News* the following day: "Cornerstone ceremonies were conducted according to the ancient Masonic rites under the command of the North Carolina Grand Master, Dr. Wallace E.

Caldwell of Chapel Hill. Attired in their traditional regalia, the several hundred Masons attending their annual communication here were present. Included in the box placed in the cornerstone were records covering the Good Health Movement from 1943, when leaders of the North Carolina Medical Society asked Governor Broughton to appoint a commission to make a study and recommend this program." Governor Kerr Scott and other speakers stressed that the ceremonies "actually and symbolically mark a new era in the good health program for the state and nation." Kay Kyser of Chapel Hill, who had been a leader in the successful effort to publicize the urgent need for the Good Health Movement in the 1940s, said, "We have won just the first leg of this race, and we'll never reach the goal unless we go the remaining laps. The whole program will be futile unless it is continually backed by the loyalty, interest, and enthusiasm of the people of North Carolina." Lennox P. McLendon, Sr., reminded those who would work at the hospital that they would be "work[ing] close to the heart of North Carolina" and challenged them to keep the hospital open for all those who "shall come here seeking the sympathetic and skillful aid of hands and hearts educated and trained by a great commonwealth."[87]

The hospital construction project gained wide attention locally and nationally. It was by far the biggest construction project in the history of Chapel Hill and the university. Roland Giduz, a Chapel Hill journalist, writing in the *Durham Morning Herald* for July 15, 1950, provided some perspective on the project's size:

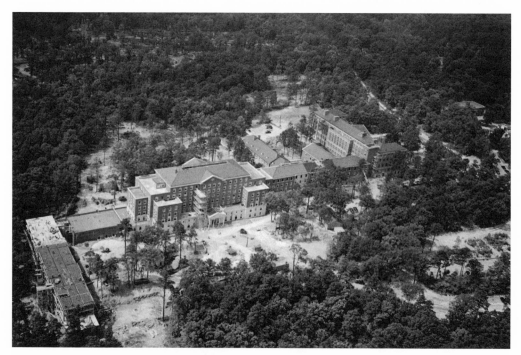

Construction of hospital and School of Nursing in progress, 1951. *(UNC Photo Lab, NCC)*

Chapel Hillians during the past few years have been rightly proud of the size of the fine five story University Medical School Building. It sits impressively in a large pine grove at the top of the Pittsboro Road hill at the town's southern limits. But this present building will be no more than a small wing of the new University Hospital and four-year Medical School—which will be about five times its size. The general clinic wing of the hospital alone will be nearly the size of the present medical school.

The actual scope and projected size of this huge building program is something still beyond the comprehension of many of the residents of this town of a scant 9,000 where the tallest building now ranges only five stor[i]es above the ground.

And the over-all projected medical center to be built in this area in the coming years is beyond the fondest dreams of what its practical-minded planners imagined only five years ago.

The 400-bed hospital, which will be about the size of the huge, sprawling Duke Hospital at Durham, will contain 1,100 rooms in its nine stories. Seven of these floors are to be above ground, while two complete stories are being constructed on basement level . . .

A visitor to the scene in late November will be able to see the brickwork completed from the ground floor to the top of the 125-foot high main building. Landscaping and construction of parking area [are] proceeding now at the same time as the building construction. Entrance to the hospital will be nearly 200 yards below the present medical building on the Pittsboro Highway, linking the hospital to the zoology building at the lower end of the hill.

When the project is finished next spring only the nucleus of the final proposed medical center will be there. In the not too distant future a dental school building will be erected—perhaps as a T-shaped connecting wing sprouting out from the west end of the present medical school. Extensions forward on the present building may bring it within a few feet of the highway, thus giving the building a huge U-shape. These would be necessary as teaching wings of the four-year school.[88]

In a more humorous vein, Giduz later retold what had become a classic Chapel Hill anecdote attributed to Jimmy Pickard, a Chapel Hill character who had worked for a number of years downtown in various stores: "When they began the massive excavations for NC Memorial Hospital . . . Jimmy went and looked at the hole and asked a friend what they were digging it for. 'That's to bury all the damn fools in Chapel Hill in,' quipped the witling. 'Well, who's gonna cover 'em up?' one-upped Jimmy, echoing his inimitable laugh."[89]

The Sunday *New York Times* for September 17, 1950, had an article about the center headlined, "Big Health Center Growing in South: $10,000,000 Construction Plan Under Way in North Carolina for State's Medical Benefit." It noted that

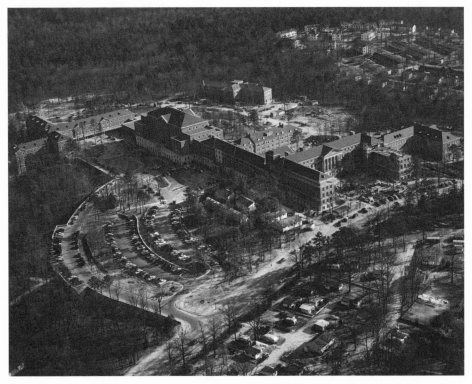

Hospital and Gravely Sanatorium construction completed, 1953. South wing of MacNider Hall under construction. Note the School of Dentistry's Quonset huts between MacNider Hall and the parking lot. Also note the married students' trailer court in the lower right (the future site of the Schools of Pharmacy and Public Health) and Victory Village in the upper right. *(UNC Photo Lab, NCC)*

one of the most comprehensive and integrated state-wide health programs and medical centers in the country is now being developed at the University of North Carolina . . . Formally established fifteen months ago as the Division of Health Affairs, it will comprise schools of medicine, public health, pharmacy, dentistry and nursing and a university hospital. Its over-all architectural and administrative design is intended to make it the focal training and service point for community-health problems throughout the state. The schools of public health and pharmacy are now fully accredited, and the school of medicine at present covers a two-year basic science course but is being expanded to a full four-year program. New dentistry and nursing buildings and the university hospital are in various stages of construction.[90]

The hospital, which was initially projected to be completed in 1951 or early 1952, actually was opened for the first patient on September 2, 1952, with seventy-eight beds. Thirteen months later, in October 1953, 210 beds were open for patients. During the first full year of operation, the hospital served 3,787 patients from some 90 of the state's 100 counties, and approximately 30,000 visits were made to the outpatient clinics.

The only other expansions to the original hospital in the first decade after its opening were the enclosures of the porches at each end of the seventh floor of the hospital for a conference room, playroom, and isolation ward for the pediatric services.[91] Significantly, the 1961 General Assembly approved funds for air conditioning North Carolina Memorial Hospital, an upgrade much appreciated by patients and staff alike during the hot summer months.[92]

By the late 1950s it was obvious that additional space was needed for various hospital services as well as for teaching and research in all the health sciences schools. Clark, the administrator of the Division of Health Affairs, initiated a comprehensive long-range planning effort for the Division of Health Affairs. This included having a national advisory committee study the situation and make recommendations. It was chaired by Jack Masur, MD, assistant surgeon general and director of the clinical center at NIH, and included directors of major national hospitals and deans of medical and other health sciences schools. William Sanger, chancellor of the Medical College of Virginia at Richmond and chair of the 1946 national committee that had recommended expansion of the UNC School of Medicine, served as a consultant to the advisory committee. The advisory committee in a 1958 report recognized the "persistent, serious problems of space shortages" at the health center "due to the growing demands of broader activities in research, teaching and the diagnosis and treatment of patients." They urged the university to "proceed as rapidly as possible in the orderly development of (a) site plans, (b) delineation of specific space needs, and (c) relative priorities for each of the components of the Division." Among the various specific recommendations were "more laboratory facilities for basic sciences and clinical investigation for the School of Medicine" and a "new building to furnish modern clinic facilities for the diagnosis and treatment of ambulatory patients."[93] Subsequent planning resulted in the building in the 1960s and early 1970s of major expansions of the hospital, the clinics, and the medical school as well as the new free-standing Health Sciences Library.[94]

Berryhill enlisted the help of Isaac M. Taylor, MD, associate professor of medicine, who took a leave of absence to coordinate the planning for the physical expansions for the hospital. Berryhill later praised Taylor for his "able and conscientious efforts" while representing the dean's office "as liaison with the faculty, the architects, and the University Planning Office."[95]

Eventually funding was obtained from several sources to build the J. Spencer Love Clinics (the Ambulatory Patient Care Facility or APCF) on the south side of Memorial Hospital. This facility increased the number of exam and treatment rooms from 50 to 164 and provided space for the clinical laboratories, radiology, and pharmacy. An addition on the north side of the hospital, finished and occupied in late 1969, provided facilities in the basement for sterile supplies; on the first floor for occupation and physical therapy; and on the second floor for new operating rooms. As part of this expansion the main entrance of the hospital was moved from the original location, facing north and the university campus, to the opposite side, facing south and Manning Drive. The 200-bed inpatient bed tower was completed above the Love clinics in 1971.[96]

Medical School Construction

Berryhill continued to stress the need for additional space as the faculty increased to accommodate the new and expanded programs. A north wing that extended MacNider Hall toward South Columbia Street was completed in 1952, and a matching south wing in 1953. These extensions provided new offices, research laboratories, and teaching laboratories for all the basic science departments.[97]

Berryhill's diligence later resulted in a Medical Sciences Research Building (MSRB) for the medical school. Approved in 1959 and completed in 1962 as an extension of MacNider Hall north toward the main campus, it provided faculty

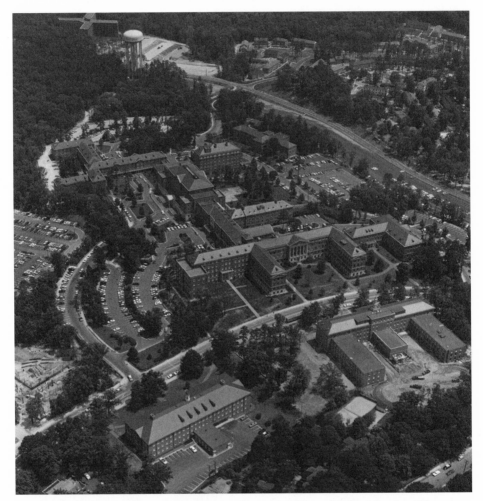

Initial medical center construction completed, 1962. Buildings for the Schools of Pharmacy and Public Health and the Medical Sciences Research Building have been completed. Manning Drive has opened, and the first high-rise dormitory has been constructed on the university's South Campus. (*UNC Photo Lab, NCC*)

offices and research laboratories for both basic sciences and clinical sciences departments, including physiology and medicine. It was the first major addition after completion of the initial construction in the 1950s and the last to match the original design of the other buildings in the medical complex. The building was financed by a $500,000 grant from the Research Facility Division of the NIH with matching funds obtained as a loan from the state's escheats fund that was paid off with the indirect costs from research grants.[98] This creative financing arrangement was one of many that would be used to finance subsequent buildings in the medical center by combining funds from various sources such as state appropriations, federal grants, private donations, and bonds and loans to be repaid with clinical income or indirect research costs.[99]

Since the late 1960s and early 1970s, with Dean Taylor's successful effort to couple expanded medical school enrollment with expanded faculty positions and new buildings, the medical school has undergone almost continuous construction and renovation projects. In the early 1970s, three major buildings for the School of Medicine were completed: the basic science educational facility (Berryhill Hall); the preclinical education building, which includes the state medical examiner's office (Brinkhous-Bullitt Building); and the clinical sciences building (Burnett Womack Building).

Today the School of Medicine occupies twenty-one major buildings on the university campus, with a total of almost two million square feet of space. These figures compare with the single School of Medicine and Public Health Building in 1939, with its 89,045 square feet and no air conditioning.

Housing for Faculty, Students, and Staff

Although Berryhill was an idealist in advocating that the medical school and the teaching hospital be located in Chapel Hill on the university campus, he was a realist in recognizing some of the practical problems that arose from building such a large enterprise in a small community. In his annual report following the initial approval of the school's expansion by the 1947 legislature, he said one of the four essentials for realizing the great potential in this expansion was to "provide adequate housing for faculty, students, and other personnel."[100] In his 1950 annual report, Berryhill restated his concern that the housing available for anticipated new faculty, increased student enrollment, and nonprofessional staff for operation of the hospital was "totally inadequate even for present needs." He concluded, "Indeed the success of the whole medical venture may well depend in large part on the adequacy with which the community is able to fill this need."[101]

The university had already begun to address the pressing need for student housing to meet the postwar explosion in student enrollment created by the GI Bill, which provided federal funding to enable veterans to obtain an education. The prewar enrollment of some 4,000 students almost doubled to more than 7,000 students shortly after the war. The university's efforts initially included placing temporary World War II Quonset huts on the varsity tennis courts. The huts were gradually replaced with permanent dormitories as funding and construction permitted.

Married university students were a distinct rarity prior to the war. With the return of the older veterans, however, the university faced the challenge of housing their families. It responded with Victory Village, located south of the medical campus and consisting of a collection of recycled wooden wartime barracks from the former Camp Butner, north of Durham. These provided 356 convenient and inexpensive housing units for married medical and other students. They were later replaced by the permanent brick buildings in Odum Village.[102] Other returning married students stayed in small travel trailers on university land on South Columbia Street across from the medical school. The small trailers soon filled the area and were embellished with porches, decks, and other additions made from lumber scavenged from the Victory Village construction site. One observer said it "soon looked like a gypsy village, each trailer differing from its neighbors. Morale was high among the occupants. They had recently won a war and having to scrounge for housing was just another challenge."[103]

These university facilities for married students supplemented the many rooms and small apartments that were made available by townspeople (including the Berryhills) for rent to students and their spouses before large commercial apartment complexes became available.

The frenzied and provisional nature of the postwar housing situation in Chapel Hill was recalled by Frederick A. "Ted" Blount, a member of the two-year medical class of 1942, who had completed his MD at Pennsylvania and then served as a physician in the navy. He returned to Chapel Hill in 1946 with Berryhill's support to fill a temporary teaching post at the medical school while awaiting an opening in a pediatric residency program. He, his wife, and their eighteen-month-old son stayed for about a week at the Carolina Inn. They then rented the second story of a house off East Franklin Street, but not too long afterward the landlord forced them to move out. When the Berryhills learned of their dilemma, the dean and his wife invited the young family to stay in a small apartment in their home on West Franklin Street, where Fowler's Grocery Store was later located. They had to enter the apartment through the Berryhills' dining or living room and had no kitchen, so they ate many meals at the Carolina Inn cafeteria. The Berryhills were most hospitable and never complained about the young couple's child, and they in turn went to great lengths to keep him quiet when the Berryhills had dinner guests. When John L. Lewis and the coal miners went on strike in the late fall of 1946, the coal supply gradually diminished in Chapel Hill and the house became cooler and cooler, but Norma Berryhill was able to find an electric heater that at least kept the child's room somewhat warm. When the Berryhills were away, they encouraged the couple to invite their friends over. On several such occasions they invited the medical students from the pharmacology class the young doctor was teaching and entertained them with a fruit punch made with 95 percent alcohol from the department. He added, "I often thought later of the irony of doing this sort of thing in the dean's house, but at the time it seemed pretty natural. That was a common sort of libation for medical students at that time."[104]

For a brief period, the medical students had a dormitory designated primarily for their usage. Whitehead Dormitory (named for the medical school dean from 1890 to 1905, Richard Henry Whitehead, MD) was completed and occupied in 1939 at the same time as the new medical school building. The two-year medical class of 1942 had some forty students (all men), and all but one (the sole married student) lived in Whitehead.[105] Immediately following the war, however, married students occupied Whitehead until Victory Village was completed, at which time Whitehead reverted to a dormitory.[106] In 1953 Berryhill stated that the need for housing for medical students was still acute. He lamented that Whitehead Dormitory, "originally built for and promised to the School of Medicine, for its students, is now used by students in Medicine, Dentistry, and Public Health. Many medical students are housed wherever they can find a haven," and "this is not good for morale." In his frustration he advocated either a new dormitory for medical students or changing the name of Whitehead Dormitory if it could not be used primarily for medical student housing.[107] Neither happened, and the medical students and their spouses continued to disperse throughout the community.

The planning for the new hospital included wings completed in 1952 as living quarters for interns and nursing students. As other university and private housing became available in the community, these two buildings were converted during the 1970s to offices for various medical school or hospital functions.[108] One floor of the former nurses' dormitory (Wing D) now houses a hospital-operated motel for patients (and their families) while they are receiving therapies that do not require them to be hospitalized.

One significant contribution to the medical school expansion and to making Carolina a research university, according to Philip Manire, PhD, in his 1986 Norma Berryhill Lecture, was the building of the Glen Lennox apartment complex by William Muirhead of Durham: "When one looks back at the years from 1950 to 1952 when more than 60 new faculty members and their families moved to Chapel Hill, the extraordinary coincidence of the opening of Glen Lennox and the four-year medical school was most fortunate indeed." The development had been announced on the front page of the *Chapel Hill Weekly* for June 21, 1949: "Work on a housing development for 300 families on a 60-acre site about a mile and a half from town . . . on the Raleigh highway . . . will begin about August 1," with "some of the apartments . . . ready for occupancy in January, more than half by the end of Spring and all of them by the following September." They were described as one-, two-, or three-bedroom apartments with heat from a central plant and with rents ranging from $60 to $80 a month.

Manire went on to describe the influence of Glen Lennox on the developing medical school faculty: "The apartments . . . were ready by the spring and summer of 1950 and very many new recruits to the Medical School in the next several years found excellent refuge in that colony. The Barnetts, Cromarties, Ellises, Flowers, Gottschalks, Schwabs, Sessions, Thomases . . . the list is long and we were all good neighbors; we shared babysitters, held regular backyard parties, and established great friendships that extend to the present. We were all much impressed when Tom Butler brought his lovely family down from Baltimore in 1950 and rented two adjacent apartments and had a door cut between. Great stories are told of those days and some have even become rituals and traditions on special occasions."[109]

Another group of young faculty members, including Judson Van Wyk, MD, in pediatrics, approached the acute shortage of affordable housing for faculty by forming a cooperative. In the mid-1950s, after many struggles, they purchased a twenty-six-acre plot of land near the university's Finley Golf Course; had it annexed by the city; negotiated electrical, sewer, and water service; and built the still-existing Highland Woods community of homes on half- to three-quarter-acre lots.[110]

FACULTY RECRUITMENT

Before recruiting the first clinical chairs, who would set the standards for years to come, Berryhill invited Alan Gregg, MD, director of the Division of Medical Sciences of the Rockefeller Foundation, in early 1950 to spend a week at the School of Medicine to discuss and to provide counsel on the school's mission and its plans for the future.[111] Out of these discussions came advice that Berryhill said was invaluable when he started recruiting the clinical chairs:

1. Don't try to become a second anything [e.g., a second Johns Hopkins, Harvard, or Michigan School of Medicine] . . . this is the University of North Carolina; it is a highly respected university. Accordingly, you should develop the University of North Carolina School of Medicine . . . [Try to] get the best man available to head each department . . . [and] try to have men from as many different institutions as possible and then develop a philosophy of the University of North Carolina School of Medicine.

2. It is wise to select chairmen with a reasonably wide range of age. There is great value in the maturity and judgment that comes with experience in medicine as well as in the enthusiasm and energy of the young men in clinical research . . .

3. Finally, if you want a particular person for a department chairman, do not hesitate to seek him just because he has recently assumed a new responsibility, even a departmental chairmanship in another medical school.

Berryhill followed this advice in recruiting individuals for the first chairs of medicine and surgery, both of whom had been chairs elsewhere for only one to three years.

Berryhill later elaborated on the criteria he used in 1951–1952 when choosing the first clinical chairs for the new clinical departments:

1. Excellence as a clinician and active participation in the care of patients.
2. Superior teaching ability and devotion to this responsibility with respect to both undergraduate medical students and to interns, residents, and fellows.
3. Competence in clinical research.
4. Evidence of a desire and motivation to work with others for the improvement of medical education at all levels in this medical school.
5. Possession of a sense of responsibility to the university and the state of North Carolina.

It is certainly not a coincidence that the characteristics Berryhill sought in the candidates for the new clinical chairs reflected many of those he had seen in his mentors at Harvard in the late 1920s—especially Peabody, Minot, and Wearn. Two decades later Berryhill admitted that these criteria might be considered outdated elsewhere—and possibly even here—but that "on the whole, the total

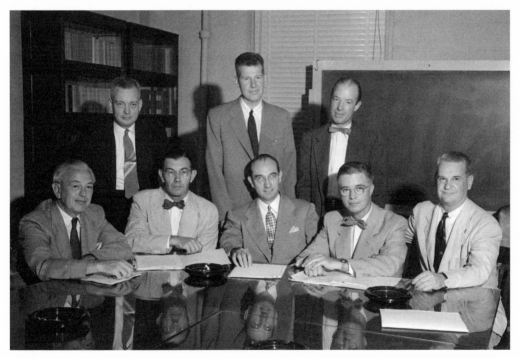

Original chairs of the clinical departments, 1952. *Seated, left to right:* Drs. Nathan A. Womack, W. Reece Berryhill (dean), Robert R. Cadmus (hospital director), George C. Ham, and Robert A. Ross. *Standing, left to right:* Drs. Ernest H. Wood, Edward C. Curnen, Jr., and William L. Fleming. *Not shown:* Dr. Charles H. Burnett. *(UNC Photo Lab, NCC)*

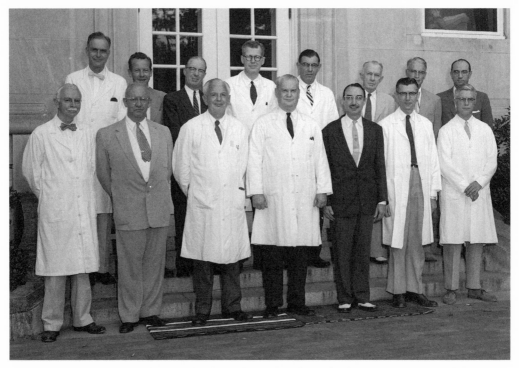

Clinical and basic sciences chairs and other School of Medicine leaders, 1957. *Front row, left to right:* Drs. Daniel A. MacPherson (bacteriology), James C. Andrews (biological chemistry), Nathan A. Womack (surgery), Robert A. Ross (obstetrics and gynecology), William P. Richardson (assistant dean), Kenneth M. Brinkhous (pathology), and George C. Ham (psychiatry). *Back row, left to right:* Thomas C. Butler (pharmacology), Charles W. Hooker (anatomy), William L. Fleming (preventive medicine), Edward C. Curnen, Jr. (pediatrics), W. Reece Berryhill (dean), W. Critz George (chair emeritus, anatomy), Charles H. Burnett (medicine), and Robert R. Cadmus (hospital director). *(UNC Photo Lab, NCC)*

of this group's accomplishments and contributions has been very significant and of a high order in the caliber of the departments they developed."[112]

Berryhill's success in this recruitment effort is reflected in a quote attributed to Duke's medical school Dean Wilburt C. Davison, who said that Berryhill recruited the best group of new clinical chairs since Welch had recruited Osler, Kelly, and Halsted to the new Johns Hopkins Medical School in the 1890s. John Graham added, "Dean Davison may have exaggerated, but the achievement was real and has been lasting. Dr. Berryhill succeeded in a single stroke in changing a small but good, regional teaching institution into one that aspired to be a comprehensive medical center with national standards in teaching, research, and patient care."[113]

A new chair who arrived at Chapel Hill in 1960 later observed:

I find it hard to imagine a more impressive group of medical academicians, and I am still awed by the fact that Dr. Berryhill was able to attract faculty of such caliber to our fledgling School of Medicine. More important than the stature of these individuals is what and how they went about their business in those early years. What I want to stress . . . is the general atmosphere of the medical school and hospital or the milieu of this academic environment . . . I found at the University of North Carolina mutual respect among faculty that I had not experienced previously. There was an openness of negotiations, easy accessibility, and low departmental barriers, which seemed to me to be almost unique. I detected a sense of humaneness and of collegiality that impressed me greatly. There was an aura about this institution which set it apart and made it a very special place to be. As we have increased in size, there are times when I fear we might be losing this remarkable characteristic; I urge those of you who are shaping the future of our school not to let this happen.[114]

A basic sciences chair later described the interest of the clinical chairs in research. "Their support in those early years of the basic sciences and the close cooperation of basic science and clinical departments were begun early and continue in an exemplary manner to the present." This "openness and collegiality in the whole school" was exemplified by the attendance from many departments at special lectures, grand rounds, and seminars during the 1950s. For instance, "the lecture series on genetics, organized by John Graham in 1959, was held on 16 Saturday mornings at 11 A.M. and the clinical auditorium was overfilled for every lecture." The next year a lecture series on viruses was attended by almost the entire medical faculty every Saturday morning.[115]

The First Clinical Chairs

Berryhill's frustration in beginning the recruitment of the clinical chairs was evident in his 1951 annual report to Chancellor House:[116] "In spite of the general acceptance of the fact that the selection of the Heads of the clinical departments and their associate staff is the key to the future of the Medical School and of the University Hospital, so many obstacles have been placed in the way of setting up these departments that we are now many months behind schedule." He attributed much of the delay to the "taking over by the Division Administrator of the funds specifically appropriated by the 1949 General Assembly for the of Medical School and the Hospital and the uncooperative attitude of the State budgetary authorities." As a result, "approval for the headships of the clinical departments was not obtained until January 1951, although requested first in the early summer of 1950." He was able to note, however, in the annual report dated June 12, 1951, that the first of the clinical chairs had been successfully recruited.

Nathan Anthony Womack, MD, the chair of surgery, was the first chair to be recruited. He was one of three native North Carolinians in the first group of seven chairs. A native of Reidsville, North Carolina, Womack was born in 1901 and received his BS in medicine from UNC's two-year School of Medicine in 1922 and his MD degree from Washington University at St. Louis in 1924. He remained in St. Louis for his graduate surgical education under Evarts Graham, MD. He joined the Washington University faculty in 1930 and conducted a private surgical practice in St. Louis. He rose to the rank of professor of clinical surgery at Washington University by 1947. From 1948 to 1951 he was professor and head of surgery at the University of Iowa before accepting the position at Chapel Hill. He served as chair for sixteen years and was succeeded by Colin G. Thomas, Jr., MD. Womack remained active in the department and medical school until his sudden death from a heart attack in 1975. In 1969 the Nathan A. Womack Surgical Society was organized by his colleagues and former trainees to honor Womack and to provide a means to "renew friendships . . . formed during residency training years," to provide "a worth-while educational opportunity," and "to provide an opportunity to meet current members of the training program." The society has held biennial meetings since 1973.[117]

Medical students and residents remembered Womack as an imposing figure with graying hair and erect stature. He could be jovial or serious as the occasion demanded. The academic highlight of a rotation on the surgery service was the pre-op conference, held each weekday at 1:30 P.M. in a room near the operating rooms. When the "Chief" walked in, the entire gathering would rise in respect and stay standing until he was seated. (This tradition disappeared with future chairs and the informalities of the 1960s.) Womack would review the operating room schedule for the next day while the resident presented a summary of the patient and the proposed operation. Woe to the resident who had not personally examined all pertinent X-rays and the microscopic slides of any biopsies or previous surgical specimens! Womack would quiz the residents and students on the differential diagnosis and alternative approaches to treatment. He used this discussion as an opportunity to comment on the latest findings in regard to the pathophysiology of the patient's condition or to provide a historical perspective on the disease or the operative procedure.

In his first annual report as chair of surgery, Womack listed some of his goals for the department: "First, the clinical staff must be able to provide the surgical care required for all lesions that may be encountered, and this care must be of the highest order. Second, this clinical staff must also be able to provide at both the undergraduate and graduate levels a form of surgical education distinctive and effective in serving the needs of the state. Third, this staff must possess the imagination and ability to advance surgical knowledge in its particular field both by observations made in the experimental laboratory and in the clinical field . . . ."[118] The department under Womack's leadership was a unified one that included as divisions many areas that today are separate academic departments in the School of Medicine, such as anesthesiology, ophthalmology, orthopaedics, and otolaryngology.

One of Womack's trainees (who later became chair of a department in another medical school) wrote that Womack's name was at the top of every list of potential candidates that Berryhill assembled as he began recruiting for the surgical chair. Furthermore, "Berryhill and Womack had been friends as students at UNC and had a high regard for each other." For Womack it was a rare opportunity to build a new department while coming home to a university and a state he loved. This experience "must have made the difficult years at Iowa and the private practice burden in St. Louis fade into obscurity." For UNC and the medical school "it was a brilliant opportunity to have a favorite son at the height of his career and productivity, an international authority in academic surgery and surgical pathology, and a loyal North Carolinian" return to a leadership position in the expanded School of Medicine.[119]

Another former trainee of the surgical program under Womack (and who would also later chair an academic department of surgery elsewhere) recounted in a tribute to Womack: "Dr. Womack's greatest contribution to surgery was and continues to be Surgical Education. He brought a broad knowledge of biology to focus on human illness and the force of his intellect stimulated thought in each of the many house officers who came under his influence. I can't define the charisma which he projected and which ignited the imagination of all of us but without doubt, it was a powerful force. He was a scholar with a deep as well as a broad knowledge of many subjects . . . He was an academic person with an abiding affection and respect for the classical tradition of the university and so influenced us, as his students."[120]

The second clinical chair recruited was Charles Hoyt Burnett, MD, the chair of medicine. A native of Colorado born in 1913, Burnett received his AB and MD from the University of Colorado. He had residencies in pathology at Presbyterian Hospital in New York City and in medicine at the Boston City Hospital and Massachusetts General Hospital. His interest in metabolism, endocrinology, and nephrology was stimulated by his work with Fuller Albright, MD, who had done pioneering studies in metabolic bone disease. Burnett served in the military in World War II, during which he participated in studies of the severely wounded and the use of blood in treatment of shock. After the war he worked with Chester Keefer, MD, at Boston University, studying the interaction of bone disease and the kidney. Burnett first described the milk-alkali syndrome (now known as Burnett syndrome) that results from ingestion of excessive amounts of milk and alkaline salts. He was also part of a team at Chapel Hill that provided the first description of vitamin D–resistant rickets. After serving thirteen years as the chair, Burnett retired in 1965 because of a chronic debilitating disease that led to his death in 1967 at age fifty-four. He was succeeded as chair in 1965 by Louis G. Welt, MD, who served until 1972, when he became chair of the Department of Medicine at Yale.[121]

Burnett was of average height and thin, with penetrating blue eyes. He was known to his faculty colleagues as Chuck, but "to the students as 'old steely blue eyes' because when [he] fixed his gaze on you his eyes were indeed steely blue and focused somewhere about your mid-brain."[122] The medical house staff would meet each morning in his office to present the new patients that had been

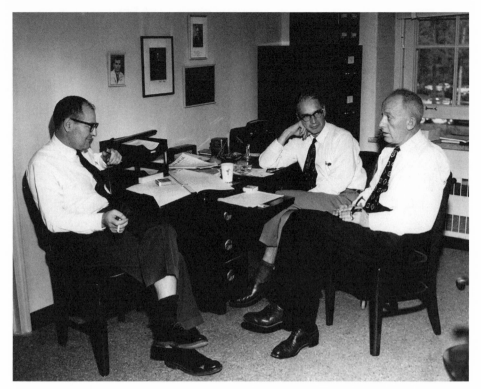

Drs. Louis G. Welt and Charles H. Burnett of the Department of Medicine with a visiting professor, Dr. Homer W. Smith, 1954. Smith was professor of medicine at New York University College of Medicine and a world authority on kidney function. *(UNC Photo Lab, NCC)*

admitted to their service. They would dread being "under the thumb" as Burnett would rotate his upward-pointing thumb around the circle to point to a resident to answer a question he had posed.[123]

A younger faculty member in medicine at the time of Burnett's chairmanship described him as "a gentle man, but a dynamic and forceful leader who had the ability to bring together diverse views." He felt strongly about the importance of the school's link to the university and believed that medical scholars should associate themselves with the humanists.[124] Floyd Denny, who came to UNC in 1960, described Burnett as "a no-nonsense guy and a nationally recognized investigator . . . He was one of the most well-rounded department chairs I have ever seen. He was a brilliant clinician and teacher, an excellent investigator and administrator, and a very thoughtful and kind human being."[125]

In his first annual report as chair of medicine, Burnett emphasized the pressing need for more faculty members because of the multiple pressures on faculty in his department owing to their heavy patient care and teaching demands and the expectation that faculty would also be investigators. In a summary in his 1957 annual report of the first five years of the department, Burnett reiterated this need while at the same time expressing the hope that the medical center "will not expand to any significant degree" and that "the pressure to increase the number of students can be resisted." He added, "One of the advantages of our entire unit has been that we are a relatively small and compact group and that 'empires' have had little opportunity to develop." While fully supporting the research activities of his faculty, he emphasized that quality of the research was the most important factor and that the department must "avoid getting too much support and too many research grants." In this review of "the very real accomplishments we have achieved since 1952," he warned "that a period of a certain amount of euphoria is probably about over. Much of the recognition which we have received as a department has been more on the basis of what we are expected to do than what we have actually achieved. The compliments we have received from visitors during periods when the dogwoods and redbuds are out have been flattering but not necessarily a true reflection of our actual ability."[126]

The clinical sciences building, completed in 1975, was named the Burnett-Womack Building in 1978 in honor of the first chairs in medicine and surgery. It was rededicated in 2006 after extensive renovations.

The third chair recruited by Berryhill was George Caverno Ham, MD, the chair of psychiatry. Ham was born in Edgewood, Pennsylvania, in 1912 and received his undergraduate education at Dartmouth College. He received the MD from the University of Pennsylvania in 1937 and had an internship, residency, and fellowship in medicine at the University of Pennsylvania Hospital. He was a Commonwealth Fund Fellow in Medicine at the University of Virginia and then served as an instructor in medicine at the University of Pennsylvania School of Medicine. During World War II he served in the army medical corps, doing research in war-related topics such as the influence of rapid changes in velocity on physiology and the effects of drugs on the central nervous system. After the war he had a residency in psychiatry at the Michael Reese Hospital in Chicago, and from 1949 to 1951 he was a research associate and then a faculty member at the Institute for Psychoanalysis in Chicago and at Michael Reese. He made his first published contributions to the field of psychosomatic medicine during this time.

Ham served as the chair of psychiatry at UNC from 1951 to 1964, when he retired to go into private practice in Chapel Hill. He was succeeded as chair by John Alexander Ewing, MD, ChB. Ham died in 1977.[127] The George Ham Society was formed in his honor in 1985 as the alumni association for the UNC psychiatry department.

Ham was a dynamic and charismatic leader and teacher. For several years he personally taught a ninety-six-hour, year-long introductory course in psychiatry for second-year medical students. He integrated the biological, social, and psychological components of illnesses and emphasized the relationship of the psyche to traditional medical problems in what was then the new field of psychosomatic medicine. So convincing was he that many of the students planned to go into psychiatry by the end of the course. Although this changed as the students had their other clinical rotations, many UNC students did pursue a career in psychiatry as a result of Ham's influence. His popularity as a speaker was affirmed when he was selected to deliver the annual Whitehead Lecture on September 23, 1952, to the medical students and faculty on the topic "Changing Concepts of Integrated Medicine."[128] In his audience were the members of the first third-year class, who would graduate in the spring of 1954 as the first MD graduates from UNC–CH.

Ham took seriously the state's mandate for the psychiatry department to help staff the expanding state mental hospitals. In this endeavor he worked closely with state Representative John W. Umstead. "Together they identified the resources and recruited the personnel to start the Department on [a course] to being recognized as one of the best in the United States. In a parallel and complementary effort, the four State Hospitals were constantly upgraded through extension of training programs from Chapel Hill and by national and international recruiting. Dr. Ham had the unusual ability to see what was needed and the talent and energy to accomplish it." The department has trained more than 40 percent of the psychiatrists currently practicing in North Carolina.[129]

The fourth chair recruited was William L. Fleming, MD, who was the first (and only) chair of preventive medicine, from 1951 to 1969. After Fleming retired, the Department of Preventive Medicine was merged into what is now the Department of Social Medicine.

A native of Morgantown, West Virginia, Fleming was born in 1905 and received his AB, MS, and MD degrees from Vanderbilt University. From 1932 to 1933 he interned at Bellevue Hospital in New York City and then returned to Vanderbilt for his residency in medicine. From 1937 to 1939 he was a Milbank Fellow at Johns Hopkins University Hospital. He became a staff member of the International Health Division of the Rockefeller Foundation in 1939 and had an appointment as a research professor in the UNC School of Public Health. During the war he established one of the nation's first research laboratories for the study of syphilis and helped conduct some of the first penicillin treatment studies in patients. He was professor and chair of the Department of Preventive Medicine at the Boston University School of Medicine from 1948 to 1952. By the time Fleming came to UNC, he was nationally recognized for his work on sexually transmitted diseases.[130]

In the early 1950s Fleming and several colleagues shared with the Department of Psychiatry the responsibility for teaching a first-year course in introduction to clinical medicine. They also taught a second-year course in epidemiology and a third-year course in preventive medicine.

Fleming, who was in charge of the outpatient clinics, obtained a grant of $160,000 from the Commonwealth Fund of New York starting in January 1953 "to support the establishment of the General Clinic . . . an interdepartmental venture in which an attempt is being made to give patients better service and medical student better instruction . . . in the Out-Patient Department of the N.C. Memorial Hospital." In his first annual report, Fleming said the department through the general clinic was developing "facilities for getting students out into the community to have contact with community agencies and to see patients in their homes and learn the importance of social and environmental factors in illness."[131] Dean Berryhill commented that this Commonwealth Fund grant was of "special significance [because] it marks the first sizable grant from a private foundation which the School has received. Furthermore, it indicates that nationally the School—because of the quality of its faculty and the uniqueness of its opportunity—is attracting attention."[132] Denny later commented that when he arrived at UNC in 1960 "there was an emphasis here on ambulatory care that was far beyond anything that I had ever experienced before. This was under Bill [Fleming]'s leadership and set the stage for the role that North Carolina has played subsequently in ambulatory medicine."[133]

Before and after his retirement from the UNC faculty in 1978, Fleming worked with both the Rockefeller Foundation and Project Hope in helping establish disease control laboratories in several countries, including Brazil, Jamaica, Ceylon, Egypt, and Tunisia. Fleming died in 2002 at age ninety-seven at a Chapel Hill retirement community.

The fifth recruit as chair, and the second native North Carolinian, was Ernest Harvey Wood, MD, the first chair of radiology. A native of New Bern, North Carolina, born in 1914, Wood graduated magna cum laude from Duke University and received the MD in 1939 from Harvard Medical School. Following an internship at the Philadelphia General Hospital and a residency in radiology at Columbia-Presbyterian Hospital in New York City, he served in the US Army during World War II from 1943 to 1946. After his military discharge with the rank of major he became an assistant professor of radiology at Columbia and was director of radiology at the Columbia-Presbyterian Neurological Institute from 1946 to 1952. During this time he authored the first book published on myelography and achieved international recognition as a neuroradiologist.

Wood served as chair of radiology at UNC from 1952 to 1965. James H. Scatliff, MD, who was then associate professor of radiology at Yale, followed him as chair.[134] In his first annual report, Wood noted that the department had three full-time faculty members, was housed in approximately 6,000 square feet of space in the hospital, and had fifteen X-ray units, two of them suitable for radiation therapy. His first faculty appointees were both assistant professors. Charles A. Bream, MD, joined the faculty in July 1952, and William H. Sprunt, III, MD, joined the faculty on January 1, 1953. In 1964 Wood co-authored with Juan Taveras, MD *Diagnostic Neuroradiology,* which came to be considered the outstanding reference book in the field at the time.

Wood returned to New York in 1965 as professor and chief of radiology at the Neurological Institute of the Columbia-Presbyterian Medical Center, a testament to his standing in the world of neuroradiology at the time. He suffered a

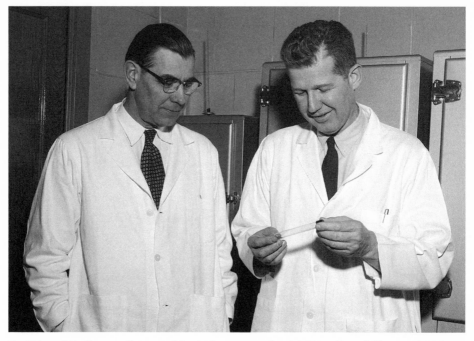

Dr. Edward C. Curnen discusses his virology research with Dean Berryhill, 1955. *(UNC Photo Lab, NCC)*

fatal heart attack in his office at the Neurological Institute in February of 1975 at the age of sixty. "His quiet charm, devotion to the highest ideals of professional integrity, and his scientific curiosity have been sources of inspiration to many," according to a colleague writing shortly after his death.[135] The UNC radiology departmental library, used daily by residents, students, and faculty, is named in his honor. The current chair of radiology now holds the endowed Ernest H. Wood Distinguished Professorship of Radiology.[136]

The sixth clinical chair recruited was Edward C. Curnen, Jr., MD, the first chair of pediatrics, a position he held from 1952 to 1960. In 1960 Curnen left UNC to assume one of the most prestigious positions in American pediatrics, that of chair of pediatrics at Columbia University and chief of pediatrics at Babies' Hospital in New York City.

Born in Yonkers, New York, in 1909, Curnen graduated from Yale College in 1931 and from the Harvard Medical School in 1935. After a year as a bacteriologist at Children's Hospital in Boston, he was an intern and resident at Children's Hospital from 1936 to 1939. This was followed by research in microbiology at the Rockefeller Institute. He served in the navy during World War II and then was a faculty member in pediatrics and preventive medicine at Yale from 1946 to 1952. His early research studies concerned the pathophysiology of bacterial infections such as pneumococcus and streptococcus, while his later investigations were in the field of virology. Curnen collaborated with some of the greatest researchers on infectious diseases at the time, including Maxwell Finland, Colin MacLeod, and Lewis Thomas. He continued his research on viral diseases while serving as chair at UNC.

Because Curnen didn't arrive until the summer of 1952, the department had little time for planning patient care and educational programs before the hospital opened on September 2, 1952. Curnen was the only full-time faculty member until Harrie R. Chamberlin, MD, arrived as an instructor in January 1953. They were ably assisted by several part-time faculty members, including Sidney Chipman, MD, from the School of Public Health, and Arthur London, MD, chief of pediatrics at Watts Hospital in Durham, who contributed two half days weekly to teaching third-year medical students. During the first year, 1952–1953, the department had forty-nine third-year students in pediatric clerkships, two pediatric interns, seventeen rotating interns, and two pediatric assistant residents.[137]

Curnen was tall and soft-spoken, and his natural shyness sometimes created awkwardness for those who did not know him well. Yet, according to an early faculty member in pediatrics, he was a leader who

> in eight short years . . . built a tradition of excellence in patient care, teaching, and research. He had done this in spite of a parsimonious budget provided by the Medical School and with resources far below those provided to the Departments of Medicine and Surgery . . . Curnen had established strong ties with pediatricians and family physicians throughout North Carolina; he had created respect among his peers because of his insistence on quality clinical care; he had established close collegial ties with the Department of Medicine and had laid the ground work for the eminently successful joint medicine-pediatric residency; and he had accomplished all this while simultaneously creating a strong tradition of excellence in research . . . Most important, Ed brought out the best in all of us and pointed out possibilities in each of us that were beyond our wildest imaginations.[138]

Curnen died at his home in New Haven, Connecticut, in 1997 at the age of eighty-eight.

The seventh and final recruit as chair was Robert A. Ross, MD, who served as the first chair of obstetrics and gynecology from 1952 to 1965. At age fifty-three, Ross was the senior member of the new clinical chairs, with Womack two years his junior. Born in Morganton in 1899, he was the third North Carolinian among the seven original clinical chairs. He earned the BS in medicine from the two-year School of Medicine at Chapel Hill in 1920 and the MD from the University of Pennsylvania in 1922. He had a residency in Philadelphia and was recruited as a faculty member in the early 1930s to the new Duke University Medical School by Bayard Carter, MD, Duke's first chair of obstetrics and gynecology.[139] Ross's career was interrupted by service in the navy beginning in 1940; he remained in the naval reserve after the war and retired with the rank of rear admiral in 1962.

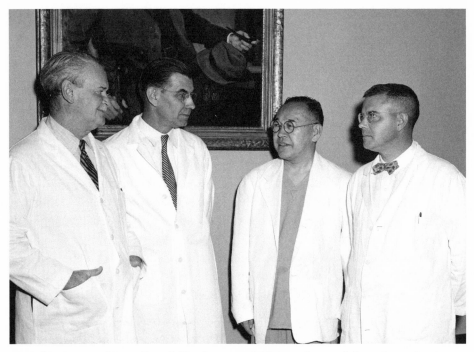

Dr. Robert Ross and Dean Berryhill welcome a visiting professor of obstetrics and gynecology from Japan, 1954. At the right is Dr. Warner Wells, assistant professor of surgery, who spent two years in Japan with the Atomic Bomb Casualty Commission. He translated and published *Hiroshima Diary,* an account by a Japanese physician of his experiences following the explosion of the atomic bomb at Hiroshima. *(UNC Photo Lab, NCC)*

Berryhill and Ross were especially close friends. In an article in a "Special Daddy Ross Issue" of the *North Carolina Medical Journal* in 1966, Berryhill stated that they had been friends for nearly fifty years and colleagues for the previous fourteen.[140] Berryhill went on to describe Ross's remarkable knowledge not only of his own specialty area, but of the Bible, history, English literature, and the English language. His appreciation for Ross's accomplishments in establishing the new department were "abundantly confirmed" during his 1964–1965 sabbatical tour of medical schools in Scotland, England, and the United States, where he found high regard for Ross and the accomplishments of his department. Berryhill added that Ross, as departmental chair, "thought first of the University, second of the Medical School, and third of his department," even though he "fought hard and stubbornly for his field and for those for whom he felt responsible." Berryhill especially appreciated the fact that after a particularly trying day Ross would drop by his office early the next morning. Even though they didn't always agree on the solution to a particular problem, Berryhill said Ross had an effective way of telling "a story about some mountain character in Burke Country or some historical figure in North Carolina, or quote a verse from the Bible, any one or all of which would be pertinent to a possible course of action or a decision which would be right and reasonable."

Ross was affectionately known far and wide as "Daddy" Ross. He was generally believed to have earned this nickname from all the babies he delivered in Durham and Chapel Hill. A former associate, however, related that it was bestowed during his undergraduate days at Chapel Hill, when he took care to see that "his classmates and fraternity brothers were tucked safely in bed when they had had too strenuous a night away from the books."[141] One former resident described Ross as "rather rotund Santa-Claus-type man (without the beard)" who was "large-framed and tall." He added that Ross "was close to his residents" but also "was a 'Chairman of the Board' type leader and not a one-on-one teacher."[142] According to Floyd Denny, Ross was "the local wag" who "always had some ready quip, and was full of homespun humor. It was with Daddy that I made a serious error in judgment. I thought at first that he was just a typical good ol' boy, only to learn that he was far smarter than I and that he was always ahead of me. Being a southern boy [from South Carolina] I should have known better, but I didn't."[143]

Ross's first two faculty recruits were Charles Fowler, MD (Johns Hopkins), and Leonard "Boom" Palumbo, MD (Duke). Because the obstetrics and gynecology space was not completed in the old infirmary wing until January 1953, the department had to operate in borrowed space when the hospital opened. For years Ross took delight in telling a now legendary story about the "first delivery" at Memorial Hospital: Early in the fall of 1952 an indigent woman from the country came to the hospital in labor, insisting that she wanted to have her baby here even though the delivery rooms weren't completed. She was delivered on her way into the hospital near the old emergency room entrance in the grassy backyard of the original hospital (where the bed tower now stands). The mother and baby were admitted and did well. When they were to be discharged, the business officer told Ross he didn't think it was right to charge them a delivery room fee because she had delivered in the hospital's backyard. After a moment's reflection, Dr. Ross suggested, "Just charge them a greens fee."

The first real delivery occurred in a surgery operating room on September 20, 1952. All twelve deliveries in 1952 were done in a surgery operating room; the mother remained in a bed borrowed from the surgery service before and after the delivery. After the renovated and new obstetrical and gynecology facilities with fifty beds were completed in January, the department had 368 deliveries during 1953, with 152 private patients and 216 staff patients. Only six cesarean sections were done, a rate of 1.6 percent, which was not unusual for the time.

For the first few years the medical students and residents supplemented their experiences in obstetrics by performing deliveries at the Robeson County Hospital in Lumberton, North Carolina, under the supervision of Hugh A. McAllister, MD, the first board-certified obstetrician in the area. The more senior residents had a six-month rotation in obstetrics at the Margaret Hague Maternity Center in Jersey City, New Jersey, where Ross's close friend was chief of obstetrics. In stark contrast to the volume at Memorial Hospital, the Hague center had upward of 10,000 deliveries a year. Since those early years, affiliations with AHEC hospitals in North Carolina have replaced these first two rotations for residents and students.[144]

In a eulogy at the memorial service for Ross in 1973, Bayard Carter stated that the Duke house officers "remember him with true love and with deep admiration. The students and house staff at Duke made him an honorary alumnus of Duke Medical School." Prior to his death his colleagues and friends endowed a chair in the UNC department in his name, as well as establishing the Robert A. Ross Obstetrical and Gynecological Society, which "has become a dynamic rallying point for the steadily increasing number of graduates of the program that Dr. Ross established." During his career Ross helped found obstetrical and gynecological societies for North Carolina and for the South Atlanta region and was elected to the presidency of all the major national organizations in his field.[145] Ross died in Chapel Hill in 1973.

Other Faculty Recruitment

Dean Berryhill delegated the responsibility for filling the other faculty positions in the new departments to the chairs, although he was actively involved in obtaining the support, interviewing the candidates, and signing off on the appointments.

The experience of one young academic surgeon revealed both the challenges facing those recruiting in the early days and the excitement and opportunities offered to new faculty members. He first visited Chapel Hill in December 1951: "En route by Eastern Airlines to Raleigh-Durham we landed in Richmond. Much to my surprise everyone else deplaned. As the sole remaining passenger, I thought, 'Raleigh-Durham must be the end of the world.' Of this I was fully convinced after finding the airport facilities to consist of a Quonset hut heated by a kerosene stove." His interest in joining the faculty, however, was soon stirred by a delicious shrimp Creole dinner with the Womacks at their temporary home in the Horace Williams House; by an interview with Dean Berryhill, "whose deep commitment to the School, the University, and the state of North Carolina was immediately apparent"; and by a discussion with Womack about his plans for the department. He was told that the hospital would open in July 1952, but "this seemed somewhat unrealistic" since at the time of his visit "the North Carolina Memorial Hospital seemed to be rising from a sea of red clay, much of which had been tracked indoors." After considering the offer, Colin G. Thomas, Jr., MD, became the second member of the surgical faculty in April of 1952, and subsequently served as the second chair of surgery, from 1966 to 1984.[146]

Ham's first recruit in psychiatry was David Hawkins, MD (Rochester), who joined the faculty in 1952. He remained here until 1967, when he became chair of psychiatry at the University of Virginia in Charlottesville. Hawkins much later related that he first thought Berryhill was a "hayseed"—especially as compared with the founding dean of the University of Rochester School of Medicine, the

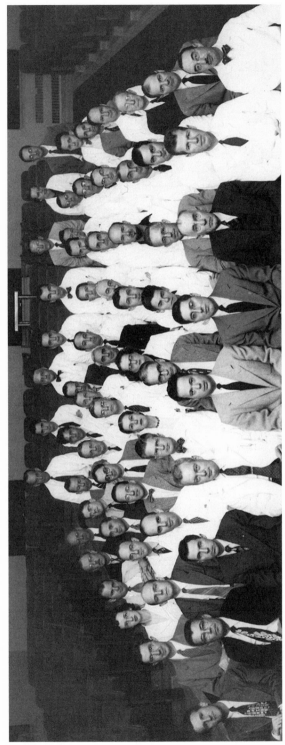

School of Medicine faculty, 1952–1953. *Column 1, front to back:* B. L. Truscott, anatomy; T. W. Farmer, neurological medicine; M. C. Swanton, pathology; G. P. Manire, bacteriology; C. D. Van Cleave, anatomy; J. C. Andrews, biological chemistry and nutrition. *Column 2:* J. H. U. Brown, physiology; I. M. Taylor, medicine; C. A. Bream, radiology; J. B. Graham, pathology; H. F. Parks, anatomy; C. W. Hooker, anatomy; C. E. Anderson, biological chemistry and nutrition. *Column 3:* W. R. Straughn, Jr., bacteriology; E. Craige, medicine; C. G. Thomas, Jr, surgery; O. J. B. Kerner, human development and psychology; R. B. Raney, surgery; J. E. Wilson, biological chemistry and nutrition; J. L. Irvin, biological chemistry and nutrition. *Column 4:* E. H. Wood, radiology; P. L. Bunce, surgery; A. Larson, bacteriology; G. C. Ham, psychiatry; S. S. Chipman, maternal and child health and pediatrics; J. A. Green, anatomy; A. P. Heusner, surgery. *Column 5:* J. G. Palmer, medicine; C. H. Burnett, medicine; L. M. Ward, medicine; J. H. Ferguson, physiology; E. C. Frank, psychiatry; G. D. Penick, pathology. *Column 6:* J. T. Sessions, Jr., medicine; D. C. Leary, obstetrics-gynecology; K. M. Brinkhous, pathology; D. A. MacPherson, bacteriology; D. R. Hawkins, psychiatry; R. D. Langdell, pathology. *Column 7:* W. C. George, histology and embryology, W. J. Cromartie, bacteriology and medicine; E. P. Hiatt, physiology; T. C. Butler, pharmacology; T. C. Barnett, medicine; J. M. Hitch, medicine; J. W. Fresh, physiology. *Column 8:* E. C. Curnen, Jr., pediatrics; M. Huppert, bacteriology; C. T. Kaylor, anatomy; J. B. Hill, pharmacology; W. R. Berryhill, medicine; W. L. Wells, surgery; J. J. Fischer, medicine. *Column 9:* W. P. Richardson, preventive medicine; L. G. Welt, medicine; J. B. Bullitt, pathology; F. W. Ellis, pharmacology; H. C. Patterson, surgery and anatomy; R. L. Peters, obstetrics-gynecology; N. D. Fischer, surgery.

New Englander and Nobel laureate George H. Whipple, MD (1878–1976). He even wondered how Berryhill had become dean, but as the years passed he was much more impressed by him. He came to realize that few people could have done what Berryhill did with the alumni and legislators; his down-home style paid off.[147]

The Berryhills' gracious hospitality was soon evident to the new faculty as they moved to Chapel Hill or moved within the town. One of the first faculty members in pediatrics recalled: "It was December 1, 1955, the long-awaited date on which we were to move, after three years in a Glen Lennox apartment, into our own house. Returning [from a trip], I was surprised to learn that Norma Berryhill had telephoned Bets and asked if she might bring us our first dinner in our new setting. It was unclear how Norma had learned of our moving day . . . Reece had not been mentioned, but they both arrived about 6 P.M." Since there was no doorbell yet, one of the children must have seen them and let them in. "In any event there they suddenly were, beaming at us from the far end of our long kitchen. Reece was bearing a goodly portion of a roast beef, clearly just out of their oven. Norma had peas in a perfectly polished Revere Ware pot, plus another vegetable and even a dessert." After a quick tour of the new house and a stop to admire the young couple's two-week-old daughter in her crib, "they were gone, leaving us to enjoy the truly fine meal that they had prepared for us." He added, "Though Reece and Norma did this for many others, it was an unforgettable event for us . . . We were part of an extended family headed by a couple who, though held a bit in awe by some, were deeply admired by all."[148]

END OF AN ERA AND BEGINNING OF A NEW ONE

As Berryhill was writing the introduction to his annual report for the academic year ending in June 1952, he could not help but be exhilarated by the fact that the university hospital was soon to open and the clinical instruction of medical students was to begin, with the prospect of the first MD graduates from UNC at Chapel Hill two years later. He declared that the 1951–1952 year "has been a most significant year in the history of the School of Medicine."

Yet in his typical pragmatic style, he recognized the ongoing challenges and stated that what should have been the most "exciting and satisfying year" since the beginning of medical education at Chapel Hill was in fact "the most frustrating in the past decade" because of "budgetary and numerous other restrictions and uncertainties."

"Nevertheless," he concluded, "in spite of what seem to be an unnecessarily large number of obstacles from within, the Medical School has made substantial progress. The high standards of teaching and the quality of research which have . . . characterized the Medical School have continued and have been enhanced by the extraordinarily competent new staff members."[149]

CHAPTER 8

Dean of the Four-Year School of Medicine

A decade after the opening of the four-year school a member of the university trustees said:

> I have laughingly told Dean Berryhill that he and I are the only two individuals in the entire history of the University, as far as I can discover, who have served as illegitimate off-springs of the University—he as Dean of the four-year Medical School and I as the Chairman of a Medical Committee of the Trustees. As for him, [he] was duly and lawfully elected by the Trustees as Dean of the two-year Medical School in 1941, but it seems never to have occurred to anyone that he needed to be elected Dean of the new four-year school. In reality this failure to act is a compliment to him for it attests the unanimous opinion of the Trustees and the Administration that he, and only he, would be considered for the new responsibility. His illegitimacy was finally cured by his official recognition by the Trustees as the Dean of the new Medical School.[1]

Berryhill's challenges and satisfactions during his first year as the dean of a four-year school were summarized in his report in October 1953 on the first year of operation of the new hospital and expanded school in the first issue of the *Bulletin of the School of Medicine*:

> Never since medical instruction began at the University of North Carolina in 1879 has so much of fundamental importance taken place in any twelve-month period as during the past year. Understandably there were problems and difficulties incident to the opening of the hospital, the organization of the clinical services, and the intern and resident programs—but on the whole the year was an exciting and genuinely satisfying one.
>
> I would like to pay tribute to the patience, the loyalty, and the understanding of the medical faculty, the intern and resident group, and the student body, all of whom carried on their work in superb fashion throughout the year.[2]

An unsigned editorial entitled "To Serve the People" in the same issue of the

Bulletin reinforced Berryhill's upbeat evaluation of the new endeavor at Chapel Hill:

> There is a spirit at Chapel Hill that must emanate for good to the entire state. It is a spirit of sincere, intelligent, untiring desire to place the facilities of medical education, medical research, and medical services within reach of all people of the State. That spirit inspires the administration, the faculty, the staff, and the students. It will be obvious to all who come to Chapel Hill.
>
> The State has given the University's medical center its mandate. That mandate is proudly accepted. Through the years its contributions must, and they will, register a singleness of purpose: to serve the people of North Carolina.[3]

Hospital

North Carolina Memorial Hospital Opens

Although Berryhill and the medical school were not then organizationally in charge of the hospital's operation, he and the clinical chairs were intimately involved in preparing for the opening of the hospital and the beginning of clinical medical student education and of graduate (house staff) medical education in the new facility. By September 1952 they had recruited forty full-time faculty members to provide the attending coverage for the hospital's clinical services. Fifty-two part-time clinical faculty members, who assisted with clinical and teaching responsibilities, supplemented their efforts. An additional thirty-six full-time faculty members were present in the basic sciences departments of the medical school.[4]

Some 108 hospital employees had been hired during the summer and were given training and orientation sessions in August 1952.[5] The newly recruited nurses were almost the only employees who had ever worked in hospitals before; most other support personnel had been recruited locally. Elizabeth (Lib) Warren, RN, a member of the nursing staff from 1952 to 1990, remembered: "The nurses had a lot of responsibility. We felt we had responsibility for the total hospital, being sure everything got together and that it was workable. When we first opened, we did everything." The first hospital director later observed, "The nurses did a remarkable job."[6] By the end of the first fiscal year of operation on June 30, 1953, the number of hospital employees (including part-time employees and house staff members) had grown to 511.[7]

While the hospital construction was being completed, many large items of equipment had to be temporarily housed in the "Tin Can," a space the size of five basketball courts that had served the university since 1924 as an indoor athletic court and the site of student dances.[8] At the end of June 1952, "Operation Tin Can" was initiated with a crew of seventeen high school boys and some trucks to move the equipment to the new hospital, starting on the seventh floor and working downward as the construction was completed floor by floor.[9]

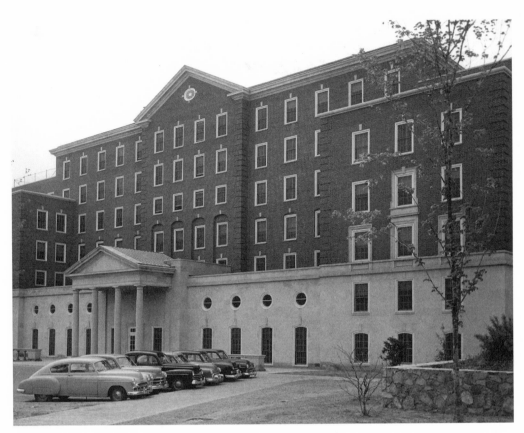

North Carolina Memorial Hospital, 1953. *(UNC Photo Lab, NCC)*

On August 8, 1952, Robert Cadmus, the first hospital director, wrote to Chancellor House: "I thought that you would like to know that after serious consideration we have decided to open the hospital for patients September 2, 1952. Because of construction delays with which you are familiar, I am sure that you realize that this is for all practical purposes an impossible task. Yet my staff and I have pledged ourselves to its accomplishment knowing full well that we have your approval and support in so doing."[10] Even though hospital construction would not be completed until December 18, 1952, planning for the September opening proceeded.[11]

In the late morning on Tuesday, September 2, 1952, the first patient was admitted to the new North Carolina Memorial Hospital and was assigned medical records unit number 00-00-01. The young woman was referred by Robert McMillan, MD, of Southern Pines, and admitted to the medicine service. Charles H. Burnett, MD, chair of medicine, was the attending physician, and C. P. Adams, MD, was the house officer; he documented an extensive history and physical examination. By the end of the first day seven patients had been admitted.[12] The first patient was still alive in 1992 on the occasion of the fortieth anniversary of the hospital's opening.[13]

Thomas Barnett, MD, a young faculty member in medicine, recalled the very first patient seen at the hospital that first day but not admitted. She arrived in the outpatient clinic very early in the morning. He saw her, recognized that her situation was out of his specialty area, and requested a consultation. Dr. Ross and his obstetrics-gynecology resident confirmed Barnett's diagnosis of "intra-uterine pregnancy, very near term." She was advised to return to the OB clinic the next week but returned earlier in labor. Because the newborn nursery and labor room were not yet completed, she returned to her local community hospital, where she was delivered of a normal child.[14]

On September 5, 1952, the hospital's seventh patient was the first patient to have an operative procedure in the new operating rooms. She was a sixty-six-year-old patient from western North Carolina, referred because of a two-year history of increasing pain in her right hip. James Manly, MD, a senior assistant resident in surgery working under the supervision of R. Beverly Raney, MD, the first chief of orthopedics, performed under local anesthesia a biopsy of a destructive lesion involving the hip and acetabular region. A diagnosis of "adenocarcinoma, papillary, moderately well differentiated, compatible with ovarian or bowel origin" was made. The patient received radiation therapy and lived until January 1955.[15]

When the hospital opened, seventy-eight beds were activated. Not only did it lack a functional labor room and newborn nursery, but the emergency room was truly a room—the treatment room on 3-West. The new labor rooms and neonatal nursery finally occupied the top two floors of the renovated and enlarged student infirmary building in January 1953, and in the interim a few deliveries were performed in the operating rooms. These temporary conditions were deemed necessary because the house staff had started their year on July 1 at various hospitals around the state and it was thought essential to get them back to Memorial Hospital as soon as possible.

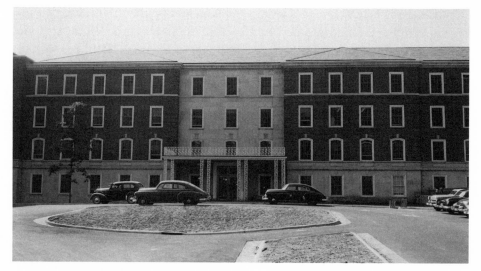

Original outpatient clinic at North Carolina Memorial Hospital, 1952. *(UNC Photo Lab, NCC)*

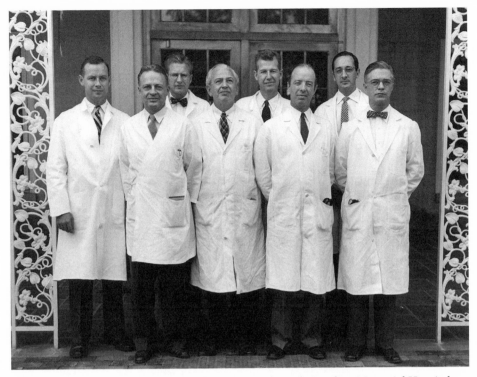

Heads of the clinics in the outpatient department of North Carolina Memorial Hospital, 1952. *Left to right:* Drs. S. D. McPherson, Jr. (ophthalmology), R. Beverly Raney (orthopedics), Paul L. Bunce (urology), Nathan A. Womack (post-operative clinic), Edward C. Curnen, Jr. (pediatrics), William L. Fleming (chairman, outpatient department, and head of the general clinic), Newton D. Fischer (eye, ear, nose, and throat), and George C. Ham (chair of psychiatry, taking the place of Dr. Edward C. Frank, director of the psychiatry clinic). *Not shown:* Dr. Robert A. Ross (obstetrics and gynecology). *(UNC Photo Lab, NCC)*

Thirteen months later, in October 1953, 210 beds were open in North Carolina Memorial Hospital. During the first twelve months the hospital had 3,687 admissions from almost 90 of the 100 North Carolina counties.[16]

The first outpatients were seen in a temporary clinic in the 3-West unit until the opening of the outpatient clinic wing, which joined the hospital with Mac-Nider Hall. There were almost 30,000 outpatient visits during the first twelve months after the hospital's opening.[17]

National attention to the new hospital and academic medical center came in various forms. Notably, the October 1953 issue of *Hospital Management: The News and Technical Journal of Administration,* published in Chicago, was devoted to "the complete story of every department of the North Carolina Memorial Hospital." The editor commented:

North Carolina is certainly in the forefront of health progress and there is no better yardstick of this enlightened point of view than this issue of *Hospital Management . . .*

We present this month an unusual view of a teaching hospital being activated. It is a brand new project . . .

What makes this story of North Carolina Memorial Hospital especially interesting and especially beneficial to all hospitals is that the staff herein makes a frank appraisal of the job that has been done. There have been problems. They have been the problems of all hospitals sharpened by a special situation.

Seen in the large, one cannot help but be impressed by the fact that the great state of North Carolina is going to be mightily benefited by this serious endeavor.[18]

The First House Staff

Berryhill described the first house staff of the North Carolina Memorial Hospital as enthusiastic and mature, in spite of the difficulties of newly organized clinical services and a relative paucity of patients. He added that the North Carolinians in this group had "a sense of accomplishment and pride in contributing to a high level of patient care and education in the hospital of their own university and in their native state."[19]

The first house staff were recruited primarily from two groups—those who were at the hospitals and medical schools from which the first clinical chairs were recruited, and those who had had their first two years of medicine at Chapel Hill. Fourteen of the original twenty-six intern staff were in the latter category; two others had graduated from the university but had not attended the medical school. The interns and the twenty-four residents made up a total house staff of fifty during 1952–1953.[20]

Although the national intern-matching program had started in 1951, the new hospital had permission to secure its first group of interns outside the match.[21]

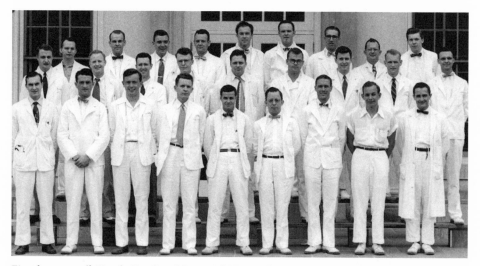

First house staff, North Carolina Memorial Hospital, 1952–1953. *(UNC Photo Lab, NCC)*

George T. Wolff, MD, a member of the first house staff, provided insight into how Berryhill utilized this flexibility to make a personal and direct approach to recruitment of the house staff for 1952–1953.

> I knew Dr. Berryhill through my father, so when I went to UNC as an undergraduate I went to visit him. My [visits with him were] brief, but pleasant. I applied to med school and was accepted at Chapel Hill and at Jefferson in Philadelphia. However Uncle Sam said he needed me for the war so I went to the navy. When I returned Jefferson said my acceptance was still good while UNC said apply again. As you can guess I went to Jeff. In my senior year at Jeff I received a four-page telegram from Dr. Berryhill. In it he said they hadn't treated the returning veterans right and he wanted to make it up to me. He then offered me a rotating internship in the first house staff at N.C. Memorial Hospital. I was delighted to accept even though I spent July and August at the High Point Hospital because N.C. Memorial wasn't opened until September.[22]

John L. Watters, MD, a 1950 graduate of UNC's two-year school and a member of the hospital's first house staff, later commented on this first year at North Carolina Memorial Hospital:

> Dean Berryhill recruited us to come back to UNC to be on the housestaff. It was quite a culture shock for most of us, because we had been busy in medical school or in internships in other hospitals. When the UNC Hospital opened, we all sort of swooped down on the first patient. But the patient load grew gradually, and I think we had more responsibility here than many of our peers had at other bigger hospitals because our housestaff was so small.[23]

In the School of Medicine's annual report for 1952–1953, Berryhill elaborated on the composition and performance of the first house staff group, to whom "the University will ever owe a deep debt of gratitude":

> It would be fair to say that no institution has ever had a more capable, interested, or loyal group of men on its intern and resident staff. Since 65% of those are our own former students, it can be safely said that they accepted positions here only because of their interest in this Medical School and their desire to contribute to its further development. The year has been a most difficult one for them and in some respects, for the intern group especially, an inadequate one. Yet throughout they have maintained the very finest sort of spirit, although at times disillusioned; they have given excellent care to patients and have worked unceasingly for the improvement of the organization.[24]

The two-month delay in the hospital's opening, originally scheduled for July 1952, provided two advantages, according to Berryhill. First, it enabled more of the essential clinical faculty and hospital staff to be in place when the hospital opened. Second, it provided a glimpse into the possibilities and problems with utilizing community and other state hospitals for the medical school educational program. These contacts and lessons would be of value in the late 1960s when Berryhill was promoting the community hospital–medical school affiliations that would provide the foundation for the highly successful NC AHEC Program.[25]

By the 1953–1954 academic year the internship and many of the residency programs had AMA approval, and the hospital had begun participating in the intern-matching program. The total house staff in the second year of the hospital's operation numbered seventy-three, including one administrative resident.[26]

Dedication of the Hospital and Medical Center, April 1953

The planning by Berryhill and many others at Chapel Hill and throughout the state culminated on a sunny spring weekend in late April 1953 as many hundreds of North Carolina health professionals, UNC alumni, and other citizens

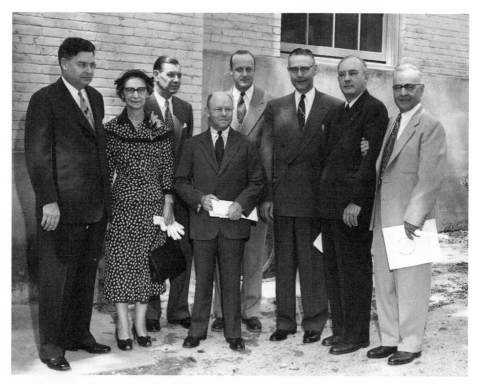

Participants in the opening day dedication ceremonies for the new medical center at UNC, April 1953. *Left to right:* A. O. Smith, president of the North Carolina Hospital Association; Josephine Kerr, president, North Carolina State Nurses' Association; Dean W. Reece Berryhill; Dr. Joseph T. Wearn, dean, Western Reserve University School of Medicine, the keynote speaker; Dr. Henry T. Clark, Jr., administrator, UNC Division of Health Affairs; the Rev. Kelsey Regen, First Presbyterian Church, Durham, who gave the invocation; Dr. J. Street Brewer, president, North Carolina Medical Society; and Dr. A. C. Current, president, North Carolina State Dental Society. *(UNC Photo Lab, NCC)*

attended a dedication ceremony at Chapel Hill for the new North Carolina Memorial Hospital, the expanded School of Medicine, and the new Schools of Dentistry and Nursing.[27] The previous Sunday's *Raleigh News and Observer* had had a special twenty-four-page "U.N.C. Medical Center Edition" section that provided an overview of the dedication events and a history of the medical and other health schools, as well as photographs of many of the new faculty and articles on most of the medical school departments and on the other schools of health sciences. A full-page advertisement taken out by "the merchants of Chapel Hill and Carrboro" invited the "men and women of the medical, dental and nursing profession . . . to come and inspect the new hospital and medical center" on Thursday, April 23. Then, on the following two days, "the remaining residents of North Carolina are extended a most cordial invitation by the hospital officials and the merchants of Chapel Hill and Carrboro to visit our fair village and also be taken on guided inspection tours of your new North Carolina Memorial Hospital."[28]

On the first day, April 23, 1953, a convocation was held in the university's Memorial Hall, at which time greetings were extended from representatives of other universities and the state's medical, dental, nursing, and hospital administrative organizations. Joseph Wearn, Berryhill's former colleague at Harvard and Western Reserve and then dean of the School of Medicine of Western Reserve University in Cleveland, gave the keynote address, entitled "The Challenge of the New University Medical Center." The afternoon was devoted to meetings

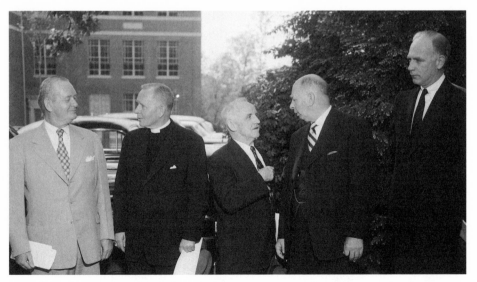

Participants in the second day of the dedication ceremonies for the new medical center at UNC, April 1953. *Left to right:* Lennox P. McLendon, chairman of the UNC Trustees Committee on Health Affairs; Edwin A. Penick, bishop of the North Carolina Episcopal Diocese, who gave the invocation; Frank Porter Graham, former UNC president and principal speaker; Chancellor Robert B. House; and UNC President Gordon Gray. *(UNC Photo Lab, NCC)*

of several professional groups of alumni and visitors, with a dinner meeting of the medical alumni in the evening.

On April 24 another convocation was held in Memorial Hall for the formal dedication of the new academic medical center. Frank Porter Graham, UNC president during the expansion of the medical center, former US senator, and then special representative of the United Nations in the India-Pakistan dispute, gave the dedicatory address. He began by expressing the view that North Carolina now had the opportunity to build "one of the major coordinated university medical centers of the modern world." Then, drawing on his training as a historian, he traced the evolution of medicine and medical centers from their Greco-Roman origins until the modern era. He observed, "America has [made] many contributions to the sciences and arts of medicine. One of the greatest is the medical center on the graduate level as an organic part of a great university." He concluded, "We dedicate this hospital and medical center for the finding of truth, the teaching of youth and the service of the people in their pilgrimage of hope for . . . freedom and health, justice and peace in the world."[29] Three days after his address Graham was tapped by the university's highest honorary society, the Order of the Golden Fleece, as its "Member of the Half Century."

The *UNC Alumni Review* characterized the dedication events as "days of celebration" that marked "another important milestone in the development of the five-school health center at the University."

Early Operational Challenges for the Hospital

Berryhill's insistence that the expanded medical school and teaching hospital be on the university campus in Chapel Hill provided some demanding challenges in the early years. Today the Chapel Hill community is accessible by four-lane interstate and US highways, and critically ill patients can be speedily transported to the medical center by helicopter. Chapel Hill has a permanent population (in addition to the some 25,000 UNC students) of some 50,000, and the population of the three counties and many communities in the Research Triangle area is approaching one million.[30] In 1952, however, the hospital was in a small community of a few thousand permanent inhabitants with access only by winding two-lane highways from Raleigh to the east, Durham to the north, Pittsboro to the south, and Burlington and Greensboro to the west.[31] Not only was the hospital census low in those early days, but more than 60 percent of patients could pay little or none of the full cost of their hospital care.

The hospital's fiscal situation was further compromised by the fact that the hospital initially used an inclusive rate plan. The daily rates ranged from $14 for a bed in a ward to $27 for a single room with private toilet and bath. The inclusive rate included "the cost of such hospital services and supplies as room, board, operating room, delivery room, anesthesia . . . drugs included in the hospital formulary, parenteral solutions, oxygen therapy, X-ray and radium, all laboratory procedures . . . [and] physical therapy."[32] This inclusive charge was structured so as to not impose fiscal restraints on those caring for the patients in a university hospital setting. This policy, however, created an unrealistic situation and rapidly led to overutilization of many ancillary services, which soon became swamped with requests. The monies were not available to add personnel or equipment because the services were generating no revenues while significantly adding to the hospital's costs.

A report a year after the hospital opened noted that in the early days of the hospital's operation, an average of eleven X-rays were taken for each patient admitted, but that this dropped during the first year to "an average of four films per patient examined, which indicates to us that requests are being self-regulated and it is not felt that unnecessary procedures are being requested." These films included "routine chest photo-fluorograms . . . on all patients . . . for the protection of both our patients and our employees [from tuberculosis]." The same report commented that "it is still a debatable question as to whether the inclusive rate stimulates unnecessary requests for laboratory procedures or whether it actually affords better medical care . . . It is our feeling . . . that very few unnecessary procedures are actually being requested. Still the line where necessity ends and luxury begins is difficult to determine."[33] These initial optimistic views did not persist, however, as time went on.

When the hospital opened it had two categories of patients, with the category being determined by hospital interviewers:

> Patients whose financial circumstances prevent payment of the full cost of medical care are called "service" patients and are not charged professional fees. They are charged in accordance with their financial resources a single daily fee (inclusive fee) to cover charges for room and board as well as necessary tests and services when hospitalized, and fees for visits and diagnostic treatment services for outpatient care. They are cared for under the supervision of senior staff physicians—in the service clinics of the Outpatient Department when ambulatory, and on the "ward services" in multiple bed units (single units only if condition warrants) when hospitalization is necessary.
>
> Private patients pay professional fees and are cared for by a senior physician of their choice or one selected by the service, if no preference has been expressed. They are cared for in the Private Clinic, if ambulatory, where in addition to professional fees, they pay fees for diagnostic and treatment services. If hospitalized they are cared for in a private or semi-private room according to their preference where in addition to professional fees they pay a single inclusive fee for hospital facilities and services.

The fees charged to service patients in the outpatient department in 1953 were "$2.00 for the first clinic visit (which includes certain routine laboratory tests) and $1.00 for subsequent visits. Separate charges are made for diagnostic procedures and treatment services other than those done routinely."[34]

Berryhill, Cadmus, and the university administration rapidly became aware of the hospital's fiscal problems. In his first letter to the hospital staff, dated February 18, 1953, Cadmus apprised them of the situation: "You have helped your hospital provide some 9,783 days of care to our bed patients and 9,355 visits to our Out Patient Department." For the period starting July 1, 1952 (even though patients did not come until September 2, 1952), "salaries, supplies and other expenses for this period have totaled $704,830," while "income from patients and other sources have only netted $213,375." He added, "The State has had to make up the difference by its very generous appropriation," but "very little of our original allocation remains." An emergency supplemental appropriation of $341,155 was being requested to carry the hospital until the end of June. Cadmus emphasized that the supplemental request was an "honest and realistic estimation of our needs, but we must live within this amount. No item of expense—salary or supply—nor any item of income can deviate from this estimate." Department heads would be held to their monthly expenditure budgets and he urged all to cooperate, just as they would in "living within a family budget."[35]

Cadmus commented after the hospital's first year of operation on the challenges of opening a new public-supported hospital: "From our brief experience it seems that hospitals are to citizen groups much like ponies are to small boys. They inherently want them and vaguely know for what purpose they will use them, but they are relatively unfamiliar and some even quite unconcerned about the cost and effort it takes to maintain them."[36] Berryhill and his colleagues commented much later on the broader problems of meeting the hospital's needs during its earlier years within a fairly rigid state university system:

> The state of North Carolina had been involved in the operation of hospitals since the opening of the Dorothea Dix Hospital in Raleigh in 1856. However, the budgeting and personnel divisions of the state government, as well as the General Assembly, had been concerned only with the costs, the personnel, and the organization involved in chronic care of the psychiatric, tuberculosis, and orthopedic hospitals. Consequently, the director of the North Carolina Memorial Hospital faced the problems of educating the university and the consolidated university business management . . . and the state agencies. For all, it was a new experience to gain an understanding of the reasons for the expense involved in operating a general hospital with the necessity for more expensive equipment, increased numbers and more experienced personnel in all areas, and the necessity of obtaining emergency supplies and equipment without waiting for weeks or months while requisitions went through channels.[37]

For instance, when the hospital opened, its purchasing department was not a separate operation but was established as a component of the university's purchasing department. Requests for some supplies had to be routed through the university's scientific supply room, which furnished supplies for the undergraduate teaching laboratories, while many of the office supplies had to be routed through the university's bookstore. Both were closed on weekends and during university holidays.[38]

William B. Aycock, UNC's second chancellor, who served from 1957 to 1964, recalled that in the early days of his administration an official in the state budget office in Raleigh would call the hospital director's office daily to obtain the patient census figure as an indication of the hospital's fiscal status.[39]

In 1958 a newspaper journalist attempted to educate the public about the costs of operating a public teaching hospital. He noted that Memorial Hospital had needed about $1 million a year of state appropriations since it opened six years previously. He compared the teaching hospital, which tended to have the more complicated cases, with the county hospital. The added complexity of the diagnostic problems seen in the teaching hospitals required "a battery of X-rays, specialists, and special treatments." The teaching hospital also had a larger staff precisely because it was a teaching hospital, responsible for educating medical and other students and young physicians. Finally, he noted that only about 30 percent of Memorial's patients paid the full bill, while the remaining 70 percent were "staff" patients who got free care from the physicians, and most of these paid little or none of the hospital's costs.[40]

Berryhill and colleagues wrote in their 1979 history of the medical school that the budget situation improved somewhat for the hospital when it came under the medical school in 1956, particularly during the administration of Governor Luther Hodges (1954–1960), a longtime friend of the Berryhills: "As a result of his interest and support and through the understanding and the helpfulness of Mr. Paul Johnson, the [state's] director of administration, a degree of flexibility never before known was most helpful. These years were the highlight of the hospital's existence in terms of administration." Berryhill added, "There was increased incentive, from the director to the ward maid, and a confidence that this hospital could thereafter develop and operate with the flexibility to meet its needs in a manner comparable to other institutions of its caliber." This hope and much of this operational flexibility for the hospital, however, were dashed during a subsequent state administration in the 1960s.[41]

Memorial Hospital's Changing Administrative Structure

Cadmus, who had been recruited by Clark in 1950 as professor and director of the hospital, directed the hospital and reported to Clark as the administrator of the Division of Health Affairs until 1956. As noted in chapter 7, the hospital director started reporting to the dean of the School of Medicine on September 1, 1956, rather than to the administrator of the Division of Health Affairs. In the spring of 1956 Cadmus asked Clark for, and received, a brief paid leave of absence "to determine what I should do in regard to the recent decision to place the Hospital under the School of Medicine." He added that he had informed his associates of his leave and had "asked them to keep all routine matters going but to refer new problems to Dean Berryhill or yourself, depending upon circumstances."[42]

Cadmus soon returned to his position as hospital director. According to Berryhill and colleagues, Cadmus "quickly found that the support of the medical faculty and of the dean was of the greatest assistance in solving some of the problems which were inherent in the hospital's operation under the original structure. Thereafter, until his request to resign from the directorship to develop a department of hospital administration in the medical school, no one could have worked more conscientiously to achieve the goals of a modern university medical center than Dr. Cadmus."[43]

In a series of letters in late 1961 and 1962 to Clark and Chancellor Aycock, Berryhill recommended the implementation of "the long planned Department of Hospital Administration" in the School of Medicine, with Cadmus as the chairman. "I am convinced the University has a very real opportunity for leadership in the general field of education, research, and consulting service in the general field of hospital administration and medical care relations, in which Dr. Cadmus has demonstrated ability and interest." The board of trustees approved his request in the spring of 1962 when they appointed Cadmus as professor and chairman of the new Department of Hospital Administration and consulting director of North Carolina Memorial Hospital, effective July 1, 1962.[44]

One of the tasks Cadmus undertook in his new capacity was to provide a detailed report on the potential for graduate medical education at Moses H. Cone Memorial Hospital in Greensboro.[45] This report provided the framework in 1967 for the formal affiliation of the UNC medical school with Moses Cone, the first of a number of medical school–community hospital affiliations for teaching purposes. Cadmus served as departmental chair until September 1966, when he resigned after sixteen years at UNC to return to his native New Jersey as president of the New Jersey College of Medicine and Dentistry.[46]

In a letter of February 11, 1962, to Aycock about the new department and Cadmus's appointment as chairman, Berryhill also recommended the "appointment of Mr. E. B. Crawford, Jr., as Director of the North Carolina Memorial Hospital as the successor to Dr. Cadmus in this important position of responsibility." Berryhill elaborated, "The years immediately ahead will be full and difficult ones . . . We will have to 'feel our way' in these developments because my own retirement as Dean of the School of Medicine will take place in this period." He thus recommended that Crawford be appointed for an initial three-year period and that the administrative relationship of Crawford and Cadmus as well as the accomplishments of Crawford as the new director be reviewed after three years.[47] Crawford served for five years, resigning in 1967 to accept a position with a hospital system in Delaware.[48]

Berryhill and colleagues recounted the medical faculty's initial concern about the original recommendations in the late 1960s to again remove the hospital from the direction of the School of Medicine and to establish a separate board to operate the hospital. When this change did occur through legislative action in 1971, however, Berryhill and colleagues stated, "Perhaps the most significant change in the hospital has been a change in its governance."[49] This change resulted in a board of directors for the hospital that included the dean of the medical school as an ex officio member. The resulting operational flexibility was the beginning of many positive developments over the succeeding years that have led to the vastly expanded and fiscally sound hospital operation know today as the UNC Hospitals within the UNC Health Care System.[50]

MEDICAL STUDENTS

Class of 1954: The First MD Graduates from Chapel Hill

Berryhill proudly noted in the fall of 1953 that the university had enrolled four classes of medical students for the first time since the Raleigh Medical Department was closed in 1910 and for the first time ever on the Chapel Hill campus. During the academic year 1953–1954, a total of 226 medical students were enrolled: 60 freshmen, 59 sophomores, 59 juniors, and 48 seniors. All but four were from North Carolina.[51]

When the medical class of 1954 entered the first year in the fall of 1950, it was still not certain that the hospital would be finished in time for them to complete their clinical training at Chapel Hill and earn the MD degree from UNC. Dean Berryhill thus gave the students the choice of staying at Chapel Hill for their clinical years or transferring to other schools, as had those before them for many decades. Only seven members of the class chose to transfer; four went to Harvard and one each to Cornell, Jefferson, and McGill.

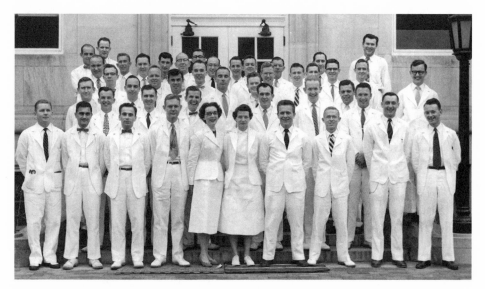

The School of Medicine class of 1954, the first to receive the MD degree from UNC at Chapel Hill. (UNC Photo Lab, NCC)

Berryhill described the class of 1954 as "an unusually able, mature, and understanding group." He later elaborated on their experiences:

> For them the four years as medical students were "the best of times, the worst of times." They were the "best" because of their pride in being the first graduating class and their motivation to set high standards of performance. Also important were the united efforts of the small but very conscientious faculty who devoted a high proportion of their time to this class, with a resulting close student-faculty relationship, which has persisted. And it was perhaps the "worst" because no class lived through four years with more physical inconveniences—crowded laboratories, noise of construction on all sides, and the inevitable frustrations in the newly organized hospital services . . .[52]

A member of this class later recalled their special bond with Berryhill: "I had a good relationship with Dr. Berryhill and had great respect and admiration for his talents as a teacher and administrator. I had been invited along with other members of my class for social gatherings in Dr. Berryhill's home by Mrs. Norma Berryhill and had met their daughters, particularly Jane, who was a contemporary." He also remembered Berryhill's meeting with their class at the end of their freshman and sophomore years.[53]

The university's 160th annual commencement on June 7, 1954, was a special event for Berryhill and the school. Seventy-five years after medical education began at the university in 1879, the MD degree was awarded to the first class of medical students educated entirely at Chapel Hill. At the university's commencement ceremony, Chancellor House introduced the speaker, Andrew Jackson Warren, MD, by noting, "It is fitting and appropriate that Dr. Warren should be our commencement speaker on this occasion when the first students graduate from our expanded School of Medicine and our new School of Dentistry." Warren, a North Carolinian who attended UNC and earned his MD degree from Tulane, had a long and distinguished career in public health and was then director of the Rockefeller Foundation's efforts in health care around the world. He concluded his address, entitled "Some Modern Health Care Problems," with a challenge to the university and all its graduates:

> The health center here at the University of North Carolina is, in many ways, the meeting ground of the challenges and the problems facing the American people today in their striving to achieve the optimum in health—physical, mental and social. There exists here a unique opportunity to acquire new knowledge of inestimable value, not only to North Carolina, but to the entire nation. This opportunity is a challenge to our professions, institutions, industry and government to unite their efforts in formulating ways and means by which sound progressive programs can be provided for the enrichment of lives. The problem is not one which can be solved by any one group, lay or professional. It is one that all of you who are graduating today, whether

in the humanities, natural sciences, social sciences, the professions, or other disciplines, must inevitably play an important role in solving.[54]

The year after the graduation of the MD class of 1954, Berryhill "reported with some pride that reports on the performances of the first graduating class from the hospitals in which they are interning indicated that they have been superior in the knowledge and in the conduct of their duties." He added that it was significant "that 47 of the 59 present seniors [class of 1955] received their first choices of internships, many in the country's most sought-after hospitals—the Massachusetts General, the Presbyterian in New York, the Johns Hopkins, to mention only a few."[55]

By 1969, Berryhill could still take pride in the fact that thirty-six of the forty-eight that graduated in the first class in 1954 were practicing in North Carolina fifteen years later; two had died, and one had not continued in medicine after graduation.[56]

Eighteen of the surviving twenty-eight members of the class of 1954 had a joyous fiftieth reunion at the annual Medical Alumni Association meeting at Chapel Hill in April 2004. At the medical school graduation ceremony later in the spring, a member of the first MD class of 1954 had the pleasure of presenting to each member of the fiftieth-anniversary class of 2004 certificates documenting their membership in the Medical Alumni Association.[57]

The next *UNC Medical Bulletin* featured a cover photograph of the Class of 1954 at its fiftieth reunion. By this time Berryhill had been dead for a quarter of a century, but his memory was still fresh in their minds. An article about the class began with the statement that "Dean Reece Berryhill liked to remind the class of 1954 . . . that what they were paying for their medical education didn't come close to covering its actual cost. Since the state was heavily subsidizing their education, he told them [that] they owed the people of North Carolina a large debt." After reviewing a sampling of what some of the class members had done since their student days and what some were still doing in medicine in the state, the article concluded that the "class of '54 set a very high standard" for subsequent classes. One of the class members, Malcolm Fleishman, MD, added, "I believe all of us tried, and everybody in our class paid their debt to North Carolina. The state made a good investment in us."[58]

The Medical Students and Berryhill

As the dean of the two-year medical school, Berryhill had made most of the decisions about admissions. With the increased class size and the many other duties for the dean during and after the expansion of the medical school, this became an impossible task for one person. The pre-expansion entering class size of 50 was increased to 60 with the class entering in 1950. More important, in the first year after the expansion, Berryhill and the medical faculty taught a total of 892 students (including medical and other health sciences students as well as

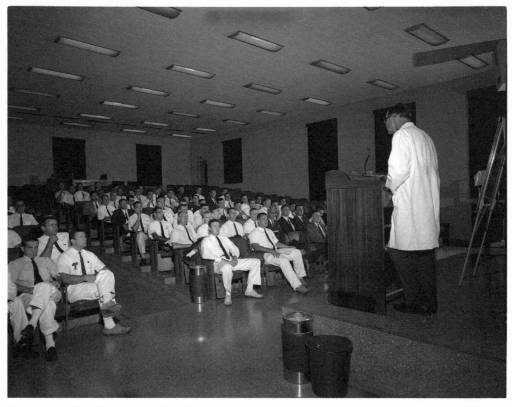

Dean Berryhill addressing third- and fourth-year students in the clinic auditorium, 1960. *(UNC Photo Lab, NCC)*

house officers). After Berryhill retired as dean, the entering medical class size increased to 75 in the fall of 1967, 85 in the fall of 1969, and 100 in the fall of 1970, to the current level of 160 by 1977.[59]

In 1949 Berryhill delegated the admission process to a faculty admissions committee under the leadership of Edward Hedgpeth, director of the student infirmary. He served in this role until 1964 and "functioned most effectively as a friend and unofficial counselor for all students" both before and after their acceptance to medical school, according to Berryhill. Christopher C. Fordham, III, MD, who would become dean of the medical school in 1971, followed Hedgpeth as chair of the admissions committee and later served as associate dean for clinical services.[60]

In spite of his vastly increased responsibilities as dean of the four-year school, Berryhill remained in charge and in touch with student affairs throughout his deanship. Noel B. McDevitt, MD (UNC 1964) related various encounters with Berryhill during his medical school and residency years at UNC that illustrated Berryhill's relationship to the students. Because his uncle had worked closely with Berryhill in setting up the Gravely Sanatorium at Chapel Hill and had praised him highly, the student said he expected Berryhill to be "a giant of a man with a halo over his head." While he later learned that Berryhill "was as human as all of us," he was most impressed when he and a group of premedical students from Davidson first visited the dean's office and saw this "tall, dark-haired, imposing gentleman wearing a long white coat . . . His eyes were sharp, his movements quick, and his thin wire-rimmed glasses accentuated his imposing features." After being admitted to medical school, he was "flabbergasted" one day when Berryhill stopped him in the hall, congratulated him on scoring so well in his anatomy practical examination, and encouraged him to keep up the good work. He was further amazed when he and his classmates visited the Berryhills' home early in the semester: Berryhill shook hands with each one and called him by name. He later learned that Berryhill "spent some time learning about each of his students as well as their families and . . . what their families' relationships had been with the university and with the state of North Carolina."[61]

During his senior year, McDevitt was elected president of the Whitehead Society (the medical student body) and had frequent discussions about the medical students and the school with Berryhill, who was completing his final year as dean. One such discussion was not so pleasant. The Student/Faculty Day was a well-attended affair in Memorial Hall on the campus late in the year. In the last class skit, a "a very direct barb" was thrown by the entire senior class at a faculty member who had been perceived by the class to be "particularly harsh with one of our fellow students [by demanding] an essay be written on a particular topic in which he thought the student was deficient, as a prerequisite to the student's graduation" three weeks later. As the curtain closed on the last scene, McDevitt received a note signed by Berryhill saying, "I will see you in my office immediately." He hurried to the dean's office, where a furious Berryhill said, "I don't care if I am retiring as dean, I'm going to talk to the new dean and if anything like this ever happens again at Student Faculty Day, there'll be no more . . . and I want you to transmit this to the new officers." Berryhill would not accept an apology, saying, "There is no way you can apologize for this kind of activity. It's unforgivable." McDevitt left the office quite shaken, but the matter was never spoken of again, and they continued to have a close relationship until Berryhill's passing fifteen years later.

After an internship at North Carolina Memorial Hospital, McDevitt left for military service and returned for a residency in surgery in 1969. He was pleased to see Berryhill still making daily rounds in the hospital as he checked on students, local residents, and friends and colleagues from around the state who were in the hospital. Several years later he had the chance to see another side of Berryhill when his young daughter had an unfortunate accident on a merry-go-round and fractured her femur. On the day after her admission, Berryhill appeared with some children's books and read to her to divert her attention from her traction and pain. He did this every day while she was in the hospital, calling her his "little girl." She never forgot Berryhill's kindness and remembered him as "the man who came to read to her." This "little girl" entered medical school in 1997.

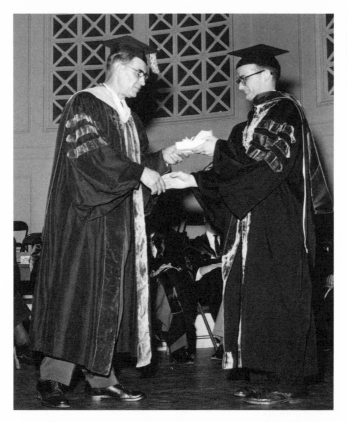

Dean Berryhill and a
graduating senior at
the School of Medicine
hooding ceremony, 1956.
(UNC Photo Lab, NCC)

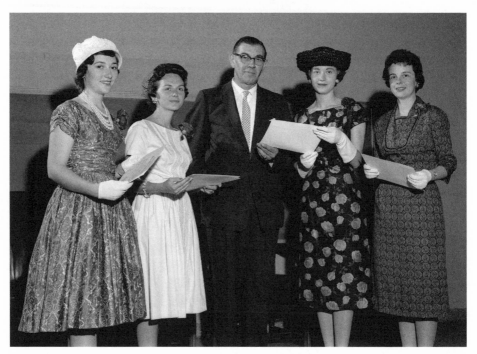

Dean Berryhill presenting certificates to wives of medical graduates, 1961. *(UNC Photo Lab, NCC)*

The medical students perceived Berryhill as all-knowing and all-powerful. A member of one of the first four-year classes recalled going to the county fair in Durham one Friday evening with some fellow medical students, where they enjoyed seeing a striptease act. On Saturday morning he received a call at Whitehead dormitory from "Peaches" Dunlap, the dean's secretary, saying that Dr. Berryhill wanted to see him right away. He hurried up the hill to Berryhill's office in MacNider Hall, wondering all the time how Berryhill knew of his adventures the night before and what he was going to say in his defense—perhaps he would claim it was a chance to learn functional anatomy. The tension increased with every minute of the some fifteen minutes he waited to see the dean. When he finally entered the office, Berryhill said, "Congratulations, Bradley, you have won the Mosby Book Award that is worth $25.00 applied to any book Mosby publishes." With a great sense of relief he left the dean's office. He picked *The Pathology of Tumors* as his book choice.[62]

Graduation of the medical classes each spring was a big event, in which Norma and Reece Berryhill actively participated. Not only did Berryhill preside at the special medical school hooding ceremonies, but he also on occasion participated in awarding the "PHT" ("Putting Hubby Through") certificates to the wives of the graduating seniors.

ACADEMIC AND FACULTY ISSUES

Accreditation

The School of Medicine was given provisional accreditation as a four-year school until the fall of 1953, when a weeklong accreditation visit was made by a team representing the AAMC and the Council on Medical Education and Hospitals of the AMA. They thoroughly studied the organization of the School of Medicine and its educational programs. Berryhill noted in his annual report, "The report of this survey as it pertained to the quality of staff, facilities, and instructional program and organization with the School of Medicine was commendatory," although the team raised concerns about the "position of the School of Medicine in the Division of Health Affairs and particularly with its relation to the North Carolina Memorial Hospital." Following the visit, the school was fully accredited as a four-year medical school.[63]

Medical School Administration

John B. Graham, MD, was a member of the medical school faculty in pathology for eighteen of the twenty-three years that Berryhill served as dean and worked with him on many projects. He said that Berryhill believed that "administration . . . should be kept to a minimum and prevented from interfering with more important matters. The fewer people involved the better. He operated the school with a minimum of assistance: Mrs. Privette, then Miss Dunlap, and finally Miss Dunlap and her several assistants, never numbering more than a half-dozen . . .

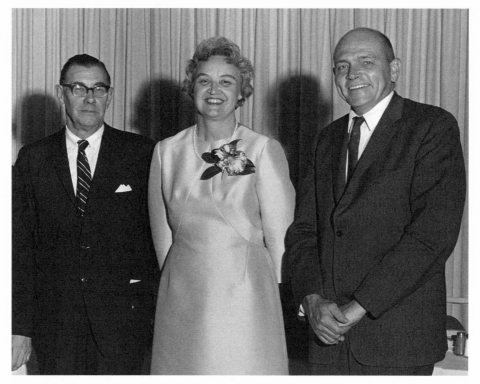

Dean Emeritus Berryhill, Sarah Virginia "Peaches" Dunlap, and Dean Isaac Taylor, 1966. *(UNC Photo Lab, NCC)*

He tried to avoid long business and committee meetings and developed an effective technique. If one asked him for an appointment, he often replied that he preferred to drop by one's office." Not only did this give him a sense of what was going on outside the dean's office, but it also "allowed him to break off a discussion whenever he wished by suddenly remembering another appointment."[64]

Berryhill himself acknowledged the "exceptionally able and loyal services of Miss Sarah Virginia Dunlap, Assistant to the Dean." While known to most others as "Peaches," she was always "Miss Dunlap" to the Dean. He said, "Her tact and understanding with visitors, students, and faculty, her close liaison with the staff in the general University offices, her intimate knowledge of the medical school and the University, and above all her high standards and her loyalty make her the one indispensable member of the administrative staff."[65]

Dunlap, who worked with Berryhill from 1942 to 1964, recalled that she first met him on the front steps of South Building on the university campus, where he interviewed her for the position of secretary in the dean's office. It was seven o'clock in the evening, and he had come back for the interview after working in his garden, which he loved; he once said it gave him "the opportunity to bury deep in the earth frustrations and even, at times, enemies." After a conversation lasting some forty-five minutes, he hired her, and she worked with him for the next twenty-two years.

According to Dunlap, "There was no small talk in Dr. Berryhill's conversation; all that he said had a point and it was not an isolated point . . . He did not pause when he spoke. There were no hems and haws. He spoke as he wrote, always grammatically correct and coherent."[66]

Berryhill's attitude toward medical administration was illustrated by an experience related by William E. Easterling, MD '56, a faculty member in obstetrics and gynecology, who was appointed by Dean Fordham and hospital director John Danielson in 1974 to be chief of the medical staff and assistant dean in the School of Medicine. Learning of this appointment, Berryhill, then retired as dean, called Easterling to his small office in a remodeled hallway in the Medical Sciences Research Building. In typical fashion, Berryhill went straight to the point. "I am very disappointed that you have decided to go into administration when your academic career has been so rewarding." Easterling recalled that his first impulse was to say, "Look who's talking." But he composed himself and replied, "You have been successful at both. Since you are such a good role model, I think I could provide good leadership for the institution in both realms." Berryhill smiled, wished him well, and "over the ensuing years was an invaluable source of advice and support."[67]

Graham related that by the mid-1950s the group of strong departmental chairs Berryhill had recruited was meeting regularly with him and was perceived by other faculty as having executive power over the entire faculty. This led in 1957 to what was then known as "the Revolt of the Associate Professors." Berryhill supported the concerns of the faculty and proposed that a constitution delineating the respective functions of the dean, the departmental chairs, and the faculty be written and approved for the medical school. The resulting document gave the faculty the right to establish or abolish departments and to be in charge of the curriculum. The document also clarified that the group of departmental chairs served in an advisory capacity to the dean. Graham later observed that the medical school constitution "has been the faculty's bulwark against arbitrary actions by a Dean or a cabal of department chairmen."[68]

Graham observed that Berryhill's "populist" view of faculty relationships was manifested in various ways. He held regular faculty meetings "as a consultative forum and educational mechanism." The agenda was short, with only important matters, and these were freely discussed. He always concluded with "Remarks by the Dean," which permitted him to comment on various current issues involving the medical school, the university, and the state. Graham concluded, "One left a faculty meeting at 5 o'clock or 5:15 to deal with personal matters feeling that the Dean had his hand on the tiller and would alert us if the need arose."[69]

Thomas Farmer, MD, first head of the Division of Neurology in the Department of Medicine, said that Berryhill "really ran the administration of the school and made decisions without delay. For example, when Dr. Burnett and Dr. Welt [chair and vice chair of medicine] were both admitted to the hospital in May 1964, Dr. Berryhill promptly called a meeting of the division heads in medicine

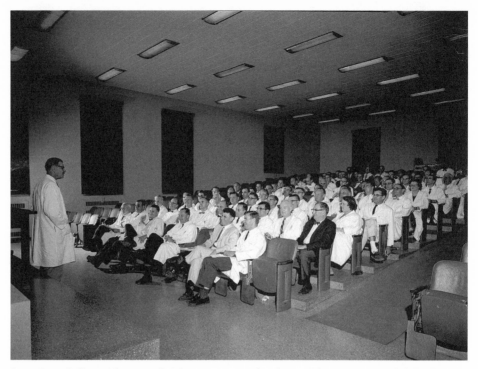

Dean Berryhill presiding at a faculty meeting in the clinic auditorium, 1961. *(UNC Photo Lab, NCC)*

in the dean's office. He outlined the problem and asked for suggestions. I said that I would be willing to serve as acting chairman. He said fine, and it was settled in a few minutes. I had his full support during the following year."[70]

In spite of Berryhill's aversion to a large administrative staff, he did find that he needed additional help to meet the challenge of operating a complex and expanding school and hospital. Berryhill said that "the counseling and guidance of medical students . . . was carried out informally over the years by members of the admissions committee and by many interested faculty members"—as well as by the dean. In 1953 he appointed F. Douglas Lawrason, MD, assistant professor of medicine, as assistant dean, with formal responsibility for this area. After Lawrason's resignation in 1956 to accept the deanship at Arkansas, Berryhill appointed Carl E. Anderson, PhD, in biochemistry, as assistant dean in charge of student affairs, and J. Mitchell Sorrow, MD, in medicine, as an assistant to the dean, with responsibilities primarily for advising senior students in regard to their internships and residencies. With Anderson's resignation as assistant dean in 1963, John B. Graham assumed his duties without the title and organized a system with a faculty advisor for each medical student class.[71]

Although the School of Medicine had been involved in continuing education efforts for practicing physicians in the state since 1916, the demand for such programs escalated in the postwar years. Berryhill thus appointed William P. Richardson, MD, professor of preventive medicine, as assistant dean for

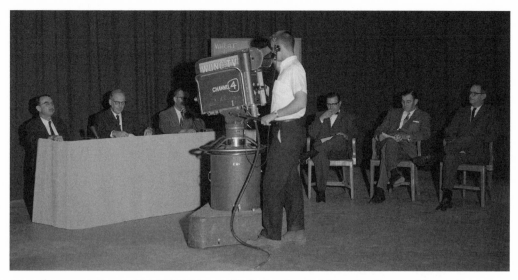

An early presentation on WUNC-TV by medical school and visiting faculty members, 1961. Chancellor William B. Aycock is seated third from the right, and Dean Berryhill is second from the right. *(UNC Photo Lab, NCC)*

continuing education in 1952, and he served until 1969. Through his and the faculty's efforts, a variety of continuing educational opportunities were offered throughout the state and in Chapel Hill. These included an annual School of Medicine symposium in Chapel Hill; other one- to three-day courses in Chapel Hill; monthly consultative and educational visits by faculty to selected hospitals; two-way radio conferences beginning in 1961 and coordinated through the university's station, WUNC-FM; and TV programs beginning in 1968 produced by WUNC-TV, which had gone on the air in 1955. Berryhill reported in 1954 that "the number of physicians attending [the formal continuing education courses sponsored by the School of Medicine] is a little more than 25 percent of the total membership of the State Medical Society."[72] Berryhill later reported that the average annual number of physicians registering for these programs was about 400 a year from 1948 to 1952, and about 700 a year from 1952 to 1969.[73]

In 1957 Berryhill tapped William L. Fleming, MD, the first and only chair of preventive medicine from 1951 to 1969, to be a part-time assistant dean in charge of the undergraduate educational programs. In 1960 Berryhill appointed Philip Manire, PhD, from the department of bacteriology, as an assistant in the dean's office to coordinate with Miss Dunlap the administration of research and training grants.

Berryhill said in the 1953–1954 annual report that for the first time it had been possible to "consolidate the admissions activities, the student counseling, the continuation education, and the work of the Medical Foundation in adjoining offices in the administrative allocation of space in the School of Medicine." He added that this had provided "for better correlation of activities and more efficiency in administrative operations."[74]

After the hospital came under the direction of the School of Medicine in September 1956, Berryhill made several unsuccessful attempts to convince the university to set up joint medical school–hospital fiscal and personnel offices. Neither proposal received the approval of the university's business officer or of the administrator of the Division of Health Affairs. A fiscal officer was provided for the Division of Health Affairs, which "was of some assistance to the School of Medicine," according to Berryhill.[75] It would not be until almost half a century later with the reorganization of the UNC Health Care System that there would be a joint fiscal officer responsible for the financial operations of the hospital, the School of Medicine, and the faculty practice plan.[76]

The addition of part-time members of the dean's office would continue under subsequent deans so that by 1977—thirteen years after Berryhill's retirement as dean and two years before his passing—there were fourteen associate or assistant deans and directors of programs who reported to the dean's office.[77]

Faculty Changes

During Berryhill's tenure as dean of the four-year school from 1952 to 1964, numerous additions were made to the clinical and basic sciences faculty in the medical school as a result of the ever-increasing volume of clinical services, expanding class sizes, and increased funding from federal research grants and the state.

During these years the school also lost some of its longtime faculty. The death of William de B. MacNider, professor of pharmacology emeritus, in June 1951 "marked the end of an era in the School of Medicine," according to Berryhill. "His kindness and his colorful personality have influenced many generations of medical students."[78]

In 1964 the school lost another longtime faculty member with the passing of James B. Bullitt, MD, professor emeritus of pathology. Berryhill noted in his final annual report:

> For thirty-three years (1913–1947) Dr. Bullitt was Chairman of the Department of Pathology and with Drs. Manning, Mangum, and MacNider exerted a lasting influence upon the character and direction of this school and its students for two generations. He was an able pathologist, teacher, archaeologist, historian—especially of medicine—a generous giver of himself to his friends and students, and of his means to the university and the School of Medicine. In the 1956 the Alumni Association of the Medical school presented him with the Distinguished Service Award, the citation of which read in part, "scholar, scientist, and friend, dear to the hearts of two generations of students, many of whose careers he has guided and all of whose lives he has enriched."[79]

Following the appointment of the initial clinical chairs in 1951 and 1952, there were relatively few turnovers among the chairs during Berryhill's deanship.[80]

W. Critz George retired as chair of anatomy in 1949 following a decade of service in this leadership role. Berryhill recruited Charles W. Hooker, PhD (Duke), from Yale Medical School as the new chair of anatomy, a post he held from 1949 to 1969. He was widely recognized for his enthusiasm for teaching and for his research.

In 1957 James C. Andrews, PhD, retired after twenty years as chair of the Department of Biological Chemistry. Berryhill appointed as his replacement J. Logan Irvin, PhD, a member of the faculty since 1950, who ably served as chair of the Department of Biochemistry and Nutrition from 1957 to 1978 while continuing his research in nucleic acids.

In 1960 Curnen, the first chair of pediatrics, was succeeded by Floyd W. Denny, Jr., MD (Vanderbilt), who came from Case Western Reserve University after having worked in infectious disease at Minnesota, Vanderbilt, and Case Western Reserve. He served as chair for twenty years, during which time the department grew from six full-time faculty members to forty-seven and became nationally recognized for its clinical, research, and teaching programs.[81]

In contrast to Berryhill's situation after the appointment of the first clinical chairs, Isaac M. Taylor, MD, who was his successor as dean from 1964 to 1971, faced the challenge of recruiting nine departmental chairs in his first five years as dean to fill vacancies owing to illness, the university's then mandatory retirement age for administrative positions, and recruitment of chairs to other centers.[82]

The Basic Sciences, the Other Health Affairs Schools, and the University

After the Division of Health Affairs was established in 1949, it was decided that the basic sciences departments of the School of Medicine would provide instruction in their disciplines for students of "the ancillary Schools of Dentistry, Nursing, and Pharmacy" rather than having each school create departments in these areas. In his 1954–1955 annual report Berryhill conceded that this arrangement had some advantages financially and otherwise for the university and noted that the medical faculty was initially enthusiastic about such an ideal. He warned, however, that it could have a devastating effect on the morale and research productivity of faculty of these departments. He emphasized that "these departments have a primary responsibility to medical students and to pursuing fundamental research" and that "additional duties can be assumed only if adequate funds are supplied [from other than medical school sources] . . . to pay for the actual cost of instruction."[83]

In the same report Berryhill took notice of the "noteworthy and encouraging" number of university graduate students now enrolled in the basic sciences departments of the School of Medicine. He cited this as "further proof of the mutual values that can accrue to the whole University when a medical school is really an integral part of its resources." He quoted Dr. Alan Gregg's comments of some years earlier to support the significance of such graduate studies and research in a university: "The chemistry, the physics and the biology of today become the physiology, the biological chemistry, the pharmacology of tomorrow and the clinical medicine of the day after." In typical fashion he also commented on the need for the school to get some "readjustment" for graduate student fees and tuition because "the Medical School bears the major cost of the instruction for graduate students—a fact which is generally unappreciated by budgetary authorities within and without the University."[84]

Research

Berryhill's tenure as dean of the School of Medicine coincided with an era of profound changes in the nation's attitude toward biomedical research. It began in 1944, when President Franklin D. Roosevelt wrote Vannevar Bush, director of the Office of Scientific Research and Development, in regard to carrying on the wartime advances in science and medicine in the postwar years. He asked Bush to make recommendations in the following areas:

> *First:* What can be done, consistent with military security . . . to make known to the world as soon as possible the contributions which have been made during our war effort to scientific knowledge?
>
> *Second:* With particular reference to the war of science against disease, what can be done now to organize a program for continuing in the future the work which has been done in medicine and related sciences?
>
> *Third:* What can the government do now and in the future to aid research activities by public and private organizations? The proper roles of public and of private research, and their interrelation, should be carefully considered.
>
> *Fourth:* Can an effective program be proposed for discovering and developing scientific talent in American youth so that the continuing future of scientific research in this country may be assured on a level comparable to what has been done during the war?[85]

Bush responded to President Truman after Roosevelt's death with recommendations that were summarized by Manire in his 1986 Norma Berryhill Lecture entitled "Carolina: A Research University":

1. [That] the federal government should accept responsibility for promoting the creation of new scientific knowledge and the development of scientific talent in our youth.
2. That new independent agencies be established which are devoted only to support of scientific research and advanced scientific education.
3. That these agencies would support research through contracts or grants to public and private colleges, universities, and research institutes outside the federal government.
4. [That] internal control of policy, personnel, and the scope of research must be left to the institutions.

Manire elaborated:

Although unstated as such, the report made clear that in the United States, the basic research enterprise in science and engineering of the nation would be a responsibility primarily of the universities and such has been the case. Based on this, my definition of a research university is a graduate institution—of which there are now 100 or 150, depending on the judge, in the United States—which has a sufficient number of highly talented investigators, a regular supply of able graduate and postdoctoral students, and adequate facilities and equipment to attract from federal, state, industrial, and private sources sufficient funds to be competitive with the best institutions across the nation—competitive for funds, competitive for faculty, competitive for students . . . Every university that I am aware of that fits this definition has a large applied science component, either engineering, agriculture, or health sciences. Some institutions have all three (Wisconsin), some have two (Johns Hopkins); and some, like UNC, have only one. There are many which I will not name that have two or three such components but have not succeeded in becoming competitive as first-class research universities . . . At Chapel Hill, we do indeed fall into the category of a national research university . . . It is my belief that this university, lacking engineering, health sciences, or agriculture (that is, no applied science) would be a much poorer place for student[s] in all disciplines, and that to be a research university is indeed good—good for our students, good for our faculty, and good for the state of North Carolina.[86]

Although the full impact of these recommendations and of the medical school's role in the blossoming of Carolina as a nationally recognized research university would not be appreciated for some years, Berryhill had in the 1940s and the 1950s laid the foundation for the explosion of biomedical research at the medical center and the university.

Fundamental to these developments in research at Chapel Hill was the decision to build the hospital and expanded medical school on the university campus, rather than in a larger city in the state, as was still the conventional wisdom at the time. Berryhill explained the conventional wisdom by noting that until then "because of economic and transportation difficulties . . . it was easier to bring students to a concentration of charity patients than the reverse." In a presentation at the Annual Congress on Medical Education in Chicago, however, Berryhill convincingly argued that "if medicine is in truth a learned profession and not a trade and if it has finally become, after a long and somewhat devious course, a university discipline, then it is logical to believe that a school of medicine whenever possible should be an integral part of a university, physically and spiritually."[87] His was one of the primary voices advocating that the state of North Carolina make this decision, which it did in 1947.

Berryhill's recruitment in 1946 of Kenneth M. Brinkhous, MD, as chair of

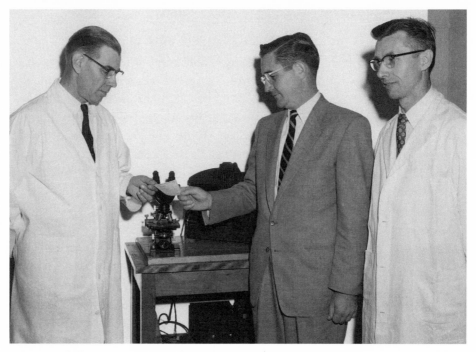

Dean Berryhill presenting a donor's check to UNC President William C. Friday for support of the coagulation research of Dr. Kenneth M. Brinkhous (at right), late 1950s. *(UNC Photo Lab, NCC)*

pathology was of critical importance in the medical school's future research endeavors. Berryhill's accomplishment is all the more remarkable because when it occurred, the location of the expanded school and hospital had not yet been determined, and Brinkhous was already a secure associate professor at Iowa with a growing reputation in his field of coagulation. Manire observed that this recruitment "was of primary value in the later recruitment of clinical faculty." Previously the sole professor and chair in a department had done the generally limited research at the medical school, with the help of an occasional student or assistant.[88] Brinkhous "introduced a new concept of research to this school; namely, the development of a critical mass of young collaborators and students to study a set of related topics. He was also the first professor in the school to have and exercise the opportunity to attract young scholars to his department and to participate actively in their growth and development as independent scholar researchers."[89] Brinkhous was highly successful in obtaining grant funding to support this venture, and before his death in 2000 he was recognized as the only researcher in NIH history to have had fifty years of continuous NIH funding.

Brinkhous also promoted joint research efforts between and among the various basic science and clinical science faculty. For example, Harold Roberts, a native North Carolinian who received his MD from UNC in 1955, was first attracted to the field of coagulation by working as a medical student research assistant with Penick in Brinkhous' group on the relationship between coagulation and cold injury, a topic of particular interest during the Korean War. Following his residency in medicine and a coagulation research fellowship in Copenhagen with the renowned Tage Astrup, he returned to Chapel Hill and rose to become Sarah Graham Kenan Professor of Medicine and Pathology by 1986. He served as chief of the hematology division in medicine from 1968 to 1993 and was the founding director of the Center for Thrombosis and Hemostasis, established at UNC in 1978. His research over the years ranged from clinically oriented problems to basic research on the nature of the coagulation Factor IX. Beginning as a deputy to Brinkhous as secretary of the International Committee on Haemostasis and Thrombosis, he became a world-recognized figure in the field and "the successor to Brinkhous as UNC's symbol for research and service in thrombosis and hemostasis."[90]

Berryhill followed his initial success with Brinkhous by recruiting an outstanding group of clinician scholars as the first chairs of the clinical departments. These chairs in turn recruited an unusually talented group of young clinician scholars. The quality of these recruits was recognized by the selection of nine young faculty members as Markle Scholars in Academic Medicine from 1949 until 1963 during Berryhill's tenure as dean, with an additional four selected from

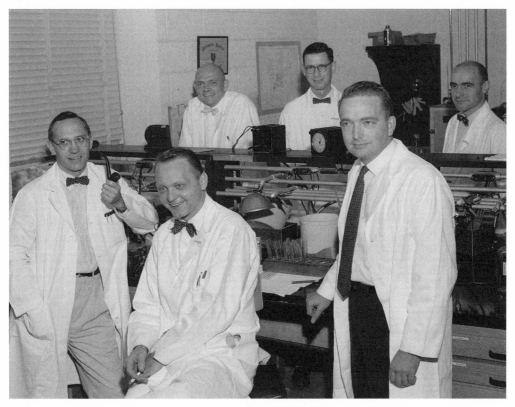

The first six Markle Scholars in Academic Medicine, 1958. *Front row, left to right:* Drs. John B. Graham, Judson J. Van Wyk, and George D. Penick. *Back row, left to right:* Drs. Isaac Taylor, Walter Hollander, and T. Franklin Williams. *(UNC Photo Lab, NCC)*

Dean of the Four-Year School of Medicine   249

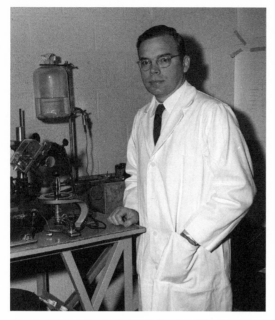

Dr. Carl W. Gottschalk in his first renal micropuncture laboratory on the fourth floor of the clinic building, 1956. *(UNC Photo Lab, NCC)*

1965 to 1968.[91] They were among some 500 Markle Scholars who were funded in US and Canadian medical schools from 1947 to 1969 by the John and Mary R. Markle Foundation and who each "received five years of financial assistance so that they might continue in academic medicine or research rather than enter more lucrative private practices."[92] The Markle Scholars at UNC had an impressive record here and elsewhere in academic medicine: John B. Graham, MD; George D. Penick, MD; Isaac M. Taylor, MD; Judson J. Van Wyk, MD; T. Franklin Williams, MD; Walter Hollander, Jr., MD; Robert Zeppa, MD; William D. Huffines, MD; William E. Lassiter, MD; Reginald G. Mason, Jr., MD; Frank C. Wilson, Jr., MD; Benson R. Wilcox, MD; and John C. Parker, MD.

Another highly productive young faculty member was Carl W. Gottschalk, MD, who carried out pioneering micropuncture studies of kidney function after his arrival at UNC–CH in the Department of Medicine in 1952. These studies confirmed the countercurrent hypothesis for renal function and propelled Gottschalk to an internationally recognized leadership position in nephrology.[93] In 1967 he chaired the national committee that recommended to Congress that Americans who suffer from chronic renal failure be provided chronic renal dialysis. His contributions were recognized with many honors, including a Kenan Professorship. He was also made a charter member of the Institute of Medicine in 1973 and was elected to the National Academy of Sciences in 1975. In addition, Gottschalk assembled one of the world's most extensive collections of publications related to the kidney and renal disease. It is now housed in the Rare Book Room at the Wilson Library on the UNC–CH campus.

The eminence of the initial faculty Berryhill recruited, the collegiality promoted by the Berryhills, and the presence of joint research activities across departmental, school, and center boundaries at Chapel Hill have been strong recruiting aids for the university and the medical center ever since.

During Berryhill's tenure as dean, the issue of space and resources for faculty research initially had to take a back seat to the building of the clinical and educational enterprise, although each of his annual reports during these years highlighted the crucial need to support the research efforts of the ever-expanding faculty in the School of Medicine.

In 1951 Berryhill lamented that

> a health-conscious State continues its short-sighted policy of providing no
> funds for fundamental research in the medical field. The entire research pro-
> gram here has to depend for financial support on outside aid, chiefly grants
> from the US Public Health Service [National Institutes of Health]. While
> these have proved life-saving in enabling the School to acquire expensive
> equipment and technical assistance, they are unsatisfactory in the long run
> because of their year-to-year basis of approval and the uncertainty and in-
> security for the staff employed on such funds, as well as in planning for any
> long range research program in a department.

He urged that efforts continue to convince the state to fund fundamental medical research, as it did for agricultural research, while at the same time building
up endowment funds for research funding.[94] In the years followed, the primary
source of research funding for the school continued to be the federal government, but increasing success was had in soliciting private donations and in tap-
ping research support from a number of other nongovernmental sources.

Berryhill's ability to listen to the faculty's concerns about the research endeavor and then act on their concerns was related by Richard M. Peters, MD,
chief of cardiothoracic surgery from 1952 to 1969. Peters said that in the early
years some faculty questioned the "degree of support by Reece [Berryhill] . . . for
the development of the research as 'opposed' to the clinical and teaching aspects
of the school." At a Christmas party at a faculty member's home, Peters and
Welt, who "in retrospect . . . had lowered our inhibitions [with martinis] more
than we realized," cornered Berryhill and "spoke strongly about how important
research was to the school and must have made it pretty clear he was not giving research enough priority." At the next faculty meeting Peters and Welt were
sitting together near the front of the auditorium when "towards the end of his
presentation Reece, while looking straight at us, described a conversation he had
had with two faculty at a cocktail party regarding research. He then went on
to say he had heard this criticism and made clear his support for this aspect of
the school" and mentioned some particular actions he was taking. Peters summarized, "Reece listened to the faculty but also heard and in doing so taught us
a great deal."[95]

Through the efforts of Charles Hooker, PhD, chair of anatomy, a $200,000
grant was obtained from the US Public Health Service along with funds from
the North Carolina Division of the American Cancer Society to equip a small
cancer research laboratory in space on the fifth floor of the clinic building,
which opened in 1952.[96] The only other research space available in 1952 was in
MacNider Hall. It was in this fairly limited research laboratory space (just down
the hall from Berryhill's former office as dean and where the student admissions
activities of the dean's office were located up until 2006) that Langdell, Wagner,
and Brinkhous did the work published in 1953 that led to the discovery of PTT

(partial thromboplastin time), today used in hospitals and clinics throughout the world to screen for bleeding disorders and monitor therapy.[97] It was also in this and in adjacent space in MacNider, and in the animal quarters then on the top floor of MacNider, that a series of studies was done to characterize hemophilia in dogs and to prove that hemophilia could exist in females.[98]

Berryhill wrote in the annual report for 1952 that "the need for additional space [for office and research laboratories for the clinical staff] is *very urgent*."[99] The upper floors of the clinic building, which opened in 1952, did provide some offices for the Departments of Medicine, Surgery, and Obstetrics and Gynecology. The opening of the south wing for psychiatry in 1953 and of the Gravely Sanatorium in 1953, and the conversion of two floors of the interns' quarters for faculty offices, provided the only additional space for clinical faculty offices and research during the early part of Berryhill's tenure as dean of the four-year school. Some additional faculty office and laboratory space was also obtained in MacNider Hall in 1963, when the School of Public Health finally vacated the basement floor and moved across the street into its new building.

As noted in the previous chapter, the first building specifically designed and designated for faculty research was the Medical Sciences Research Building (MSRB), a $1 million addition to MacNider Hall that was approved in 1959 and completed in 1962. Berryhill appointed a small committee chaired by Welt to recommend space assignments in the new research building in view of the tremendous needs and the rather modest size of the building. Each faculty member was asked by their chair to apply for space for his or her needs while keeping in mind the needs of others. According to Manire, "To the delight of everyone, all requests were met on the first round, although several departments had need of at least half the building."[100]

A major step forward in clinical research occurred during Berryhill's deanship with the establishment of the first clinical research unit for the medical center.[101] Faculty planning for this unit occurred in 1960–1961, with Burnett, Welt, and Brinkhous providing the leadership. The medical school was one of first in the nation to obtain federal funding for an institutional general clinical research unit. The initial grant of $897,528 was for three years with a later grant of $2,491,000 for a seven-year extension. On the basis of the coagulation research by Brinkhous' group in pathology and Ferguson's group in physiology, an additional seven-year program grant for $1,573,435 was received for a clinical research unit in hemorrhage and thrombosis. Ham and his colleagues in psychiatry moved their offices to the interns' quarters to provide space in the south wing for the initial Clinical Research Unit, with twelve beds and associated support services. Three Markle Scholars provided the initial leadership for these units. Hollander and Zeppa were the initial director and assistant director of the general Clinical Research Unit, while Penick was the director of the Hemorrhage and Thrombosis Clinical Research Unit. William Blythe, MD, in medicine, and Campbell MacMillan, MD, in pediatrics, became the director and assistant director of the Clinical Research Unit in 1966. In the early 1970s the unit moved to a larger facility with expanded laboratories in the Spencer Love Clinic building (Ambulatory Patient Care Facility) as a result of a generous gift from the R. J. Reynolds Company.[102]

In 1953 Berryhill proudly announced, "The research efforts of our entire staff are expanding rapidly. In the past year there were 112 [published] reports of research projects prepared by members of the faculty and 104 papers presented by the staff at various medical meetings. This is only as pointer as to what we may expect in the next few years."[103] This contrasted with 57 publications and 30 presentations at medical meetings in 1950–1951, before the expansion of the school had begun.[104] These statistics are reflected in outside funding received in support of research and of teaching and training programs. These totaled $106,355 for the 1950–1951 academic year and had more than tripled to $384,674 for 1952–1953, the first year of the expanded school.[105] In Berryhill's final annual report as dean, he said that the outside research and training grants had increased to a total of $4,256,614 for the academic year 1963–1964.[106]

The Research Triangle Park

Frank Porter Graham, in his 1931 inaugural address as UNC president, anticipated the development of North Carolina's Research Triangle in the second half of the twentieth century: "With the University today stand all the state and denominational schools, colleges, and the neighbor university [Duke]. Not in antagonism but in all friendliness and rivalry in excellence we would work in this region and build here together one of the great intellectual and spiritual centers of the world."[107]

Graham's dream began to materialize in the 1950s when a remarkable group of business, government, and university leaders developed the Research Triangle Park in an area located between Duke University, North Carolina State University, and the University of North Carolina at Chapel Hill. The hub of this enterprise is the nonprofit Research Triangle Institute, founded in 1959 and now the nation's second-largest independent research organization. The arrival of IBM and the National Institute of Environmental Health Sciences in 1965 started a phase of rapid growth that has continued to this day.

Although Berryhill had little, if any, direct involvement with development of the Research Triangle Park, the research endeavor he helped create on the UNC campus has continued to play a vital role in the Park, which is anchored by the three major research universities in North Carolina's Triangle area.

Racial Integration of the Hospital and Medical School

Berryhill, in keeping with his upbringing in a rural North Carolina community during the early years of the twentieth century—when memories of the Civil

War and Reconstruction were still vivid, and when white supremacy movements and Jim Crow laws were at their height in the South—initially had great difficulty facing the prospect of an integrated hospital and medical school student body. One young faculty member remembered a faculty meeting in about 1950 when Berryhill was discussing the possibility of integration of the school's student body. The faculty member said that he had never seen Berryhill so "visibly emotional" and that "there were tears in his eyes."[108]

Most of the younger faculty members, especially those recruited from Harvard, Yale, and elsewhere, however, were not at all troubled by the prospect of desegregation, and some were politically active in promoting integration of the public school system. Berryhill's devotion to his faculty and his belief that an academic community must preserve freedom for responsible discussion and action by the faculty overrode his personal views of the integration issue. For example, a young surgery faculty member from Yale, who was elected to the local school board in the early 1960s and who helped lead the desegregation of the Chapel Hill public schools, recalled, "On more than one occasion Nathan [Womack] and Reece [Berryhill] told me that they thought we were going too fast, but never did more than express their opinion." Furthermore, when a very influential and prominent local citizen came to Dean Berryhill's office demanding that he tell his faculty members to cease their agitation to integrate the public schools in Chapel Hill, Berryhill reminded the visitor that "the request was improper," that the faculty "had a constitutional right to their opinions," and that their "activities did not affect their medical school obligations."[109]

At the far extreme from the younger faculty members, or even from Berryhill, was Wesley Critz George, PhD, professor of histology and embryology at the medical school from 1924 to 1949 and chair of the department from 1939 to 1949, who taught embryology into the early 1950s. George promoted throughout the South the theory that science proved the inferiority of the black race. He also was politically active as the founding president of the Patriots of North Carolina, a large and influential segregationist organization.[110] One of the early black medical students later recalled that George was well known for his belief that blacks were inferior, "but when it came to teaching in the classroom, I didn't see any favoritism. Even though he had his private views and expressed them out of the classroom, I didn't have any problems [with him] in the classroom."[111]

North Carolina Memorial Hospital served patients of all races when it opened in 1952, but many of the services were segregated within the hospital, in keeping with state law and local customs. Black medical and surgical patients were admitted only to the 3-West ward in the hospital. Although black and white patients were on the same floor in the pediatrics and ob-gyn services, they were placed in separate rooms according to race.

The decades following World War II saw major changes in attitude and laws with regard to segregation, although these changes were widely resisted and protested in many areas of the South. In 1948 President Harry Truman ordered the desegregation of the armed forces. In 1954, with the *Brown v. Board of Education* decision, the US Supreme Court struck down segregated public schools as "inherently unequal" and ordered that desegregation proceed "with all deliberate speed."

When Congress passed the Hill-Burton Act in 1946 to fund hospital construction, it contained compromise wording with regard to segregation of hospital facilities, so that segregated hospitals continued to receive federal funding until the 1960s. In a case against Moses Cone Hospital in Greensboro concerning a qualified black dentist, George Simkins, DDS, who was denied hospital privileges because of his race, the US Fourth District Court of Appeals ruled in 1963 "that any hospital that received public funds yet discriminated on the basis of race in either admitting patients or granting staff privileges violated the Fourth Amendment rights of African Americans."[112]

Segregation in publicly operated facilities became illegal with the passage by Congress of the 1964 Civil Rights Act. Title VI of this act prohibited segregation in any public facility receiving federal funds, which covered hospitals such as North Carolina Memorial that had received Hill-Burton or other federal funding. Further financial incentive for hospitals to do away with segregation came in 1965 with the passage of the Medicare law, which provided federal funding for health care for citizens sixty-five and older—but only in nonsegregated facilities.

As the Jim Crow practices and laws from the early 1900s were challenged and struck down throughout the country in the 1950 and 1960s, there was a gradual integration of health care services in Memorial Hospital and its clinics. Improving patient care generally motivated these efforts; desegregation was simply a desirable side benefit. For instance, Cadmus told of an episode involving a little girl in a private room on the pediatric floor who, while in recovery from a tonsillectomy, was discovered by the nurse to have a blocked airway. She was saved because of the nurse's prompt action, but this and other experiences led to the establishment at North Carolina Memorial Hospital of what were probably the nation's first pediatric and adult special care or intensive care units where critically ill patients could be closely monitored around the clock. Blacks and whites were admitted to these units because of their medical needs, without regard to race or sex. As Cadmus said later, "The patients in the units were too sick to care, and their relatives were so thankful for the care the patients were receiving that they were going to be the last person to worry about a little thing like that [i.e., the race of the patient in the next bed]."[113]

An early faculty member in surgery recalled, "Over the seventeen years that I was on the faculty there was no time that a major decision was made to desegregate the hospital. Rather, a change in patient needs and methods of care had the first priority, and this led to a steady erosion of the barriers between races. One example is that the first ICU [intensive care unit] was developed by using two four-bed wards on 3-West as a post-surgical ICU. This was dictated by proximity to the operating rooms."[114]

Thus, by the late 1960s Memorial Hospital was essentially desegregated, without the court challenges or major protest marches faced by some facilities in the South and elsewhere.

As the pressure to integrate hospitals and other public facilities increased during the 1950s and 1960s, a parallel effort was under way to eliminate the unequal opportunities for minorities to receive education in colleges, universities, and professional schools.

Following the closure of Leonard Medical School at Shaw University in Raleigh in 1910, North Carolina blacks had few opportunities to attend medical school other than at historically black medical schools—Howard, founded in 1868 in Washington, DC, and Meharry, founded in 1876 in Nashville, Tennessee. The Murphy Act was passed by the North Carolina general assembly in 1939 to assist qualified black students with "an expense differential if they enrolled in an out-of-state university for graduate courses that are offered in the University of North Carolina and not offered in the State's Negro Colleges." One of the subcommittees of the Poe Commission was on "Special Needs of Our Negro Population." The commission's final report documented the poor health care the black population was receiving and acknowledged "the high moral duty of the state to provide greatly improved opportunities for enabling capable Negro youths to become physicians serving their race." The commission members recommended that North Carolina take the lead in cooperating with neighboring states to establish "a Regional Medical School for Negroes . . . [with] as prompt action as possible to [allow] reasonably adequate time for study and investigation."[115] Fortunately, the perceived need to support a segregated regional medical school became irrelevant in the 1950s and beyond as universities and medical schools were integrated.

An article in *Collier's* magazine in 1947 reported that US medical schools (other than the traditionally black schools) in the North and West admitted only some eight to ten black medical students a year, and some also had quotas for admission of Jewish students. Medical schools in the South (including the three then in North Carolina) did not even consider applications from black students.[116]

In the 1930s the university successfully defended its segregated admission policy in a suit filed in a state court by a black student who was refused admission to the School of Pharmacy. Legal challenges to UNC's refusal to admit black students into the professional programs began in federal court in 1950 with applications to the School of Law. The university argued that the state was providing a "separate but equal" law school for blacks at the nearby North Carolina College in Durham (renamed North Carolina Central University in 1969). This was before the 1954 *Brown v. Board of Education* decision of the Supreme Court, so that university President Gordon Gray argued, "The doctrine of 'separate but equal' educational facilities is still the law of the land."[117] A federal district court initially upheld this argument, although in March 1951 the Fourth US Circuit Court of Appeals reversed the decision on the grounds that the college's law school did not offer an educational opportunity for blacks equal to that at Chapel Hill. The university trustees in April 1951 voted to process graduate and professional school applications "without regard to color or race." UNC–CH thus became the first historically white Southern university to admit blacks without a direct court order, although clearly the pressure from the courts had a profound effect on the university's decision.[118]

Four black students were admitted to the law school in 1951. In June 1952, one of them, Harvey Beech, became the first African American to graduate from UNC. In the fall of 1955 the first black undergraduates entered the university, although none of the three stayed to graduate. David Dansby was admitted in 1957 and in 1961 became the first black undergraduate to graduate from UNC; he returned to UNC, graduated with a law degree in 1964, and practiced law in Greensboro. Dansby said later that during his student years "the hospital had segregated waiting rooms and bathrooms." He recalled that he and some other activists protested a School of Public Health dedication ceremony in order to call attention to the segregated facilities. He added, "After we announced that we were going to picket, they removed every sign segregating the facilities, and those signs never came back."[119]

When Edward Diggs, a native of Winston-Salem, applied for entry to the UNC medical school in the fall of 1951, his application was considered by the faculty members of the admission committee, the majority of whom felt he was qualified. However, Hedgpeth (the committee chair) and Berryhill initially rejected his application on the grounds that "had Diggs been a white man rather than a Negro in his particular circumstances he would not have been found competently qualified." The six faculty committee members who had recommended Diggs's admission countered with a letter they wished included in his file. They reiterated that "Mr. Diggs' academic accomplishment[s] were outstanding—well above the accepted standard of this school."[120]

In his annual report for 1950–1951 Berryhill reviewed the integration situation in the medical school in detail. Seven applications for 1951–1952 were received from black applicants residing in the state and all "were processed in the regular fashion." The faculty members recommended one as "competitively qualified," but Hedgpeth and the dean, "after careful study of all applicants," initially disagreed. They reversed this decision, however, "in view (1) of the decisions of the Board of Trustees in regard to the admission of qualified Negro students in those graduate and professional schools for training in which no opportunity was provided at the Negro colleges within the State, (2) that the applicant did appear to have the qualifications to enter Medical School, and (3) because of the suit already pending for admission of Negroes to the Medical School, it seemed wise and certainly expedient to approve the admission of this applicant." Berryhill added that the trustees, the university administration, the chair of the admissions committee, and the medical school dean all agreed with this decision.[121]

Berryhill predicted that admission of this student would "raise many problems should the Negro student do satisfactory work and eventually reach the clinical years" but felt that "undoubtedly these problems can be solved if patience and understanding prevail." He added, "The problem now is not one of discrimination against the minority but a consideration of all the safeguards to prevent discrimination against the majority group among the applicants. It is essential that exactly the same standards be followed in the selection of students for admission and in evaluating their performance as students in the School."

After the admission of Diggs to the class of 1955 and the second black student, James Slade, to the class of 1957, Berryhill wrote Chancellor House in 1953, "There has been no difficulty as long as the [two] Negro students were in the basic science laboratories and dealt only with other students, faculty and laboratory animals."[122] The situation was more complex when the students entered the third year and had direct patient contact with patients from a still segregated society. A letter of September 16, 1953, from Curnen, chair of pediatrics, to Dean Berryhill highlighted the problem:

> Early in September, at the beginning of the fall term of medical school, you instructed me that white patients were not to be assigned to our third year Negro student, Edward Diggs. After some reflection on this, which I understood to be a statement of policy, I expressed to you the opinion that it could not be carried out unless Diggs himself was informed of the ruling and agreed to abide by it. In answer to my question as to whether Diggs had been informed, you said he had not.
>
> This arrangement seemed to me to be untenable, and to impose the obligation of both execution and explanation upon members of the house staff who were neither qualified nor prepared for this responsibility. I therefore requested that you discuss the matter as soon as possible with the chiefs of the various clinical services and with Diggs himself. I understood that this would be done. In the meanwhile, I have attempted to avoid situations which might call attention to the matter until questions concerning it could be giver consideration and settled.
>
> This afternoon Diggs came to me and asked whether a special policy existed regarding the assignment of patients to him. He stated that as an applicant for admission to the medical school he had been assured that if accepted as a student he would be treated as other students and that in his experience to date he had not been aware of any special restrictions. He expressed deep

concern over the possibility that this treatment was now being altered and wanted to know where this policy originated.

I was obliged to acknowledge that I had instructed residents on the Pediatric Service not to assign new white patients to him. I did not tell him or my residents that this was done in accordance with your instructions. I did not offer an opinion as to where the policy originated, as I do not know myself.

I expressed the view that I and, presumably, all members of the medical faculty wished to help him to obtain a fine medical education and to become established as a competent and effective physician. We discussed these objectives and various possibilities for disagreement on how they might best be achieved.

. . . I agreed to speak to [the chiefs of the other clinical services] and to you concerning the matter and assured him that he could expect us to give it prompt and thoughtful consideration and to let him know the result of our deliberations.

I should like to request that we meet for this purpose soon. I believe that this is important and fairly urgent.

Judson Van Wyk, MD, several months later attended a meeting for Curnen and noted his understanding of "the policy re Negro medical students as laid down by the chancellor:"

1. We are obliged to give our Negro students "equivalent" but not "identical" experience.
2. We are not obliged to have our Negro students handle white patients unless clearly they can get equivalent experience in no other way.
   a. "Trouble" should be taken to provide equivalent experience with Negro patients as far as possible.
   b. Where it be documented that circumstances made it necessary for colored to handle whites, e.g., inpatient psychiatry, the chancellor will back the med school fully.
   c. Individual value judgment left to the various departments.

Van Wyk added, "I see no mandate for the dept. of ped. [pediatrics] to revise our policies. In fact, it was generally agreed that ped. is not a delicate area."[123]

Berryhill later reported to President Friday that he had met with Diggs and that "after a very frank discussion with him on the mores of this State at this time and probably for years to come he appeared to accept the policy in a realistic fashion."[124] Although the situation and policies in the various clinical services varied, it was some time before all student assignments were made without reference to race.

After graduating from UNC, Diggs interned at Kate Biting Reynolds Hospital, a black hospital in Winston-Salem; practiced for a few years in High Point; and then practiced in Washington, DC, until his retirement in 1978. When contacted in 1998 by phone by a student writing about the integration of medical facilities in North Carolina, he said he had "fond memories of [my] days at UNC. It wasn't the easiest thing in the world—I had my problems—but most of my experiences were good. My classmates were all gentlemen except one—[long pause]—and she was a gentle-lady . . . [As a woman] she was a minority, too."[125]

James Slade, a native of Edenton, North Carolina, and a graduate of North Carolina Agricultural and Technical State University in Greensboro, in 1957 was the second African American to receive the MD from UNC. After internship at the University of Pittsburgh, military service, and pediatric training at Los Angeles County Hospital, he returned to Edenton, where he practiced pediatrics and general medicine for almost four decades. He said much later that he had been accepted at both UNC and Meharry but wanted to go to UNC because it was closer to home and less expensive, and because "I felt I could do the work as well as the guys from Duke and Carolina and Davidson." The first time he went to the hospital cafeteria,

> the [serving] girls were a little skeptical about serving me. I guess they didn't know what to do. I went and talked to Diggs, and he told me that he hadn't had any problems there—he was lighter skinned and that may have made a difference. So I went back . . . and told them it was OK . . . I got down to the cashier. She told me, "You'll have to sit over there in the corner." I started toward the corner, but then I stopped and I sat dead center. We didn't have but two girls in my class, and one of the girls came and sat down at my table. Then some of my other classmates came and sat down, too, and that was the end of that.

In a recent interview Slade said he had had little trouble in the first two years. At the beginning of the third year, the chief of surgery talked with him and "said they didn't particularly think it was right, but they wanted to know if I would consent to work just on the black patients' ward . . . At that time, even Chapel Hill was separated by color. I went along with it. It wasn't anything I would have put a stamp of approval on, but, by the same token, I was willing to go ahead, at that point in time, and see what would work out. My white patients didn't resent my taking care of them; but the administration just wasn't ready for it. They were in the growing stages of integration." Slade added, "Obstetrics was hardest. OB was strictly divided down the line by race. On OB, where I should have been learning to do pelvic exams, they never let me do them on white patients. I could only do them on black. And I only got called in when the black ladies were in labor. On the medicine service, though, they would let me do pelvic exams on anybody, white or black. It just depended on who was the attending physician." Slade concluded the interview by saying, "Everything wasn't perfect in Chapel Hill, but . . . I have never really regretted going to Chapel Hill . . . My senior year, I didn't know anything about the Alpha Omega Alpha honor society [the medical school equivalent of Phi Beta Kappa]. They could easily have passed me by and I wouldn't have known the difference, but they invited me in." He added, "So I thought that spoke well for the faculty at Chapel Hill."[126]

By 1959 it was reported that since the first admissions of blacks in 1951, UNC had enrolled twenty-three black undergraduates, sixty-nine graduate students, twenty-three law students, five medical students, and a few in other professional schools.[127] Through the efforts of Dean Christopher Fordham and subsequent deans, the School of Medicine made steady progress in recruiting both women and African Americans to the medical school. As a result, the UNC medical school has ranked in some recent years as having more African American graduates than any medical school in the nation other than the historically black medical schools.[128]

The medical classes of 1954 and 2004 provide an interesting perspective on the changing demography of the state and of medical education at the university. The forty-eight graduating members of the first four-year class of 1954 were all from North Carolina, and all were white males, with the exception of two white females. In contrast, the fiftieth-anniversary class of 2004 was representative of the rich diversity of the School of Medicine and other university programs in the early part of the university's third century of service to the people of the state and nation. The class of 2004 entered medical school in the fall of 2000 with 160 students, 140 (88 percent) of whom were from within the state and 20 (12 percent) of whom were from out of state. At the time of graduation in 2004, the class of 153 students was composed of 79 men and 74 women. Of the class, 115 members were white, 16 were African American, 11 were East Asian, 7 were Indian or Pakistani, 2 were Hispanic, 1 was Native American, and 1 person's race was unreported.[129]

MEDICAL ALUMNI

Berryhill always recognized the vital role of loyal alumni in supporting the school during the different stages of its growth and the various crises dating back to its opening. He was unequivocal in stating "that the alumni were the most important force in initialing and carrying to a successful conclusion the fourth move to develop the four-year medical school during the years 1943–1947."[130]

The UNC medical alumni had met for lunch at the annual meetings of the Medical Society of North Carolina beginning in the 1930s, but the first annual meeting of the Medical Alumni Association in Chapel Hill was held on March 5, 1952, six months before the hospital opened. Berryhill had organized the meeting as a way to thank alumni for their support and to involve them in the ongoing needs and concerns of the medical school. He said that the turnout of almost 250 alumni and the "evident interest in and enthusiasm for the faculty, the hospital, and the whole development was most gratifying." He added, "This fine and active group with proper guidance can be of tremendous help throughout North

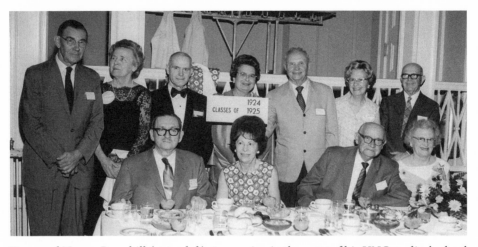

Reece and Norma Berryhill *(upper left)* at a reunion in the 1950s of his UNC medical school classmates from the 1924 and 1925 classes. *(UNC Photo Lab, NCC)*

Carolina and many have already shown their willingness to contribute annually to the financial support of the School."[131]

The administrator of the Division of Health Affairs vetoed an effort by Berryhill to establish a public relations office for the medical school and hospital in the early 1950s. As an alternative Berryhill supported the founding in 1953 of the *Bulletin of the School of Medicine,* which was co-sponsored by the Whitehead Society (the medical student body) and the Medical Foundation.[132] The first issue contained a condensation of the Whitehead Society address delivered to the entering class on September 18, 1953, by Brinkhous, who hoped they would be able to be "in line for many feasts of medical knowledge" throughout their careers and that they would "continue all your professional life as a scholar—the real meaning of the word Doctor." Hedgpeth provided a brief summary of the admissions policy for the school: "Definite preference is given to North Carolina students and the Admissions Committee tries diligently to select students they feel will make good physicians in North Carolina." This was followed by a compendium of the accomplishments and challenges of the new school by Dean Berryhill in an article entitled, "Medical Progress at Chapel Hill: A New and Yet an Old School."[133]

The annual Medical Alumni Association meeting in Chapel Hill on April 12–13, 1954, was of special significance for Berryhill and the School of Medicine. Not only would the first class of medical students be graduating with the MD degree later in the spring, but also it was the seventy-fifth anniversary of the beginning of medical education at the university in 1879. The latter was celebrated the next year with two days of events "geared to future plans, responsibilities and ambitions rather than past accomplishments." The anniversary program brought "to the campus a number of men prominent in the state and nation as well as a panel of distinguished members of the University faculty." The first panel discussion, held in the campus's Hill Hall, looked at "Medical Education at

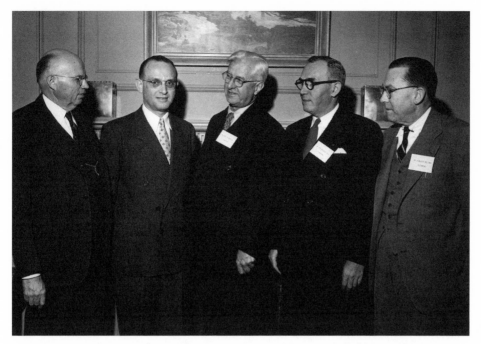

Speakers at the first annual Medical Alumni Association meeting in Chapel Hill, March 1952, included *(left)* Dr. W. T. Sanger, president of the Medical College of Virginia at Richmond and chair of the national committee that produced the 1946 Sanger Report and *(third from left)* Dr. John A. Ferrell, a 1907 MD graduate of the UNC Medical Department at Raleigh and executive secretary, North Carolina Medical Care Commission *(NCC)*

the University of North Carolina, Past, Present, Future" and was followed by an open house at the School of Medicine, where the laboratories and other facilities in the basic sciences were open to the public. One panel the next day focused on "Financing Medical Education" and included panelists from New York Hospital, the Yale University School of Medicine, and the National Heart Institute. The participants in the third panel, "Humane Letters and Human Illness," consisted of Nathan Womack and a group of UNC faculty that included Professors Hall in philosophy, Howell in English, Holmes in romance philology, Lyons in English, Leavitt in Spanish, and Ullman in classics.[134]

A Distinguished Service Award was initiated at the annual Medical Alumni Association meeting in the spring of 1954 and has continued to this day. Berryhill wrote that the initial awards were intended to recognize the contributions of alumni and others to the expansion of the medical school, while subsequent awards were to go to alumni and others for their exceptional achievements in medicine or their unique contributions in support of the school.[135] A 1950 graduate of the two-year school recalled a discussion about a candidate for this award when both he and Berryhill were serving on the selection committee. The candidate had practiced primary care in a small town for years and was an outstanding example of the physician-citizen, "which then, as now, was held to be the desirable product of a medical school." Berryhill rejected him, stating simply, "That's what we trained him to do." The alumnus added later, "In retrospect and somewhat older I have to confess to agreeing with him."[136]

Another special medical alumni celebration occurred in March 1963 with the celebration of the tenth anniversary of the hospital opening and the expansion of the School of Medicine. The theme was "A Decade of Achievement—Opportunities for the Future." Chancellor Aycock led off with a discussion of future developments at the university and the role of the medical center, while Lennox P. McLendon, Sr., reviewed the highlights of the years from 1944 to 1952. Kenneth Brinkhous reviewed the previous ten years from the point of view of the pre-clinical departments, while Nathan Womack did the same for the clinical departments. John S. Rhodes, MD, a 1927 graduate of the two-year school and a past president of the Medical Alumni Association, reviewed the contributions of the School of Medicine from the point of view of the medical alumni, while Holt McPherson, editor of the *High Point Enterprise,* discussed the changes in and contribution to the state of the School of Medicine and North Carolina Memorial Hospital from the point of view of the public. Berryhill concluded with a "look to the future."[137]

In addition to attending the medical alumni events held in Chapel Hill, Berryhill was frequently on the road to make presentations to county and district medical societies throughout the state. In 1951–1952 he made ten such presentations. He was also in demand to consult with other states that were contemplating expanded or new medical schools. In 1951–1952 this included a "conference with a committee from the New Jersey Medical Society and N.J. legislature concerning establishment of a medical school" and a "conference with West Virginia state and University officials concerning expansion of their medical school."[138]

Although membership in the Medical Alumni Association initially was confined to graduates of the School of Medicine, it was later expanded to include all who had had house staff training at Memorial Hospital and UNC Hospitals. In keeping with Berryhill's desires, the Medical Alumni Association has never had membership dues.[139] By 2004 there were 9,599 living members of the association, including 5,934 medical school alumni and 3, 665 hospital house staff alumni.

Quite characteristically, Berryhill concluded his final remarks as dean at the annual Medical Alumni Association meeting in Chapel Hill in the spring of 1964 by reflecting on the sometimes contentious role of the alumni in the medical school and university:

> It is important to remember that in our society the institutions which are more nearly lasting and eternal are the church and the university with its many schools. It is very easy as humans to confuse an individual, a very temporary force in the church or the university, as [sic] the institution itself and when one becomes vexed or irritated or worse with a particular person

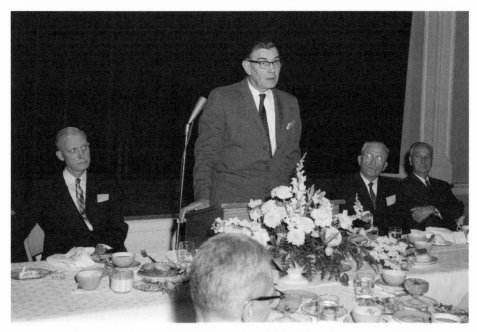

Dean Berryhill giving one of his annual reports to the Medical Alumni Association meeting, 1961. *(UNC Photo Lab, NCC)*

for doing or not doing any of a hundred things, to vent one's unhappiness by criticizing the institution far and wide, which may and frequently does [do] a great deal of harm. I would hope that more and more of the alumni of this University could develop the feeling and adopt the philosophy so well stated in the famous toast of the naval officer, Stephen Decatur, which, with no apologies for my paraphrasing, "Our University! May she always be right, but our University right or wrong." And again, a paraphrasing of the now famous dictum of the late Francis Weld Peabody, "The secret of the care of the University, is to care for the University."[140]

RESIGNATION AS DEAN

Berryhill and colleagues related that "in the autumn of 1962, Dean Berryhill had informed President Friday and Chancellor Aycock of his intention to resign from the deanship at the end of the 1963–1964 academic year, two years in advance of the [then] mandatory retirement age for administrative officers in the university."[141] This must have been a verbal communication, because the first preserved written documentation of his resignation is a letter in Berryhill's personnel file from Berryhill to Chancellor Aycock (with a copy to H. T. Clark) dated May 15, 1963.[142] He submitted his resignation "effective June 30, 1964, or as soon thereafter as it may be possible to effect an orderly transfer of administrative responsibility for the University Medical Center to whomever may be selected as my successor, but in any event I would hope this could take place not later than the autumn of 1964." By this time he said that "(1) my responsibilities in connection with decisions relating to the final plans for the southward expansion of the Hospital will have been completed and I hope as satisfactorily discharged as will be possible in view of what will almost certainly be inadequate funds to provide the space most urgently needed; and (2) the current fund-raising drive of the Medical Foundation will probably have accomplished about all it can."

Berryhill elaborated that he could have remained dean through the 1965–1966 year, but "after several months of very thoughtful and, I hope, objective consideration, I am taking this step at an earlier date for the following reasons:

1. The School of Medicine is beginning its second decade of development as an expanded school and as a University medical center in the true sense of the meaning of that designation. It has great potential in terms of a superior faculty and in its opportunity to become a truly great center . . . in medicine for the State and the Nation. It would seem appropriate that as early as practicable in this period the person who will have the responsibility for guiding future developments be selected. Hopefully, this will provide younger, abler, and more imaginative leadership, which is essential at this time.

2. While the above is a very important reason . . . for this decision at this time, in all honesty to you and in fairness to my successor I must state that of over-riding importance—and indeed the determining factor—is that it is impossible for the dean of the School of Medicine to continue to function administratively in the Division of Health Affairs. This applies both to the structure and, of more fundamental importance, to the unrealistic and illogical philosophy—both administrative and operating—of an organization which is fundamentally divisive throughout and not of University caliber in attitudes, in goals, and in performance . . . For more than a decade those of us in the Medical School, while captives in this unhappy environment and in effect the "whipping post" for the other Schools and the Administrator, have struggled to develop an excellent medical school and in spite of these adverse conditions have in large measure succeeded. To continue this struggle for the foreseeable future raises the question as to whether the goal is worth the price, when at comparable universities there is more encouragement, more assistance, and fewer obstructions . . .

3. For obvious reasons the greatest service I could render my successor would be an absence from the scene during the initial year of his tenure . . . Accordingly, I wish now to request my first leave of absence in thirty years' service, with whatever financial support from the University which may seem appropriate.

Berryhill included with his resignation letter a copy of his appointment letter as dean from R. B. House, dean of administration, dated August 27, 1941. He stated that this letter "carried the approval of President Frank Graham," and called attention to item 8: "In case of necessary relinquishment of the Deanship you will continue as Director of the Student Health Service at least at your present rate and share in any general advance in salary scale." In his 1963 letter Berryhill stated, "At that time neither of the three of us could possibly have predicted the events of the next two decades nor that I would continue as Dean of the Medical School for this length of time. As you are aware, I resigned as Director of the Student Health Service some time ago in fairness to Dr. Hedgpeth and the organization which he has so ably directed." He emphasized that discussion in the context of the university's commitment in 1941 was now required with regard to his continuing salary and "future work as a member of the Medical School Faculty until the usual retirement age." He added, "A satisfactory solution of these [questions] obviously has an important bearing on the implementation of this resignation."

Berryhill concluded his resignation letter: "I think you know that the welfare of the University and that of its School of Medicine have been—next to that of my own family—my chief interest and concern for the past thirty years." In his typical uncompromising style, he added, "I shall always give you and my successor all the possible support so long as the objectives and goals sought are those which I feel are to the best interests of the university and this medical center."

After other correspondence and discussions, on June 21, 1963, Aycock wrote to Berryhill telling him that "President Friday and I will honor your request to resign from the Medical School Deanship effective August 31, 1964. A leave of absence for the period September 1, 1964–August 31, 1965, is richly deserved and we will recommend it to the Executive Committee of the Board of Trustees . . . If necessary, your full salary will be paid from Medical School funds," but it was understood that he would apply for a foundation grant to pay part of his salary during his sabbatical. Aycock added, "We look forward to your return to full time University duties after the leave at a salary appropriate for a person of your training, experience, and seniority . . . I shall at a later date, express to you more fully my deep appreciation for all you have done for the University in the past; and I am confident that you will continue to work effectively and fruitfully in some other capacity. Please accept my personal good wishes and warmest regards."[143]

Clark acknowledged Berryhill's resignation in a brief letter dated July 9, 1963:

In reflecting today over your resignation as Dean of the School of Medicine, I am mindful of the great energy, dedication and singleness of purpose you have brought to the position for almost twenty-five years. I congratulate you on your many accomplishments during this period and wish for you a happy and satisfying experience in the years ahead.[144]

In his resignation letter, Berryhill appended "additional statements in support of the Medical School's position and some suggestions as to possible solutions" about the Health Affairs administrative structure in the university. Although he recognized that such suggestions had not been requested by the chancellor, he presented them "nevertheless in the hope that a different administrative and functional environment can be provided for the next dean of the Medical School." In this six-page statement he reviewed the recent history with such organizational structures in universities and noted that both Johns Hopkins and the University of Iowa had abandoned such structures because of the belief that "such an organization was both unnecessary and in a more important sense divisive and harmful to the larger interests of the institution."

He noted that "superficially there might appear to be some justifiable reason for such an administrative structure and such a grouping of professional schools" because "all schools [in the Division of Health Affairs] in one way or another are concerned with the education or training of personnel for the health professions." On the other hand, "the School of Medicine is more and more dependent upon and has established more mutually helpful relations with the Biological, Physical, and Social Sciences and with the Humanities in the University than with the schools in this Division."

Berryhill then cited statistics to show that the medical school faculty represented some 57 percent of all the faculty in the five-school Division; that the medical school had more than two-thirds of all the research and training grant support in the Division; and that the total operating budget for the medical school and hospital in 1961–1962 was 75 percent of the budget for the entire Division and 38 percent of the budget for the entire University of North Carolina at Chapel Hill. He cited these statistics "not in a boastful fashion but to indicate the real importance of the Medical Center in the operation of the University as well as its magnitude. Yet in spite of this, in actual fact, in the Division Board and in operating philosophy the Medical Faculty comprises a minority group in a very real sense." As a consequence, he said, this structure has interfered with the planning for needed expansion in the Medical Center, because the

> internal operations, policies or projects of the School of Medicine have to be reported to and reviewed by the Division of Health Affairs Board [more often] than those of any other school. This has been true for a long time. One can only conclude from this practice that the Administrator and Deans of the other schools either have little or no confidence in the School of Medicine or what is more likely, they fear the greater potential of the Medical School and wish to take every opportunity to get into every activity or to "control" the Medical School's development. This is for the most part a petty annoyance, although in reality it can be and indeed has been a serious handicap to the Medical School.

Because of the medical faculty's lack of confidence in the Division's administration and its advisory committee, Berryhill urged that the chancellor appoint a search committee for his successor composed of representative members of the medical faculty along with "any other appropriate representation but especially I would hope from the Graduate School and the College of Arts and Sciences. It would be reassuring also if you would make it clear that the appointment [of the new dean] would be yours and not that of the Administrator and that the Advisory Committee of the Division would have no part in this appointment."

Berryhill concluded this statement with recommendations that would require several decades before they were partially or fully realized:

1. That the designation, the *University of North Carolina Medical Center* comprising these units [School of Medicine and North Carolina Memorial Hospital] and the Gravely Sanatorium for teaching, research and patient care be officially approved. This is a simple, dignified, and meaningful designation and is in keeping with present thought and nomenclature in major universities.

2. That this important segment of the University be removed administratively from the Division of Health Affairs, and that hereafter the Dean of the Medical School be designated Dean and Director of the Medical Center, responsible directly to the Chancellor and the Business Manager of the University.[145]

He amplified on the second recommendation: "The contributions and accomplishments of the Medical School in education and research in the past ten years would appear to have now earned for it a definite place in the academic life of the University and to merit inclusion within the General University in what is currently designated 'the academic division,' a status which it occupied from approximately 1900 to 1949." He also argued that

in large measure the fiscal problems of the Medical School and Hospital can, with adequate and competent assistance which to date has never been available, be handled internally within the Medical Center. Those which cannot are of such importance and complexity that the [university] Business Manager and Chancellor are inevitably involved. In my experience, such problems can be presented more effectively and accurately by those intimately concerned with the day to day operation of the Medical Center than through a "third party" [that is, the administrator of the Division] . . . In general, therefore, the Division organization is of limited assistance, either to the School of Medicine or to you [the chancellor], in matters of major importance both financial and educational.

Berryhill elaborated on these 1963 recommendations to Chancellor Aycock in remarks he made as his last report as dean to the Medical Alumni Association meeting in the spring of 1964:

He said his call to remove the Medical School from the Division of Health Affairs is not intended as a criticism of the Schools of Dentistry, Nursing, Pharmacy, and Public Health, all of which are performing well in terms of their professional roles and responsibilities. At the same time, at this stage in their evolution as professional schools, they are primarily concerned with vocational training, as important and indeed invaluable as this is in the health fields. The fact remains that these schools depend upon medicine and its excellence and the problem we have to struggle against constantly in this administrative structure is to prevent medicine from being equated with the other schools. I am convinced medicine will continue to be in trouble until there is a definite and clear concept with implementing policy that medicine has a different role in a university and must have the opportunity and the freedoms within the general policies of the university to work out its own future.[146]

In a reflection of the ever-increasing complexity of the medical school administration and his own changing attitudes about this endeavor, he advised:

Aside from removing the Medical School from the Division of Health Affairs the new dean of the Medical School, to preserve a reasonable degree of equanimity and sanity, must have: A larger group of full-time, or nearly so, able administrative assistants. This will cost money but it would be a small outlay in terms of results in a more effective and pleasant administration. Among others these include: (1) A combined financial office for the Hospital and Medical School. (2) A joint personnel office for Hospital and Medical School. (3) Three or more Assistant or Associate Deans essentially full time. (4) A full-time, competent public information, public relations and development officer and office.

I should make it very clear that in recommending these assistants, as I have said over and over again, that for an effective University and Medical School administration, the fiscal office, the personnel office and the public information and development should be branches of the University's main undertaking in these areas. Everyone in the Medical School is striving to get back into the University not to secede from it.

Berryhill's readiness for retirement is well documented in his twenty-third and last annual report as dean for 1963–1964. He begins with a lament that "there is little evidence that many of the major problems of the Medical Center which have been presented repeatedly in these reports and elsewhere for almost a decade, together with suggestions for possible solutions, have received any serious consideration by those in the University who could have been helpful." He then provides a list of nine "frustrating and disappointing events of the year," the last of which repeated his concern about "the increasing evidence over the past six to eight months that the Administration of the Division of Health Affairs has been moving in to undermine and indeed take over the administrative responsibilities of the Medical School in policy-making decisions of the utmost importance to the future of the Medical Center without discussion or consultation." This list was only partially balanced by eight developments "on the brighter side" that included a state Medical Care Commission award of $2,487,375 for the addition to the hospital and his recognition of "the able and conscientious efforts of Dr. Isaac M. Taylor," who had represented the dean's office in coordinating the planning for this major hospital expansion.[147]

An article in the *Raleigh News and Observer* in September 1963 about Berryhill's planned retirement the following summer both praised him and his accomplishments and addressed some of the continuing concerns about the supply of doctors in the state's communities, an issue Berryhill would try to address after returning from his sabbatical year.[148] It began:

> The dean is not retiring.
>
> Dr. Wallace [*sic*] Reece Berryhill, 63, dean of the medical school of the University of North Carolina, is merely going back to his first love, teaching.
>
> His monumental work in the development of the four-year medical school at Chapel Hill has brought praise from his colleagues over the length and breadth of the State.
>
> Development of the school and the great medical center of which it is a part has been a struggle, rife with tug-of-war politics and varied controversy. But now it is there in high splendor on a hilltop, dominant in the pastoral setting of the graceful old campus.
>
> In his efforts toward the establishment of the four-year medical school, Dr. Berryhill moved over the State, talking, persuading and even begging. The tall doctor with the big, powerful hands at last saw the dream rise in brick, granite and concrete.

After relating several stories about Berryhill and his role as a teacher and leader, the reporter concluded: "Dr. Berryhill is a friendly man without pretensions. Recently a visitor to the medical center who had occasion to talk to the dean, summed up his impression in his own homespun way: 'You know, the bigger they are, the plainer they are.'"

The reporter cited a number of statistics to show the growth of the school under Berryhill's leadership. The first class in 1954 had forty-eight graduates with MD degrees; just eight years later, in 1962, the school graduated sixty-two MDs. Berryhill "proudly cites the UNC school of medicine as the largest single source of doctors in the State." The total enrollment of medical students had grown to 264, in addition to 41 students working toward graduate degrees in the medical school. The full-time medical faculty had grown to 190, with an additional 193 physicians providing part-time teaching services. "This seemingly large faculty" was justified because it provided instruction not only to medical students, interns, and residents but also to students in the other health sciences schools of dentistry, nursing, pharmacy, and public health as well as to students in the allied health sciences programs, such as medical technicians and physiotherapists. In addition, more than 1,000 practicing physicians took postgraduate courses provided by the medical school, while the medical staffs of a dozen community hospitals in the state had continuing education programs from the school conducted by two-way radio. Thus, in all there were some 2,800 who received instruction from the medical faculty in the previous year.

In spite of these accomplishments, the reporter noted, "medicine and medical care are in controversy in legislative halls and among the citizenry generally" because of the continuing shortage of physicians at the community level. Berryhill recognized the inevitable question posed by these shortages: "Does the medical center with its vast program of teaching and research tend to siphon off doctors who would otherwise set up practice throughout the State, thus contributing to the shortage of doctors rather than alleviating that shortage[?]" While agreeing that "it is difficult to keep in proper balance the three vital components of teaching, patient care and research" with the large sums of federal monies now available for research, Berryhill maintained that "the overwhelming majority of graduates of the medical school go into private practice." He added, "92 per cent of all the graduates of the four-year medical school since its inception have remained in North Carolina. He said that of these a relatively small number have gone into research and teaching, while the majority are practicing in 70 counties."

In contrast, the reporter noted that "many doctors are outspoken in their views on federal research grants and private foundations" and commented that "the immensity of the payroll of one large organization professing dedication to the eradication of a certain disease provoked a physician to remark that the ailment is 'supporting more people than it's killing.'"

The president of the North Carolina Medical Society, John Rhodes, MD, a graduate of the UNC two-year medical school who practiced in Raleigh, pointed to the fact that the NIH, which was supporting most of the research grants, had grown in fifteen years from a budget of about $600,000 to its current budget of some $973 million. He saw this as a problem for the younger physician, who "might be influenced a lot by the size of the grant he gets rather than zeal and dedication." Nevertheless, Rhodes emphasized "the continuing need for genuine medical research. We (the practicing physician and the medical researcher) are both working for the same end."

Another physician, John Morris, MD, a University of Virginia graduate who practiced in Morehead City, was more outspoken about his perception of the problem. He believed that the current emphasis on research was based on "competing for money rather than research":

Many of the researchers picked during their time in medical school would benefit more spending their summers with doctors in practice, particularly in small communities. They wouldn't feel they had to gravitate to the big medical centers where they would to stay too close to the ivory tower. There they get to the place where they don't want to leave, they have a fear of getting out into practice and taking the really hard knocks. They get a salary and don't have to do a lot of things they don't want to do. Yet we in the field see a shortage of doctors and it's getting worse than a lot of medical schools like to admit.

Morris conceded that the "medical centers offer a tremendous amount of help in difficult cases . . . but more doctors are needed in the field . . . Were it not for large amounts of money, boys would not be kept on with grants, but would have to get out and practice."

The reporter concluded that this "controversy [of researchers vs. practicing physicians] isn't likely to subside. It is also unlikely that the research program in the medical school of the University of North Carolina will diminish. Both teachers and practitioners agree the goal to be achieved is proper balance."

Following his sabbatical leave during 1964–1965, Berryhill would return to North Carolina with the goal of helping to restore this balance by focusing on the university's role in community medical education and thus on educating more physicians for community practice.

PART IV

Taking Medical Education to the Communities
of North Carolina, 1964–1979

Dr. Berryhill firmly believes that "with the active cooperation and participation by the [then] three medical schools in the state, many educational and service opportunities will become available to the medically isolated communities throughout the State."

> —Tar Heel of the Week citation, *Raleigh News and Observer,* February 26, 1950

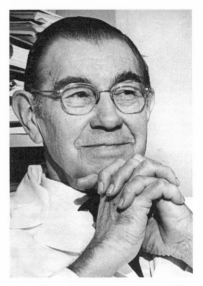

Dean Emeritus W. Reece Berryhill, 1973. *(Berryhill Family)*

What colleges of agriculture once did for a rural society can now be done for an urban society by the health sciences centers [a medical school, other health sciences schools and the associated teaching hospital]—and that is to improve the quality of life for nearly all people in their areas.

We recommend 126 area health education centers to serve localities without a health science center. Each of these centers would be at a local hospital. The centers' educational programs would be administered by university health science centers. They would train medical residents and M.D. and D.D.S. candidates on a rotational basis; they would carry on continuing education for local doctors, dentists, and other health care personnel . . . We consider this development of basic importance. It would put most of the local advantages of a health science center into many localities which do not warrant a full-scale center. This proposal would put essential health services within one hour of driving time for over 95 percent of all Americans and within the same amount of time for all health care personnel. Much of the nation would be served by a higher level of expertise than is now locally available.

Carnegie Commission Report, 1970

CHAPTER 9

Community Medical Education
and the Final Years

After completing his first career as university physician in 1941 and his second career as dean of the UNC medical school in 1964, Dean Emeritus Reece Berryhill launched a third one as an advocate for bringing medical education to the community level, with the goal of further improving the distribution of physicians and the quality of medical care throughout North Carolina. He began this new career with a well-deserved year-long sabbatical, during which he studied trends in medical education and medical practice abroad and in this country.

Berryhill's appointment in 1966 as director of the UNC medical school's new Division of Education and Research in Community Medical Care provided him the staff and resources for the finale of his long and dedicated service to the university and to the people of the state. He served as director until 1969 and remained a full-time member of the Division until 1971. He served as a half-time member of the Division from 1971 to 1973 and then as a consultant to the Division until 1975. He then continued as Sarah Graham Kenan Professor of Medicine Emeritus and remained an interested observer of the events in the university and medical school until his death in 1979.

Glenn Wilson followed Berryhill as director of the Division in 1970. He led the highly successful effort to obtain federal Area Health Education Center (AHEC) funding in 1972 and was the dynamic and innovative founding director of the NC AHEC Program from 1972 to 1978.

The creation of the Division in 1966 came at a time of great social and political changes in the nation and state and of intense ferment in medical education circles. The 1960s were a time not only of national unrest due to the Vietnam War and the assassinations of John Kennedy, Robert Kennedy, and Martin Luther King, Jr., but also of the War on Poverty and of major new federal programs in civil rights and health care. Medicare for citizens over age sixty-five was enacted in 1965 over the opposition of many physicians, who feared that it would lead to socialized medicine. The Regional Medical Program (RMP) attempted to establish regional medical education centers, with a particular focus on dealing with the three major fatal diseases at the time—heart disease, cancer, and stroke.

The Office of Economic Opportunity (OEO), through its declared War on Poverty, initiated a nationwide program of community health centers particularly oriented to the needs of poor and minority communities.

From the local and national developments in health care delivery and medical education in the 1960s and early 1970s came a number of changes that have had a lasting impact on health care education and delivery in North Carolina:

1. The establishment in 1966 of the Division for Education and Research in Community Medical Care at the UNC–CH School of Medicine; the establishment in 1966 of the Department of Community Health Sciences at the Duke University Medical Center; and the founding in 1974 at the Bowman Gray School of Medicine at Wake Forest University of a Department of Family Medicine.

2. The establishment in 1968 at UNC–CH of the Medical Air Operations program to provide air transportation for various outreach programs in the state.

3. The establishment in 1968 of the Health Services Research Center on the UNC–CH campus. The center, now known as the Cecil G. Sheps Center for Health Service Research, is one of the oldest and largest of such centers in the nation.

4. The establishment of physician extender programs. The Duke University Medical Center was a pioneer in training physician extenders when the Physician Assistant Program was established in 1965.[1] Initially the students were former military medical corpsmen who entered an academic and clinical curriculum to prepare them to work as assistants to practicing physicians. The Bowman Gray School of Medicine established a Physician Assistant Program in 1968. A Nurse Practitioner program was established in 1970 at UNC–CH to train nurses to work as primary care providers in rural communities under the direction of area physicians. This program continues today as one of several tracks toward the degree of Master of Science in Nursing, although the requirement for a sponsoring physician and practice site as a prerequisite for admission to the program has been dropped.

5. The founding in 1970 at UNC–CH of the new Department of Family Medicine, the only UNC medical school department that was mandated by legislative action. Today this department is ranked among the top of its kind in the nation and has educated numerous physicians for both practice and academic positions.

6. The establishment with federal funds in 1970 of the Orange Chatham

Comprehensive Health System (OCCHS) to provide health services for the poor and minorities in local communities. This continues today as Piedmont Health Services, with clinical facilities in four counties in the Chapel Hill area.

7. The development in the late 1960s and early 1970s of UNC medical school affiliations with community hospitals in the state for the purpose of providing undergraduate and graduate educational programs in community medicine.

8. The establishment in 1972 of the North Carolina AHEC program, which now covers the entire state and is in partnership with all four of the state's medical schools: Duke University, East Carolina University, the University of North Carolina, and Wake Forest University.

9. The establishment of a second state-supported medical school at East Carolina University. From 1972 to 1975 this was a one-year program, with the student transferring to UNC–CH for the last three years of medical school. It became a four-year medical school in 1977 and graduated its first MD class in 1981. The ECU medical school was one of twenty-five new community-based medical schools that state legislatures funded around the nation in the 1970s to address the shortage of primary care physicians. Most (like ECU, which utilized the expanded Pitt County Memorial Hospital as its teaching hospital) used community hospitals for teaching rather than constructing new university hospitals. These new schools almost doubled the number of MD graduates in the United States, from 8,367 in 1970 to 15,113 in 1980. See Appendix C.

10. The establishment in 1973 of the Office of Rural Health as a branch of the state government in Raleigh, the first in the nation. The office has developed more than eighty rural community health centers across the state, many of which serve as educational sites for students and residents; has helped recruit more than 2,500 physicians, nurses, and other health care personnel for rural communities; and administers several other programs to strengthen health care in rural areas.[2]

Background

Berryhill's vision of the university's role in improving the health of all North Carolinians was strongly influenced by his exposure as an undergraduate at Chapel Hill during 1917–1921 to the views of the young and vibrant UNC president, Edward Kidder Graham, whose own dream was "to make the campus co-extensive with the boundaries of the State, and while keeping the standards of university instruction and scholarly research on the highest plane, to put the

University—as head of the State's educational system—in warm, sensitive touch with every problem in North Carolina life, small and great."[3]

The medical school, under the leadership of Dean Isaac H. Manning and with the encouragement of the state health officer and the leaders of the Medical Society of the State of North Carolina, put Graham's dream into practice as early as 1916 by sponsoring circuit-riding, community-based courses for physicians who had neither the time nor the money to attend courses at distant academic medical centers or national meetings. The first summer courses were offered in pediatrics one day a week for sixteen weeks in six eastern communities and for twelve weeks in six central and western communities. The visiting experts would repeat their program each day for a week as they made the circuit—usually by train—from one community to another; the next week the speaker would visit the same circuit of communities with a new program. This unique approach reached some 185 practicing physicians the first year and was "believed to be the first such statewide effort in the country."[4]

The earliest published evidence of Berryhill's and the state's commitment to a statewide approach to medical care and education is found in a paper entitled "A Proposed Program for More Adequate Medical Care and Hospitalization in North Carolina" that he read in the Section on Medical Education and Hospital Training at the Southern Medical Association's Annual Meeting in Cincinnati in November 1945, only three months after the conclusion of World War II.[5] Berryhill described how in 1943 he and a group of North Carolina's medical leaders had held a series of meetings to determine what steps could be taken at the community and state levels to address the inadequacies of medical care in North Carolina.

He told the Cincinnati audience about the first two steps made in addressing the state's health needs. The first was taken when the recommendations for action by the committee of physicians received the enthusiastic support of Governor J. Melville Broughton.

The second step was taken in early 1944 when Broughton, with the approval of the university's board of trustees, appointed an ad hoc Hospital and Medical Care Commission to study the health problems in North Carolina and to make recommendations to the state legislature. Berryhill and the other members of the commission worked for almost a year on this task and produced a comprehensive report that formed the basis for his presentation in Cincinnati.[6]

Berryhill summarized for the Cincinnati audience some of the ad hoc commission's recommendations in its 1945 report:

> To meet the need for more medical personnel, and especially as an essential part of the foundation for a comprehensive statewide hospital and medical care program, it was recommended that the present two-year medical school of the University of North Carolina be expanded into a four-year school with the construction of at least a 400-bed general hospital, available for patients

from all economic levels throughout the state but especially for the low income groups . . .

The University Medical Center was visualized as an integral and essential part of any program designed to provide better medical care in the state (1) in providing opportunities for training state residents in medicine, nursing, medical technology, dietetics, hospital administration, and possibly later in dentistry; (2) in improving the quality of medical care through a program of continuation courses for practicing physicians in the state, at the center but especially through carrying postgraduate instruction to the small hospitals and health centers in the more rural and medically isolated areas; and (3) in supplying, as a part of a medical care and an educational program, a consultation and teaching service by members of the university staff to the smaller hospitals . . . It was believed that through these services the quality of medical care can be improved and standards maintained and that younger physicians will be better satisfied to locate and to remain in smaller communities with assurance of this type of professional stimulation and aid.

Berryhill concluded his presentation in Cincinnati, "For a conservative Southern state like North Carolina to have done as much as this in one year in the midst of a world war is definitely encouraging." See Appendix G.

The third step in taking a statewide approach to health education and medical care came in July 1945, when the state legislature established a permanent Medical Care Commission to succeed the ad hoc Hospital and Medical Care Commission of 1944–1945. Its mission was to coordinate the planning and implementation of the statewide plan for improved health care for North Carolinians.

The new commission took the fourth step when it assembled the National Committee for the Medical School Survey to study and make recommendations about the need for, and the feasibility of, expanding the medical school at Chapel Hill. Five of the seven members of the committee, led by William T. Sanger, PhD, president of the Medical College of Virginia, made a majority recommendation in 1946 supporting the expansion of the medical school and the building of a teaching hospital at Chapel Hill, with various stipulations. (See Appendix I.) Two other recommendations of the majority Sanger Report emphasized the need for a statewide approach by the university to improving medical care:

That such a school of medicine and associated services of the medical center, responsive to the will of the people, be integrated effectively and continuously with a State-wide network of hospitals and health centers in so far as these volunteer to cooperate; merely to expand the two-year medical school at Chapel Hill in order to graduate a greater number of physicians is not regarded as sufficient justification for such expansion . . .

That the University of North Carolina develop a philosophy of medical education, research, and medical care which will make it a service facility for the whole State.[7]

This goal of a statewide health program integrated with the expanded medical school was ridiculed in a minority report by two members of the national committee: "The comprehensive educational and service program recommended in this [the majority] report has not been attempted in all its details anywhere in the world."[8] See Appendix J. In the heated debate that preceded the Medical Care Commission's adoption of the majority report, Paul Whitaker, MD, cited this sentence as indicating the "complete lack of comprehension and imagination which characterizes this minority report." He called instead for the state "to engage the cooperative efforts of all agencies and institutions—public and private" to solve its health problems. "What North Carolina acutely needs is more cooperation and less appeal to religious, denominational, and 'interest' rivalry and prejudice."[9]

The unique opportunity that UNC had to take a leadership role in developing a statewide approach to medical education was reiterated by Andrew J. Warren, MD, a UNC graduate and a director of the Rockefeller Foundation's efforts in medicine and public health, in an address at the university's 160th annual commencement in June 1954 on the occasion of the graduation of the first MDs from the expanded School of Medicine and of the first DDSs from the new School of Dentistry:

> The recommendation "that the University of North Carolina develop a philosophy of medical education, research and medical care which will make it a service facility for the whole State" is unique in the experience of health-care programs at the present time [1954], and yet this uniqueness is rather surprising in view of the obvious logic of a concept which provides for the close integration of teaching and health service. This concept has proved successful in the Institute of Government, the Institute for Research in Social Science and in the field of agriculture. And if methodology for its application to the health field can be developed, an outstanding contribution to the solution of the problem of medical care will have been made . . . Pioneering always offers the opportunity for contributing something of value along a path previously undeveloped or even unknown. This is an opportunity which the University is now well equipped to develop.[10]

Although Berryhill never wavered in his commitment to this statewide approach to medical education, when it came to the timetable he was a realist. Several papers in the April 1955 issue of the *Bulletin of the School of Medicine* commemorated the first seventy-five years of medical education at Chapel Hill. Berryhill's contribution to this review of the history of the school was entitled "What About the Road Ahead?" and concluded:

It must be pointed out that the National Committee realized that an education program with such broad and far-reaching objectives would take time and thought to effectuate if it were to be done wisely and in a lasting manner. The wording [in the final summary paragraph of the Sanger Report] is "... *ultimately* develop a philosophy ... which will make it a service facility for the whole State." No institution can become full grown overnight. The faculty is unmoved in its determination to build soundly in reaching the goals outlined even though with the facilities available this may be a slower process than we would have hoped.[11]

The fifth and final step toward achieving the statewide approach recommended by the Hospital and Medical Care Commission in 1945 and by the Sanger Committee in 1946 came two and a half decades later in the 1970s with the medical school's outreach across the state through the North Carolina Area Health Education Centers (AHEC) program. This federal- and state-funded effort has the mission of improving the quality and distribution of medical care by providing medical and other health-related educational programs in communities outside of academic medical centers.

Further Evolution of Thinking about Community Medical Education and Practice

Another stimulus for Berryhill's personal commitment to the concept of a statewide approach to medical education undoubtedly was the indignant reaction of some in his home community of Charlotte to the recommendation of the Sanger Committee that the expanded school and teaching hospital be located in Chapel Hill. Although other state newspapers were generally supportive of the Sanger Report, a July 1946 editorial in the *Charlotte Observer* entitled "Virtually an Absurdity" had this to say:

> If the recommendation of the Survey committee comes to fruition, the largest city in the state with the greatest density of population within its environs and already recognized as a foremost medical center of the Southeast will be ignored with all of its admitted assets and indisputable claims as the site of this development in favor of the village of Chapel Hill, which has little to offer except intangible traditions and institutional pride.[12]

A follow-up letter entitled "A Rural Doctor Protests" in the *Charlotte Observer,* by Grady Dixon, MD, of Ayden, noted that many of the leaders in the North Carolina health care effort were not UNC graduates (and thus were not motivated by "institutional pride"). He concluded:

> I speak as a rural doctor who has done rural practice for over 30 years and one who knows the untold benefits that will come to all of our people when

this program is successfully inaugurated. I know as a rural practitioner the value that a State supported medical teaching institution will be to all of our people. The rural doctors and the rural people say to you, "Forget your local disappointments and join us in the general interests of all the people."[13]

The next edition of the *Charlotte Observer* carried a defensive editorial stating that it was "not opposed to the general better health program" for all the state but "does not believe a THIRD four-year medical school, with the adjunct of a 500-bed hospital, is the most important part or even an essential factor in such a program, or that it would necessarily provide needed hospital facilities and adequate medical care for the rural people of the State, whose views Dr. Dixon says the *Observer* does not express."[14]

Berryhill could appreciate Charlotte's continuing desire to have a medical school after the loss of its own school in the aftermath of the 1910 Flexner Report, but he must have been shocked at the bitterness of this reaction and frustrated by his own inability to address the issue at the time. It would take another two decades of building the home base at Chapel Hill before he was able to establish UNC affiliations for medical student and residency training at Charlotte and to make the Charlotte medical community a vital player in the university's state-wide medical education endeavor.

These earlier activities clearly had shaped Berryhill's vision of the role of the university's medical school in improving health care in the communities of the state. Further developments in the later years of his service as dean galvanized his determination to accomplish these goals.

A critical development supporting the move of medical education to the community level in North Carolina was the remarkable change in the hospitals of the state in the decades of the 1950s and 1960s. This was in good measure because of North Carolina's Good Health Movement and the concomitant availability of federal Hill-Burton funds for hospital construction.

At the beginning of the Good Health Movement in the mid-1940s, the state had only two hospitals of any size with significant educational programs—Duke Hospital and medical school in Durham and Baptist Hospital and Bowman Gray School of Medicine in Winston-Salem. By the late 1960s the state had three academic medical centers—in Chapel Hill, Durham, and Winston-Salem. Another nine community hospitals of more than 200 beds each were located in all the major geographic regions of the state. Although none of these nine hospitals had a formal affiliation with a medical school at the beginning of the 1960s, by the end of the decade six of the nine already had physicians as part-time or full-time directors of medical education, while a seventh was recruiting one. The community hospital and medical staff leadership had clearly recognized the importance of an educational environment in their hospitals for successfully recruiting physicians and providing the best medical care for their patients.[15]

Another motivation for the community medicine educational effort came in the 1960s as citizens and political leaders throughout the country began to complain about the "ivory tower" approach of many academic medical centers, with their dedication to research funded by seemingly inexhaustible NIH grants and their education of specialist physicians to the exclusion of any others. Residents of smaller communities and rural areas saw their old general practitioners (GPs) dying out.[16] These citizens had the perception that they had been abandoned by the academic medical centers in which the public had made such a tremendous investment and began demanding that they provide doctors to care for the people's basic medical needs. However, because the specialists being trained by the leading academic medical centers were in such demand, many faculty members were slow to change their ways.[17]

What the general public could not see was that a small group of physicians and others in academic medicine were beginning to focus on the importance of primary or generalist physicians. Notable among these were three faculty members at Chapel Hill: Kerr L. White, MD, and T. Franklin Williams, MD, both in the Departments of Medicine and Preventive Medicine, and Bernard Greenberg, PhD, in the Department of Biostatistics of the School of Public Health. Beginning in the late 1950s, they and their colleagues obtained grants to study patients seen in the practices of some ninety general practitioners in North Carolina. These included tabulation of the number of patients referred to other physicians and the number referred to the three teaching hospitals then serving North Carolina's four million citizens. Among their findings was "massive miscommunication" among the patient, the referring physician, the medical student, the resident, and the attending physician. For example, one patient wanted help for her depression; her GP referred her for "back pain" and the attending physician at the medical center found a thyroid nodule. White, Williams, and Greenberg published several articles on their findings, which today would be called health service research but at the time were looked down upon by those engaged in the more prestigious biomedical research.[18]

In 1961 White, Williams, and Greenberg published in the *New England Journal of Medicine* a now-classic article entitled "The Ecology of Medical Care." They showed—based on their data and other literature—that out of 1,000 adults in a typical population, the vast majority of the patients having symptoms in a particular month would be seen and handled by primary care physicians at the local level; only a few would receive specialist or local hospital care. Only approximately 1 of the 1,000 symptomatic adults would be treated in a university hospital. The corollary to this study—which initially was bitterly criticized by many academic physicians but since 1961 has been confirmed by other studies in different populations—was that educating medical students and resident physicians only in university hospitals was not realistic, and that training only specialists was not meeting the future health care needs of the people. They coined the term "primary medical care" and argued that the miscommunications they found in their earlier studies pointed to the need for well-trained primary care physicians who could coordinate the management of patients' problems and referrals.[19]

A memorandum of May 18, 1963, to Dean Berryhill from three junior faculty members—Williams, Dan A. Martin, MD, and Robert R. Huntley, MD—outlined "a proposed systematic approach to the study and development of facilities for medical care in the Chapel Hill area."[20] As background they cited a 1961 study that showed that 25 to 50 percent of clinic patients (depending on whether the clinic was a specialty clinic or a general clinic) seen at North Carolina Memorial Hospital were from Chapel Hill, Orange County, or adjacent areas, yet the plans for the new outpatient facility (which opened a decade later as the Spencer Love Clinics) did not include space for primary or family medical care for local patients. They noted that this was related to the fact that the stated policy of the hospital was that, with certain exceptions, it was a referral institution. (This policy had been adopted when the hospital was being planned to assuage the fears of the physicians of Durham and Chapel Hill that the teaching hospital would "put them out of business.")

Williams and his colleagues continued by summarizing the lively discussions held at a recent Department of Medicine conference about training UNC medical students and residents in internal medicine. These discussions included the need for affiliations with other hospitals for training purposes and the issue of whether in years to come North Carolina Memorial Hospital or a new community hospital would be providing medical care for the local community of Chapel Hill, Carrboro, and Orange County. The memorandum also observed that the university administration was showing increased interest in new approaches to financing and delivering health care for its faculty and employees. Another factor that needed to be addressed was the rising numbers of physicians trained at UNC or elsewhere who desired to go into practice in Chapel Hill and wanted to have a relationship with the hospital and its teaching functions. (At the time only physicians with full-time faculty appointments had admitting privileges at the hospital.) Finally, they cited the growing interest on the part of various university faculty members in studies of health care delivery and how it could be improved.

Williams, Martin, and Huntley proposed a systematic study of these issues by the hospital, the medical school, and their clinical departments. They stated that their interest was "not aimed at achieving any single, pre-conceived plan or program"; rather, they urged a public discussion of the problems and possible solutions after preliminary studies are completed. Because of the interrelationship of the issues, they stated, "it is essential that we work towards decisions in all these areas simultaneously if we are to arrive at a rational approach to our needs within the next 2–4 years."

Berryhill was acutely aware of these growing local and national demands for primary care physicians at the community level. In the annual Whitehead Lecture, his final address as dean to the graduating class of 1964, Berryhill observed that

> when a community is unable to secure a physician—more often a general physician but frequently also one in a particular specialty—the blame must be placed somewhere and most generally it is upon the medical school and its faculty . . . Further, it is alleged by some that the medical schools are interested only in research and in inducing or seducing their graduates to remain in the ivory towered institution instead of entering private practice in communities where the need for them is desperate . . . The modern medical graduate is "too scientific" and the "art" of medicine is being lost because of the over-emphasis on research in the medical school–university hospital environment. In short, for reasons sometimes difficult to understand, American medical schools are becoming to a degree the "whipping post" for a segment of the public and, unfortunately, also of the medical profession.[21]

Berryhill proposed as the solution to this dilemma the education and training of an adequate number of "family physicians of tomorrow" whose interest and competence would be in "providing (primary) continuing medical care of a high order of excellence to individuals and families in their communities." He believed "this specialist [would] be primarily an internist and pediatrician . . . [with] the training and competence . . . to 'hold his own' with the consulting internists and pediatricians in his community and on the hospital staff." His vision is not surprising in view of his background as an internist and of his support of North Carolina Memorial Hospital's mixed internship and residency program, which rapidly evolved into the innovative medicine-pediatrics residency program that serves as a national model to this day.

In his 1964 Whitehead Lecture Berryhill was recognizing the dilemma facing medical educators in the 1960s with regard to the best training for future primary care physicians. First, the traditional GP, who typically went into practice after a one-year rotating internship or sometimes with no internship, clearly did not have adequate postgraduate education for modern medical practice. Things had gotten so bad that Dean Wilburt Davison at the new Duke medical school in the 1930s was said to have put the MD diplomas of his new graduates in a safe so that they could not go into practice until they had proved to him they had had at least one year of postgraduate training. Second, the early graduates of the medicine-pediatrics residency program at North Carolina Memorial Hospital suffered from the lack of specialty board certification and specialty organizations in the increasingly specialty-oriented practice community. (This was later corrected so that physicians who completed the combined four-year program were eligible to become board certified in both medicine and pediatrics.) Third, the proposed new specialty of family medicine—which ultimately had its own academic departments, training programs, specialty board, continuing medical education requirements, organizations, and journals—was not yet well defined.

Berryhill concluded his Whitehead Lecture with a preview of what was to become his mission for the next several years:

> Two things seem very clear to me—the first is that schools of medicine and university hospitals can and must provide leadership by example for developing graduate education for what I believe will become a specialty of the future. This will inevitably necessitate some innovations or perhaps experiments in most current undergraduate and house officer education . . . The second is that with all their obligations university hospitals alone or within their own walls can never provide opportunities for the education and training of sufficient number of these physicians to meet the needs adequately.
>
> Accordingly, I am convinced we must now in the fairly immediate future, but at the same time wisely, undertake one or more pilot projects, perhaps not necessarily identical, in affiliation with one or more of the good community hospitals best equipped with clinical faculty, physical and financial resources, and motivation for education. This could be one of the exciting and worthwhile ventures over the next five years.

Having spent the years from 1941 to 1964 building a sound clinical and academic base of operations for the medical school on the university campus at Chapel Hill, Berryhill's retirement as dean provided him the freedom and opportunity to lead a community medicine initiative that had taken root years earlier. His new mission was later described by David Citron, MD, who had been associated with the development of the AHEC in the Charlotte area:

> Dr. Berryhill had repeatedly expressed the concern that he had not fulfilled [the] expectation [of the Sanger Report] and that this was a debt he owed to the state. His sense of mission to meet the needs of the people of NC for health care became an unflagging drive which was to define the remainder of the trajectory of his life. Now he would express it not as architect and leader of a great medical school but as a missionary with a constituency far beyond the boundaries of Chapel Hill . . . he would extend medical education to the community hospitals of North Carolina, challenging the physicians of those communities and the faculty at Chapel Hill to envision the potential of such an initiative.[22]

A Well-Deserved Sabbatical

Berryhill's resignation as dean was effective August 31, 1964. He was succeeded by Isaac (Ike) M. Taylor, MD. Taylor was a former Markle Scholar in academic medicine and a professor of medicine whose initial appointment in 1951 by Charles H. Burnett, MD, the founding chair, was the first in the new Department of Medicine. Taylor had been introduced to medical administration during 1962–1964, when as a special assistant to Dean Berryhill he was given the responsibility for planning a new ambulatory patient care facility and bed tower for North Carolina Memorial Hospital.[23]

Before tackling this new mission, Berryhill had a sabbatical leave—his first since joining the university thirty-one years earlier in 1933—to relax, to provide his successor some freedom of action, and to survey current trends in medical education and patient care abroad and in the United States.

Berryhill obtained a Commonwealth Fund Traveling Fellowship for 1964–1965 to provide partial salary support and to contribute to his travel and subsistence expenses. In his application to the Commonwealth Fund, he summarized his interests and how this year would contribute to his plan for his final years as a faculty member:

> In giving up the heavy responsibilities of the Deanship, I hope to spend the period 1965 to 1970, when I shall reach the University retirement age as a member of the faculty, actively participating in the planning and implementation of changes in the undergraduate, graduate (house officers) and continuing education of physicians.
>
> Today one of the most important concerns of the public and of the medical schools is the education of the physician (regardless of the name given him) who will render primary continuing medical care in the future . . .
>
> The faculty at the University of North Carolina School of Medicine has been concerned about this problem for some years. In our own University Hospital we have tried several experimental types of house officer training designed for the family physician of the future [including the mixed pediatrics-medicine residency]. No one is happy with our own efforts or results to date.
>
> Furthermore, our faculty has committed itself to undertaking a critical restudy of the entire medical undergraduate curriculum and graduate training of house officers in all areas of clinical medicine . . .
>
> For many reasons this is an appropriate point in time for this Medical School to undertake a curriculum study. As a part of this larger undertaking it would seem important also to include a specific study relating to the total education of the family or personal physician of the future.[24]

He outlined in the application his plans to obtain "the firsthand information and experience that would enable me to make a worthwhile contribution to the development of the educational projects outlined above at the University of North Carolina School of Medicine." He proposed spending the year visiting and learning from individuals and institutions. He listed eleven people in England and Scotland, including Sir Theodore Fox, editor of the *Lancet;* Dr. John Hunt, president of the College of General Practitioners, London, "who has pioneered the concern of this body for academic standards and participation in epidemiological research"; Dr. John Ellis, London Hospital, and secretary of the Association for the Study of Medical Education; Sir Robert Platt, University of Manchester, "who has just completed a year's study of 'good' general practice as Rock Carling fellow"; Dr. John Brotherston, chairman of the Department of Social Medicine and Public Health, University of Edinburgh, who was "shortly to become Chief Medical Officer for Scotland"; and Dr. Richard Scott, "originator of the first family practice teaching unit and now the Sir James MacKenzie Professor of General Practice, University of Edinburgh." He listed another eleven individuals he proposed visiting in the United States, including Dr. Robert Ebert, Massachusetts General Hospital, Boston; Dr Robert V. Haggerty, medical director, Family Health Program, Boston Children's Hospital; Dr. Lenor S. Goerke, professor of preventive medicine and Dean of the School of Public Health, University of California, Los Angeles; Dr. Ward Darley, executive director of the AAMC, Chicago; Dr. J. Wendell McLeod, Association of Canadian Medical Colleges, Ottawa; and Dr. Kent W. Deuschle, Department of Community Medicine, and Dr. Edmund D. Pellegrino, professor and chairman of medicine , both at the University of Kentucky in Lexington. Berryhill suggested that to prepare for the general curriculum restudy, it would be useful to spend some time at five four-year medical schools in the United States (Western Reserve University, Johns Hopkins University, the Jefferson–Penn State Program in Philadelphia, Northwestern University, and Boston University) as well as in three basic sciences schools (Brown University, Rutgers University, and the University of Arizona).

Berryhill concluded his proposal to the Commonwealth Fund with the hope "that the information, general background and experience gained in this year's study and observation will enable me to be of very real assistance to the faculty of the University of North Carolina Medicine" in its general curriculum review as well as in their efforts in planning and implementing "realistic graduate education . . . for the family or personal physician of the future." He added, "It seems clear that this critical problem needs the leadership of university medical centers in attempts at its solution. We believe the University of North Carolina School of Medicine is in a position to make some contributions toward this end."

In addition to the Commonwealth Fund support, before they departed the Berryhills received a check for $9,000 raised by alumni and other friends in appreciation of their dedication to the School of Medicine.

Reece and Norma Berryhill left in September 1964 for a three-month working vacation in Europe. He studied the British National Health Service in depth, for the United States was then debating federal support for health care. He interviewed many teachers, physicians, and politicians about the British system and was astounded that some of the prominent members of the Royal College of Physicians only grudgingly accepted the GP as worthy of being included in the National Health Service.[25]

Berryhill was not interested in sightseeing and spent most of his time abroad studying health care systems and medical education programs for community

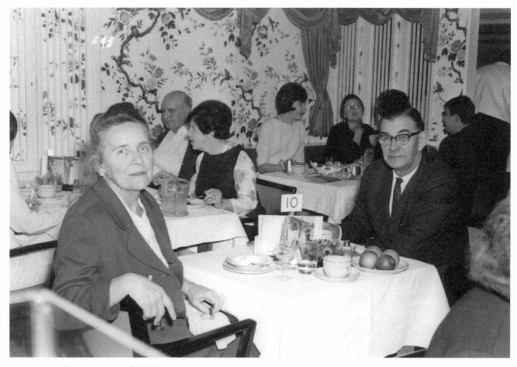

Norma and Reece Berryhill aboard RMS *Franconia* on their way to Europe, September 1964. *(Berryhill Family)*

practice. At the same time he anxiously awaited the arrival of newspaper clippings and the almost daily letters from Sarah Dunlap, his former secretary in Chapel Hill, telling him about what was going on at the medical school. The story is told that he had decided to eliminate a stop in Rome during a visit to the Continent in order to get back to his interviews in the United Kingdom, but then relented when he realized that letters from Chapel Hill might be waiting there. Someone commented that he was probably one of the few tourists who first visited Rome solely to pick up mail.

Berryhill began visiting US medical schools after his and Norma's return to the United States in December 1964. In an address given shortly after his return from the sabbatical year, Berryhill summarized the year by stating that he had visited "a number of medical schools from Boston to Seattle and in Scotland and England."[26]

Norma Berryhill did not accompany him on most of the trips in the United States because "money was still hard to come by then." She further commented, "Reece wanted to stay home" following the sabbatical travels. After his death, however, Norma made many trips abroad with companions. Someone asked her when she was almost ninety, "Why are you going on a trip up the Amazon River when you could visit London or Paris?" She responded without a pause, "At my age I can't afford to waste time going places I have already visited!"[27]

The Division for Research and Education in Community Medical Care

When Taylor became dean in September of 1964, it was clear that the medical school needed to respond to public pressure to provide more practicing primary care physicians in the communities of the state. For example, in a memo to Taylor dated April 21, 1965, Martin suggested that UNC was suffering from the perception in the state that "we not only are not encouraging family physicians, but that we are thwarting those students who have a natural desire for that type of practice." He elaborated on three related matters. First, he advocated that the proposed affiliations with community hospitals begin with family physician residencies, because such residencies have difficulty competing with the straight residencies in pediatrics and medicine at university hospitals. He believed such residencies would provide good training for medical students interested in family medicine. Second, he discussed some difficulties with the current mixed internship and residency in medicine-pediatrics at Chapel Hill but strongly encouraged that it continue to be supported as another way to train family physicians. Third, he shared his frustration with the discussions at a national meeting he attended about the future of family practice. He agreed with the advice given by one speaker that the proposed new specialty of family medicine needed to be better defined and that there should be board certification for family practitioners, a proposal that received divided support from the members of the Academy of General Practice at the meeting.[28]

Under the leadership of Dean Taylor, in the mid-1960s the medical school started the first review of its mission and the first long-range plan since the hospital opened and the expanded medical school was implemented in 1952. A resulting policy statement of the medical faculty was adopted in January 1966 to guide these planning efforts.[29] It began, "As a State University, we have a special opportunity and challenge for leadership and service in meeting the health needs of the State," and confirmed a commitment to a broad-based student body and faculty who would provide educational opportunities for "both those who will deliver primary care to the public as well as those who will be the next generation of educators and investigators."

The 1966 faculty policy statement also indicated its commitment to the development of new approaches to primary care, as had Berryhill in his 1964 Whitehead Lecture. The faculty stated:

> We believe that a properly trained family practitioner is among those qualified to deliver primary medical care. Such a practitioner should have essentially the same degree of training and the same status as specialists. He should be trained in depth in both internal medicine and pediatrics, and should have an understanding of the emotional needs and psychology of the

individual as well as the psychology of the family in its relationship to society. We recognize that in certain settings primary medical care may be more effectively given by groups, internists or pediatricians.

Formation of the Division and Appointment of the Director

On June 22, 1965, William J. Cromartie, MD, associate dean of clinical sciences and chief of staff of North Carolina Memorial Hospital, sent Dean Taylor a "Proposal Regarding the Establishment of A Division of Health and Medical Care Research in the School of Medicine of the UNC."[30] Cromartie stated that a number of recent activities in this area had led him to conclude that a new administrative structure was long overdue to consolidate responsibilities "that are now in the hands of various individuals and committees." These activities included "those relating to the education of family physicians, the establishment of model medical care units in rural areas and in Chapel Hill, the development of affiliations with community hospitals, and selected current programs relating to health and medical care research." He felt that the Departments of Medicine and Pediatrics were the logical places for such an administrative structure because, "in spite of their good intentions, Schools of Public Health, Departments of Preventive Medicine . . . Hospital Administration . . . Community Medicine, etc., do not offer attractive academic homes for programs that are concerned with the delivery of health and medical care to individuals." He suggested that the proposed Division be led by an "outstanding pediatrician or internist and medical statesman, who would be responsible to both the Chairman of the Department of Medicine and the Chairman of the Department of Pediatrics." He advocated that funds be allocated to support sufficient faculty positions and a small support staff.

Apparently stimulated by some concerns expressed about the original proposal, Cromartie submitted a revised proposal concerning the Division to Taylor two weeks later.[31] Cromartie agreed that the proposed structure "could operate satisfactorily as a division of the Dean's office with the staff member holding appointment in Pediatrics or Medicine." He added that he believed the proposal was in keeping with the deliberations during the summer by a joint ad hoc committee of the Schools of Medicine and Public Health concerned with promoting research in medical care.

Williams, in a memorandum to Dean Taylor dated July 29, 1965, summarized a meeting held several days previously with Berryhill, Cadmus, Cromartie, Denny, Fleming (consulted but not present), Huntley, and Welt to discuss the proposed new Division.[32] They agreed that a new assistant dean for education and research in medical care was appropriate, but that support from the department chairs, especially those of medicine and pediatrics, was critical to its success. Williams added that in his opinion the "need for decision and action in this area is urgent. We as a school are already later than we should be in a number of these developments . . . Unless we undertake, promptly, the leadership in this area which it is appropriate and important for us to undertake, clearly the leadership will be taken by others."

Dean Taylor followed up these proposals and discussions with a letter to Berryhill dated December 27, 1965. He said he "will not apologize for the length of this letter because of the importance of its subjects, [but] I will ask your understanding for my lateness in preparing it."[33] Taylor stated, "I am establishing in the Medical School as part of the Dean's Office a division for development and administration of our increasing educational service and research activities in the general area of community medicine . . . I want you to accept the position of Director of this new division, which I suggest we call the Section of Community Medicine." (Taylor was appropriately sensitive to Berryhill's status as the former dean and thus suggested that he be made director, rather than being demoted to an assistant dean.) He emphasized that Berryhill's appointment to this position had the unanimous approval of the medical school's advisory committee (composed of the departmental chairs) and had the approval of UNC Chancellor Paul Sharp. He stated that Berryhill would have the full authority to develop the Division, to operate it, and to control the budget, which would include funds for one or more faculty members and appropriate staff. He gave the completion of the affiliation discussions with Moses Cone Hospital a high priority but urged that other affiliation agreements be pursued. The Division would also be responsible for existing affiliations such as those with the Dorothea Dix and Charlotte Memorial hospitals. Among the other responsibilities would be the relationship of the medical school and hospital with medical care at the community level; the coordination of the school's relationship with the federal Regional Medical Program and its heart disease, cancer, and stroke initiative; and the school's liaison with the federal Appalachian Regional Commission and with the federal Office of Economic Opportunity's War on Poverty program.

Taylor also asked Berryhill to become the director of alumni affairs for the school, because the medical alumni would obviously be vital to the success of any outreach efforts in the state. Taylor also wanted to enhance the identity of the alumni association as distinct from the medical foundation's fund-raising activities with the alumni.

In his reply, Berryhill declined the offer to be head of alumni affairs but accepted the offer to direct the new administrative unit, which came to be known as the Division of Education and Research in Community Medical Care.

Funding the Division

Dean Taylor provided the limited original funding for Berryhill and the Division from sources available to him in the medical school. By 1966–1967 monies from the federal Regional Medical Program (RMP) in North Carolina provided some support for faculty, although the clinical departments continued to carry most of the faculty salary support in the early years of the Division. The RMP funds were limited to faculty support for continuing-education efforts in the community hospitals and for Medical Air Operations, but they lasted only several years. Through the efforts of Dean Taylor, a new ongoing appropriation of $395,000 was obtained from the state in 1969, the first specifically designated for the Division.[34]

Further expansion of the funding of the Division and of the expansion of the medical school's role in the state came through the far-reaching efforts of Dean Taylor and his colleagues in working with university and state political leaders to define the course the medical school would follow in the coming years. In response to the state and national shortage of physicians, the school agreed to increase the entering class size from around 65 members to some 160 members by the late 1970s. These efforts resulted in funding for new faculty and for much-needed new buildings, including the Health Sciences Library, a preclinical teaching building (later named Berryhill Hall), a clinical sciences building (later named the Burnett Womack Building), some research buildings, and an ambulatory patient care center and bed tower for North Carolina Memorial Hospital.

Dean Taylor also obtained from the 1971 legislature an additional ongoing appropriation of $1.5 million to support community medicine efforts. Because the facilities at Chapel Hill were not sufficient to provide clinical instruction for the larger classes, the faculty agreed that one-third to one-half of the clinical teaching would be done within the state but outside Chapel Hill.[35] The increased funding for the Division was thus justified on the basis of the need for new sites to teach clinical medicine to the increased number of medical students in each class and of the need to provide residency training for primary care physicians in communities where they might stay to practice. The fact that North Carolina already had these state-appropriated funds for community medicine played a major role in the state's successful bid in 1972 for federal funds to promote community medical education efforts through the proposed NC AHEC Program. Dean Taylor deserves recognition for this major accomplishment.

Establishing and Staffing the Division

The Division—which Berryhill led from 1966 to 1969 and of which he was a full-time member until 1971—was described by an active participant in the early years as a think tank where numerous discussions were held concerning the health care needs of the people. These deliberations focused especially on the poor status of medical care in the rural areas of the state and on how to marshal the political support and resources to address their needs. He observed that Berryhill's unique contribution was to recruit bright young people and then let them address these problems without arbitrary restrictions. Although his political and medical wisdom was solicited by the members of the Division, Berryhill did not dictate outcomes and on several major issues ultimately supported approaches that were opposed to his own personal views.[36]

The Division, which was created as a section within the dean's office, had its beginning when Berryhill assumed the leadership position in early January 1966. Berryhill's office was constructed by closing off a hallway entrance on the ground floor of the Medical Sciences Research Building (now Bondurant Hall). The other members of the Division staff were located in a temporary office trailer across Manning Drive from the dental school.

At the time the Division was formed, Carl B. Lyle, Jr., MD (Columbia 1957), assistant professor of medicine, was on leave to the Appalachian Regional Commission, a federal and state partnership created in 1965 to promote the development of the mostly rural thirteen-state Appalachian region of the eastern United States. He was promoted to associate professor and assumed the position of assistant director of the Division upon his return to full-time status with the university in August 1966. In this role he was involved with all the Division's activities and played a key role in founding the Medical Air Operations program. Lyle remained in Chapel Hill with the Division until he moved to Charlotte in the early 1970s to join an internal medicine practice.

Robert R. Huntley, MD (Bowman Gray 1951), assistant professor of medicine and of preventive medicine since joining the faculty in 1959, was also on leave with the Appalachian Regional Commission when the Division was established. He returned to the university full time in August 1967 as an associate professor and worked with the Division on a number of fronts. He left in 1968 for a position with the federal government and then became the founding chair of the Department of Family Medicine at Georgetown University.[37]

Berryhill later made contacts with C. Glenn Pickard, Jr., MD (UNC 1962), who had started his training in internal medicine at Columbia-Presbyterian in New York and was completing a residency in internal medicine at UNC, as well as with Lawrence Cutchin, MD (UNC 1962), who was completing his residency in the combined medicine-pediatrics program at UNC. They were included in many of the Division meetings and field trips while still residents. Pickard joined the Division in 1968 with an academic appointment in the Department of Medicine and became responsible for the primary care activities of the Division in Orange County and the immediate surrounding area.[38]

Cutchin moved to Tarboro to practice in 1969 and was followed the next year by George Hemingway, MD, a fellow resident in the UNC medicine-pediatrics program. They joined the Tarboro Clinic, a small, multispecialty group practice. This was a radically new practice pattern for small North Carolina towns. Cutchin continued to have appointments in the Division and in the Departments of Medicine and Pediatrics. He flew to Chapel Hill weekly to teach and consult about the development of the clinic and about the health services research being conducted there. Berryhill was supportive of their move and made several trips to Tarboro to help negotiate the arrangements. Cutchin also received considerable support from Cecil G. Sheps, MD, the first director of the Health Service Research Center at UNC. Medical students from Chapel Hill were flown to Tarboro to demonstrate to them how a multispecialty clinic could operate in a small community and to encourage them to consider practicing in the smaller communities of the state. By 1972 Tarboro and the surrounding area had regular medical student rotations from Chapel Hill, active health services research projects, a medical library, and a well-organized continuing medical education program for local physicians.[39]

By 1969 the Division included Drs. Berryhill, Cutchin, Huntley, Lyle, and Pickard, as well as Robert A. Shaw, MD (Ohio State 1963), and Robert Smith, MD (Trinity College, Dublin 1945). Shaw, who had a faculty appointment in pediatrics, had been recruited from Alaska, where he had been the medical director of an Indian Health Service clinic that provided primary care to a large Eskimo population. Smith, who had an appointment in preventive medicine, had been recruited by Berryhill and Huntley from Guys Hospital in London, where he "had been planning primary care services for a new town southeast of London, while working to upgrade training for British GPs by utilizing teaching practices to demonstrate excellent primary care."[40] Smith became the founding chair of UNC's new Department of Family Medicine in 1970.

John B. Wilson, MBA, was an early administrator of the Division. John A. Payne, MPH (UNC 1968), joined the Division in 1968 as an administrator and served the Division and then the NC AHEC Program until his death in 1996. Payne, whose father was a general practitioner in Hertford County and a close personal friend of the Berryhills, was encouraged by Berryhill to follow a career in medical administration. He served with distinction for many years in several positions, including as deputy director and then as interim director of the NC AHEC Program.

The First Months in the Division

Berryhill went right to work in January and by early March 1966 had an approved budget for the rest of the fiscal year. He had also recommended members for an advisory committee, who were then appointed by the dean; visited Moses Cone Hospital with Robert R. Cadmus, MD (chair of the Department of Hospital Administration), to begin a study in preparation for the hospital's affiliation with the medical school; visited Charlotte to discuss future possibilities there; and proposed further discussions with Cape Fear Valley Hospital in Fayetteville. In addition, he was setting up appointments with the administrator at Wake County Hospital and planning to meet with Ed Monroe, MD—a practicing physician in Greenville who was a medical school alumnus and the first chief resident in medicine at North Carolina Memorial Hospital—concerning Pitt County Memorial Hospital.[41]

The growing interest among the state's three medical schools in teaching community medicine in North Carolina was reflected in the minutes of a meeting held at North Carolina Memorial Hospital in Chapel Hill in March 1966. Berryhill was not in attendance, but there were representatives of the Department of Preventive Medicine at Duke; the Departments of Medicine and Preventive

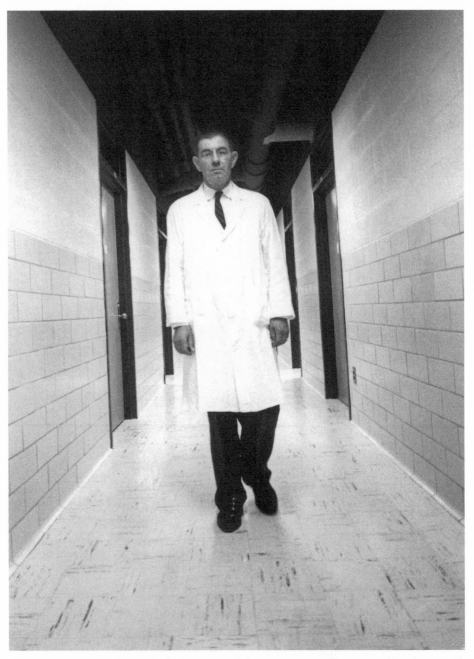

Dean Emeritus Berryhill in the hallway outside his retirement office, created by closing off a hallway in the Medical Sciences Research Building, late 1960s. *(Berryhill Family)*

Medicine at Bowman Gray; and the UNC Departments of Pedodontics (dental school), Preventive Medicine (medical school), and Epidemiology (public health school). All gave brief summaries of their activities at the community level and of their attempts to educate students about community medicine. The minutes included the statement that "Dr. Lyle, of the UNC Department of Medicine, mentioned that he was working with Dr. Berryhill in planning a Division of Teaching and Research in Community Medical Care." In conclusion, Huntley stated, "There was consensus that firm, long-term financial support is now required if teaching and research in all these areas are to receive the attention they require. A 'categorical' approach [for example, the heart disease, cancer, and stroke approach of the federal Regional Medical Program] to supporting these activities will no longer suffice."[42]

The first meeting of the advisory committee to the Division was held on June 24, 1966, with Berryhill presiding.[43] Thirteen of the nineteen members were in attendance. These included several medical school faculty members and Dean Taylor as well as a practicing physician from the local community, Kempton Jones, MD; the state health director, Jacob Koomen, MD; and an alumnus and pediatrician from High Point, John Lynch, MD. Taylor began by discussing the reasons for establishing the Division and his hopes for it. He explained that the school had had an interest in community medicine for some time, but only now was there was sufficient momentum at Chapel Hill to permit expansion elsewhere in the state. He thought it was a good sign that the Departments of Medicine and Pediatrics were giving "careful attention" to the proposed affiliations with Moses Cone Hospital in Greensboro and other hospitals.

Dean Taylor said he hoped that "this Division can provide [both] the opportunity for young men and women as interns and residents to have experience to prepare them for practice in community medicine" and "an environment in which we can send our medical students for this experience." He hoped that research into community medical practice would be possible through the Division's activities. Finally, he hoped that the "Division will help to provide a good relationship between this medical center and local communities, including the Orange County community." He concluded his remarks by assuring the committee that the Division had his full support.

Discussion was held about the family care unit in the local community and the fact that North Carolina Memorial was becoming a community hospital as well as a referral hospital for the state. It was observed that it would be better for the community and county to support more beds for Memorial Hospital than to attempt to fund an independent community hospital for Chapel Hill and Orange County. It was indicated that two internists who were UNC medical school graduates would be establishing a group practice in Chapel Hill in July 1967, and that they would be members of the faculty and have staff privileges at Memorial Hospital.[44]

As a final item of business at the advisory committee meeting, the status of affiliations was reviewed, as were efforts to obtain grant support for the Division. The affiliation discussions were going on with Moses Cone Hospital in Greensboro, Charlotte Memorial Hospital, Wake Memorial Hospital in Raleigh, and several others.

Getting appropriate publicity about the Division to the public through the newspapers was one of Berryhill's major frustrations during the first eight months with the Division. Various drafts of a proposed news story had been circulated between the UNC News Bureau, Chancellor Lyle Sitterson, Dean Taylor, and Berryhill, but nothing had been published when Berryhill read a report about Duke's efforts in community medicine in the newspapers in the summer of 1966. A similar report about the Duke program also appeared in a news note in the September 1966 issue of the *North Carolina Medical Journal*:

A program to help meet the need for well-trained physicians devoted to family and community health is being launched by Duke University Medical Center.

A key step in the program is changing the department of preventive medicine to the department of community health sciences.

"Our aim," said Dean W. G. Anlyan, "is to create a new physician—one who will bridge the gap between the exciting advances being made at the research level of medical sciences and their application at the family and community level."

Dr. E. Harvey Estes has been appointed chairman of the new department.

Dr. Estes, who also is secretary-treasurer of the Durham–Orange County Medical Society, played a major role in setting up the North Carolina Regional Medical Program, now in the planning stages as part of the President's war on heart disease, cancer, stroke and related diseases.[45]

Berryhill's legendary but usually well-controlled temper was clearly evident in the letter he wrote Dean Taylor following the appearance of a newspaper article about the new Duke program:

Yesterday when I read the attached I was so disgusted and furious at the ineptitude in this University I just said to hell with all of you and went home.

It is obvious that our neighbors across the [New Hope] creek have again outsmarted and outscooped us which I think could have been predicted once they knew that we were entering this field. You may recall that I tactfully suggested that this announcement be made last January (a) because the University needed to have some publicity of a constructive nature in the light of all the other kind of publicity we were receiving and (b) from my thirty years experience with our neighbors I felt fairly certain that if it was humanly possible they would and as quickly as possible come up with something that would be in this field.

Please understand that I am not criticizing the people at Duke. They are smart. We have the capacity for smartness but we don't act that way too often unfortunately. All of this adds up to the fact that the "togetherness" may not be as much in fact as is being talked about and second, regardless of what it costs, I do hope you will insist upon having an able writer with some knowledge of medical affairs on your staff.[46]

It is likely that the "togetherness" Berryhill referred to concerned the meetings of Duke, UNC, and Wake Forest faculty—such as the one in March 1966—to discuss the teaching of community medicine in North Carolina.

A belated report concerning the new Division at UNC did appear shortly thereafter in newspapers throughout the state.[47] A news note in the October issue of the *North Carolina Medical Journal* stated:

> A new Division of Education and Research in Community Medical Care has been established at the UNC School of Medicine to plan and coordinate the increasing activities in community medicine more effectively.
>
> Dr. W. Reece Berryhill, professor of medicine and dean emeritus, has been appointed director of the division, and Dr. Carl B. Lyle, assistant professor of medicine, will serve as assistant director.
>
> Dr. Berryhill said the new division would have three major objectives. It will establish affiliations with a few of the larger community hospitals in working toward the development of regional medical educational centers.
>
> It will establish one or more demonstration centers in rural areas in as [*sic*] effort to improve the quality and availability of medical care and to provide training opportunities for medical students.
>
> And it will provide opportunities for members of the UNC medical faculty interested in medical care research to study disease patterns and the medical needs of North Carolina communities.[48]

Berryhill's challenges didn't end when the publicity issue was settled for the moment. In his efforts to expand medical education to communities statewide, he soon found that he was fighting a battle on two fronts. The first was at the community level, where both political and medical leaders had been overwhelmed in recent years with various federally mandated programs, including those in civil rights, the War on Poverty, and Medicare. They were understandably very suspicious of anyone—even from the state's university—who approached them saying, "We are from the government and we are here to help you."

Berryhill's second front was in Chapel Hill with the medical school faculty leaders, whom he had recruited from some of the best medical schools in the country to build strong academic programs at UNC. Many of them quite naturally perceived the community medical education efforts as a threat to both their academic mission and their funding. As an example, Louis G. Welt, MD, who became the second chair of medicine in 1965, wrote Berryhill in April 1967 that they needed to have a conversation about "who is going to be involved in the final value judgments as to what the Department of Medicine will and will not be doing" about proposed monthly sabbaticals at Chapel Hill for community internists whose practices might be covered by second-year medical residents. Welt emphasized, "I can assure you at this particular moment in time it is not our intention to send our assistant residents out to cover these practices."[49] Berryhill's temper rose again when he responded a week later, with a copy to Dean Taylor: "Most particularly because of its unreasonableness, your letter . . . made me so furious I have not as yet completely recovered my composure. I am gaining on this, however, and if you should be in town next week let me know when you want to talk with me. The letter has been destroyed [*sic:* it wasn't] because I did not wish to have this in a file of otherwise pleasant correspondence between us over the past fifteen years."[50]

A young faculty member in the Division in the early days had this to say later about Welt's initial opposition to these outreach efforts:

[Welt] said that the only service that an academic medical center provides to its constituency is teaching and research. Patient care is a derivative of the above two, and you should never focus on patient care. We fought that and argued with him, but in a sense in the end we came to agree with him. There was just no way that the university could or should take on the direct patient care responsibilities. Our job was to train people to go out there and do it. And to try to train them with an orientation and a mindset that would be more egalitarian, that would be more willing to get into community health centers, that would be more willing to move out and change the way care was delivered . . . [Direct patient care in the communities] was not something that we were good at, not something we should do, and it would be a major political liability.[51]

Another faculty member in the Department of Medicine, who had the first full-time faculty appointment in an affiliated community hospital in 1967, related that Welt's view of the affiliation was initially impractical, "but, to his credit, he changed his viewpoint entirely." He added that Welt's "views evolved honestly and I never felt that I lacked his personal support. He took his responsibility on the Joint Education Committee [the medical school—hospital oversight committee for the affiliation] seriously and supported me in promotion and salary enhancement unstintingly."[52]

As much as five years after the Division was established, two articles in the *Medical Alumni Association Bulletin* in 1971 revealed the excitement but also the continuing concerns on the part of faculty members about the community medicine efforts of the medical school. A senior faculty member, in a tribute to Isaac Taylor, who was retiring as dean after seven years, commented on one of "the three great issues on which he has initiated action and which will require [the faculty's] understanding and response: . . . [this is] our role as a center for study of health as a community service, an area which could rise to dominate us and inundate our other activities, but one in which we must provide wise leadership."

A new faculty member, Glenn Wilson—who, as the new associate dean for community health services, would soon be the leader in a major statewide effort in community medical education—concluded an article on the UNC medical center's comprehensive medical care program for Orange and Chatham Counties in the same 1971 *Medical Alumni Association Bulletin* with this perceptive observation:

> Twenty years ago this country poured its resources into the field of biomedical research. Unfortunately, the arguments to do research both in health care delivery and in biomedical sciences did not prevail. The nation [now] knows a great deal more than can be delivered. It would be unfortunate should society again make a violent swing on the pendulum to devote all efforts to the delivery of medical care and find in 1990 that while able to deliver something, there is nothing new to offer.
>
> The faculty at the University of North Carolina is persuaded that a university can successfully address community health service problems. This new and challenging adventure will be based in large part on the ability of the faculty to harness its energy and talent, focus its resources on an appropriate role, and develop a clear written understanding with its community.
>
> Sir Oliver Lodge is quoted as saying that the last thing in the world a deep sea fish could discover would be salt water. Medical schools and health sciences schools have discovered the need for their participation in the evolution of new forms of adequate health care delivery. Having discovered this need, it is to be hoped they will not drown in it.[53]

Primary Care for Chapel Hill, Orange County, and the Surrounding Area

Members of the Division for Education and Research in Community Medical Care realized that the provision of primary services at North Carolina Memorial Hospital and in the local community was essential if they were to be successful in other communities.

Although Berryhill was not directly involved in most of these activities, he kept up with developments and provided advice and support when needed. One Division member later observed, "His name and influence served us well in our relationships with the community and the political structure . . . once committed to an idea, he was ever faithful and helpful as the political battles inside and outside the Medical Center waxed and waned."[54]

The initial bylaws of North Carolina Memorial Hospital precluded primary care activities by faculty members and specified that all patients were to be referred by outside physicians in order to prevent the teaching hospital from competing with physicians in the surrounding communities. In practice, however, many patients received continuing care in various clinics once they were inside the system. By the late 1960s local physicians recognized that there were more than enough patients to go around and appreciated having an institution that would take some of the "charity" patients out of their practices. At the same time primary care activities were being recognized as essential for the teaching, service, and research missions of the medical school and the hospital. The bylaws of the hospital were thus changed to permit the faculty and house staff to provide primary care.

An initial attempt by the medical school to develop a primary care educational program in the Chapel Hill–Carrboro area was the Home Care program, established by William L. Fleming, MD (Vanderbilt 1932), chair of preventive medicine, and Sarah Lou Warren, MD (Virginia 1949), in the 1950s. Senior medical students, under the supervision of the faculty members, visited patients in their homes to provide care and to learn about community medical care.

In the mid-1950s White, Williams, and Fleming established a general medicine clinic at North Carolina Memorial Hospital with support from the Commonwealth Fund, the Rockefeller Foundation, and the state. White later described this clinic and its operation:

> Undergraduates [medical students] and residents, as well as all faculty members in the department of internal medicine, had extended rotations and assignments in the General Clinic coping with the problems of general medical patients. The goal was to expose all faculty, medical students and residents in the department of medicine to the problems faced by "generalists." In addition, we were committed to preparing adequate numbers of "general physicians" for North Carolina as promised to its state legislature in return for the funding of UNC's new medical school.[55]

In the late 1960s Pickard and James A. Bryan II, MD (Pennsylvania 1957), a faculty member in the General Medicine Division of the Department of Medicine, established at North Carolina Memorial Hospital a continuing care clinic that was partially funded by a federal grant from the Bureau of Community Health in the Department of Health, Education and Welfare (HEW). An essential feature of this clinic was the presence of a nurse coordinator who knew all of the patients and could provide immediate care when the physician was not available, much as office nurses stand in for busy physicians in community practices. The Division also provided partial support for a physician in this clinic in an "effort to test some of the concepts of a comprehensive program and the use of new manpower" and noted that approximately 3,400 patient contacts were made in the clinic during 1969.[56]

Glenn Wilson, after joining the Division as its director in 1970, led the effort to establish a university-community partnership to provide comprehensive medical care for indigent persons in and around Orange and Chatham counties. A community corporation composed of consumers—no health professionals participated—provided one component of the effort. This group contracted for professional services with "a University Committee composed of the deans of the five health schools plus departmental chairmen whose departments have an interest in the program." A federal planning grant was obtained from the Office of Economic Opportunity to help establish a network of community health clinics in the local area. These efforts led to the establishment of Orange Chatham Comprehensive Health Services (OCCHS), whose mission was to provide comprehensive services to those receiving inadequate health care and to train indigent individuals to work in the clinics.[57] This effort continues today, though without the anti-poverty objectives, as Piedmont Health Services, with clinical facilities in Alamance County (Burlington), Caswell County (Prospect Hill), Chatham County (Moncure and Siler City), and Orange County (Carrboro and Chapel Hill).[58]

An important component of OCCHS was the clinic that opened in 1971 at Prospect Hill in southern Caswell county. The entire community medicine effort benefited "when it became apparent that the community leader from Prospect Hill who had initially invited us into the community was a long time ally and colleague of the Scott family of nearby Alamance County. This family included two governors, the long time chairman of the North Carolina Senate Finance Committee and a US Senator. Such political connections were extremely helpful [in getting] funds and [in changing] the Medical Practice Act, the Nursing Practice Act, and the Pharmacy Practice Act to legitimize and legalize . . . the Nurse Practitioner role and the system of satellite clinics that developed."[59]

The activist medical students of the 1960s established their own free primary care clinic in 1968 to provide care for the medically underserved in the Chapel Hill area. Huntley and Bryan initially provided physician coverage for this organization, named the Student Health Action Coalition (SHAC), and ran interference for them in the hospital and medical school.[60] SHAC still operates today as the oldest student-run free clinic in the nation and involves students from all of the UNC health sciences schools in a weekly free medical clinic, a free dental clinic, a Habitat for Humanity building project, and a home health education program.

Medical Air Operations

As affiliations were being planned and implemented with various community hospitals throughout the state, it quickly became apparent that automobile travel for university faculty visiting the communities and for community physicians and others visiting the medical center at Chapel Hill was going to be a limiting factor in the success of these programs, because at its farthest points the state extends more than 500 miles from the Atlantic Ocean to the Tennessee border and more than 180 miles from the Virginia border to the South Carolina border. One department chair emphatically stated, "I will not have my faculty killed on the highways of North Carolina" going back and forth to these affiliated sites.[61]

A small group of the faculty headed by Carl Lyle, MD, himself a licensed commercial pilot, recognized the value of air transportation for these two-way contacts. The Medical Foundation purchased the first medical school airplane in 1968, the result of a gift from a Charlotte donor in appreciation for the affiliation efforts with Charlotte Memorial Hospital. This and the other planes acquired later for the Medical Air Operations program were based and operated out of the university's Horace Williams Airport, which was within the Chapel Hill city limits, except when bad weather forced them to use the better-equipped Raleigh-Durham Airport.

Lyle took a leave of absence from his faculty duties to pilot the medical school plane during the first year of operation.[62] The following year Colonel Earl Provancha, a retired US Air Force pilot, joined the program as the director of air operations. Berryhill later observed, "The excellent service which has been provided to the University, the School of Medicine, and the state . . . has been largely due to his initiative, his devotion to this opportunity, his enthusiasm, and his wise selection of experienced pilots." Provancha served until the fall of 1977, when he resigned and returned to Salt Lake City.[63]

The early impact of the Medical Air Operations program was noted in a 1970 report to the Division's advisory committee:

Air transportation has provided essential support to all of the Division's activities. It has demonstrated the concept that air transportation can greatly increase the productivity of scarce manpower . . . and has played a valuable role in the organ transplant program. Physicians from most all specialties

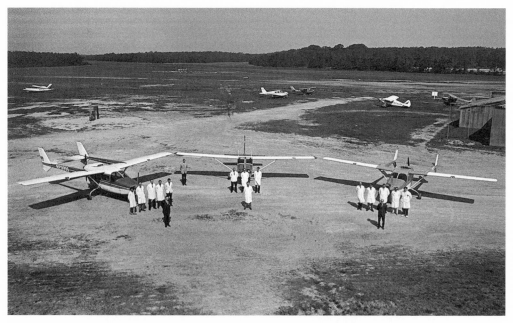

Planes of the Medical Air Operations program at Horace Williams Airport in Chapel Hill, 1970. The residents and faculty members who would be conducting clinics or CME programs around the state are shown with the pilots who would fly them to and from their destinations for the day. *(UNC Photo Lab, NCC)*

have been transported throughout the state to provide medical services during the past year [including staffing bi-weekly otolaryngology clinics in Morganton and Tarboro and monthly orthopedic clinics at Elizabeth City, Jacksonville, and Tarboro]. In addition, physicians have been transported throughout the state in order to consult with and provide continuing educating for practicing physicians.[64]

A second plane was purchased in 1968 and a third in 1969. By 2005 there were six twin-engine planes with three certified mechanics to maintain the aircraft and pilots who have flown an average of 10,000 hours in both civilian and military aircraft. They use state-of-the art weather-avoidance equipment and satellite navigational systems, similar to those found on commercial airliners. Most locations in the state, including those not accessible by commercial airliners, can be reached in an hour or less. In 2003–2004 these planes logged more than 500,000 passenger miles while transporting more than 4,000 passengers to more than eighty destinations in the state. The program has had an exemplary safety record with no major accidents on the ground or in the air during more than thirty-five years of operations.[65]

Affiliation Agreements with Community Hospitals

For many years the medical school had informal arrangements with community and state hospitals for the clinical education of medical students. Berryhill himself had negotiated some of these arrangements in the 1930s when he was the university physician and a junior faculty member in the two-year medical school. He had accepted the challenge to improve the clinical experience of the second-year medical students before they transferred elsewhere for their clinical years and MD degrees. Because the university's student infirmary did not provide the necessary number or variety of patients, he had to take the students elsewhere for their clinical instruction.

Even with the availability of the patients at North Carolina Memorial Hospital, which opened in 1952, the school still needed other sites for both medical student and residency education, as noted in a response by Berryhill to a 1966 inquiry by Dean Taylor. Berryhill related that more than a dozen state and community hospitals were serving as sites for medical student instruction in medicine, psychiatry, obstetrics, and surgery and as sites for intern and residency training in surgery and obstetrics. These included the Gravely (tuberculosis) Sanatorium at Chapel Hill (on the university campus but at the time still operated by a separate state agency); the state mental hospitals in Butner, Goldsboro, and Raleigh; and community or specialty hospitals in Burlington, Charlotte, Durham, Gastonia, Lumberton, and Raleigh. Berryhill told Taylor that so far as he knew, only two of these affiliations (Gravely Sanatorium and Dorothea Dix Hospital) had a "rather firm written agreement" with the medical school; the others were based on a "more general agreement" or "a gentlemen's agreement" between the involved parties, without anything in writing. Berryhill elaborated that "these arrangements are not actually affiliations in the ordinary sense," but they "are known to and approved by the Boards of Trustees of the hospitals involved as well as the staff of these institutions."[66]

A report prepared for the meeting of the Division's advisory committee in December 1970 noted that the Division's original charge in 1966 was "to develop and strengthen cooperative arrangements between the medical school and community hospitals and community medical care programs," the specific objectives being to "develop affiliations with selected community hospitals," to "provide continuing education for physicians in these settings," and to "carry out research activities that would help the communities to improve their medical care delivery system." In meeting these goals, the Division in its first several years had "explored in some depth affiliations with eleven hospitals throughout the state" and relationships with seven regional health planning councils, as well as with eight individual practices in the state. It was noted that "the Medical School, through the Division, has shown some foresight in working in these specific areas. In its special report this year, the Carnegie Commission on Higher Education recommended the establishment of area health education centers in local hospitals. Wilmington and Charlotte were suggested as two of the three centers in this state [along with Asheville]."[67]

Glenn Wilson, who became the new director of the Division in 1970, reported in the spring of 1971 that formal affiliations existed between four of the ten non-university hospitals with more than 300 beds in the state: Charlotte Memorial Hospital, Moses Cone Memorial Hospital, New Hanover Memorial Hospital, and Wake Memorial Hospital.[68] He noted that these affiliations had become essential for the clinical training of the vastly expanded medical school student body, which had grown from 60 entering students in the 1950s to 85 in 1969 and 110 in 1971.[69]

The transition from these informal affiliation agreements to more structured agreements began in 1965, when, in a nine-page statement concerning the goals and requirements for the affiliation of community hospitals with the School of Medicine, Cromartie stated that the school "includes among its obligations the extension of its educational influence into all areas of the state [and that] cooperating in the establishment of regional medical educational centers in the larger community hospitals is considered one appropriate way of meeting this obligation." Among the mutual benefits he enumerated were the school's provision of postgraduate medical education programs for practicing physicians; the education of the faculty about the "realities of the practice of medicine and the health problems of the community"; the development of additional sites for education of medical and other students from the university; the development of new types of educational programs for house staff, such as for family physicians;

the provision of opportunities for university faculty to do medical care research in the community; the provision of an environment in which advances in medical care could be introduced into the community; and the opportunity for local physicians to plan changes for their own community rather than having such changes "come from other sources and with very undesirable results." Cromartie then outlined in detail a suggested approach for such affiliations, including the development of a clear agreement on educational goals (for example, house staff programs in some areas); the appointment of full-time faculty as chiefs of each teaching service, with one of these appointed chief of the hospital's teaching program; the recruitment of part-time teaching staff from the hospital medical staff; the appointment of appropriate committees; the formulation of an annual budget, with the hospital responsible for most of the cost of the faculty and all of the resident positions; the furnishing of office and lab space for the teaching faculty; and the setting aside of a specific number of beds for the teaching services. (It was soon realized that laboratory bench research for community-based faculty members was impractical, so this requirement was eventually dropped.) He suggested that the hospital and the school commit to a minimum trial period of six years, with a review of the program after four years to determine whether the agreement was to be renewed.[70]

Two divergent approaches to the organizational structure for new community health programs were being advocated nationally and locally at the time the new affiliations were being developed between the medical school and community hospitals in the state. One group in Washington, led by individuals active in the operation of the federal Regional Medical Program, advocated establishing entirely new community boards to be responsible for these programs. The boards were to have representation mirroring the population of the community. In theory such a structure was attractive to many, but in practice it often resulted in relatively weak boards that were subject to pressures from vested interests and thus found themselves unable to accomplish their stated goals. Other groups advocated working through existing community health care organizations such as the existing boards at the community hospitals. Traditionally these boards were composed of local business, professional, and political leaders and thus represented the established power structure of the community.

Berryhill's success as dean had to a large measure been due to the fact that he knew and understood the political and medical establishment in North Carolina and was a master of the technique that today would be called "networking." As a result he strongly advocated working with the established health care organizations in the community whenever possible rather than establishing new structures. Berryhill advocated letting the "ownership" of the affiliated program reside with the community while the university maintained control of the affiliations' academic content, as Edward Kidder Graham had advocated many years before. Graham had emphasized that "the university can be a part of the community, a partner if you will, but never a dictator."[71] Berryhill frequently used a medical analogy: just as a foreign body introduced into a human being is rejected, a foreign organization introduced into a community would also likely be rejected.

Berryhill's success in dealing with community hospital issues was also due to his own experiences with such hospitals. In a talk he gave in 1974 on community medicine, he reminded the audience that he had served on the medical staff at a "very good community hospital" (Watts Hospital in Durham) and had served on the boards of two community hospitals. Thanks to these experiences, he said, he could fully understand some of the misgivings and insecurities felt by community hospitals as they considered affiliating with a university medical center: the availability of enough beds for the patients of the hospital's medical staff, the impact of students and residents on patient care, and "perhaps most importantly, the fear of university control of the policies of the cooperating institution." He reiterated that it had been his and the university's policy that replicating academic medical centers at the community level was not the goal of the affiliations. Furthermore, while the university was responsible for the academic standards, all other matters were a joint decision of the community hospital medical staffs, the hospital administrators, and hospital trustees with the university. The ultimate goal of such ventures was "to develop new, different, and better methods of providing improved health care" in the community.[72]

Berryhill's way of defusing ownership issues was illustrated in a meeting he had with the board of trustees of the Moses H. Cone Memorial Hospital in Greensboro during the final stages of negotiating the affiliation agreement between the hospital and the university. One of the authors (McLendon) was then a medical staff member serving on Moses Cone Hospital's Education Committee and remembers vividly an exchange that occurred during the meeting. Ben Cone, the president of the board (and a UNC classmate of Berryhill), said, "Reece, we don't want you to come over here and run *our* hospital." Berryhill replied with a twinkle in his eyes, "Ben, we can't even run the hospital we have at Chapel Hill, and we are not about to come over here and run your hospital." His honesty and openness in response to a serious and legitimate concern of many local trustees and physicians defused an issue that could easily have blocked the affiliation.

Affiliation Agreement with Moses H. Cone Memorial Hospital

The Division's first formal community hospital affiliation was with Moses H. Cone Memorial Hospital in Greensboro because of several favorable factors. First, Moses Cone was located only fifty miles west of Chapel Hill and was a relatively easy hour's drive, making it the closest major hospital in the state outside the Research Triangle area of Chapel Hill, Durham, and Raleigh. Second, it was unique among community hospitals in the state because of a sizable endowment that permitted it to be more innovative than other comparable hospitals.

Bertha Lindau Cone had established this endowment in 1911 in memory of her husband, Moses H. Cone, a textile industrialist who had died suddenly in 1908 at the age of fifty-one. Upon Mrs. Cone's death in 1947, the funds became available to the community of Greensboro to build a hospital. In the interval other Cone family members had contributed, and the endowment had grown to some $15 million, so that the hospital was initially constructed without invading the principal. Third, the university at Chapel Hill, North Carolina State College at Raleigh (now North Carolina State University), and the Woman's College at Greensboro (now UNC–Greensboro) had been administratively consolidated by the state legislature in 1933 as a money-saving approach during the Great Depression, providing a university presence in Greensboro. Finally, a detailed review had been conducted in 1947 to determine the feasibility of consolidating on the same site in Greensboro the proposed teaching hospital for UNC and the developing Moses Cone Hospital. The conclusion was that the restrictions of the Cone bequest (a hospital that would primarily serve the people of Guilford County) and the requirement that the university hospital serve all the people of the state, as well as other state policies, made it impossible for the two institutions to honor their commitments in a consolidated hospital setting.[73] Concerning the Moses Cone–UNC discussions, Dean Berryhill's annual report for 1947 concluded prophetically: "This end of negotiations, we hope, does not preclude close professional cooperation in the future between the two hospitals and an arrangement which would aid in better undergraduate and graduate training between the Moses Cone and University hospitals."[74]

In spite of the mutual interest in an affiliation between Moses Cone and the medical school, these negotiations crept along for some time. Cromartie related how the logjam in the negotiations was finally broken. While the dream of affiliated teaching services in community hospitals had existed for some time, the Division of Community Medicine was then operating on a shoestring budget, and the medical school had no monies available to support new faculty positions and other expenses incurred in implementing such programs. The impasse was broken when Caesar Cone, at a meeting with Berryhill and Cromartie, said he was tired of talking about the affiliation and wanted to know how much it would cost to fund the program. Berryhill replied, "$100,000 a year." Cone committed the hospital to this sum, and the pace of the affiliation negotiations accelerated.[75]

The medical staff at Moses Cone approved an affiliation in December 1965, and the executive committee of the hospital trustees added their approval the next week. Harold Bettis, the hospital director, wrote Dean Taylor on December 22, 1965, telling him that the executive committee had "approved the proposed affiliation in principle, and authorized funds for the immediate employment of the Chief of the Teaching Services . . . to work with representatives from the Medical School and the Hospital to develop details of the program along the guidelines of the plan submitted by the Medical School faculty committee." Taylor responded on January 11, 1966, with thanks for his letter and added:

> Dr. W. R. Berryhill, Dean Emeritus, has assumed administrative direction of our developing affiliations programs, and he will be in touch with you about further plans. He will, of course, be working with Drs. Cromartie, Denny and Welt. Dr. Berryhill has, as you know, been interested for a long time in an affiliation between the Medical School and the Cone Hospital and I am sure he will do everything possible to bring our plans to early fruition.[76]

A committee at Chapel Hill then prepared a draft affiliation agreement in the spring of 1966. This was followed by a study by Robert Cadmus, MD, the first director of North Carolina Memorial Hospital and then chair of the Department of Hospital Administration at UNC. His report, made in August 1966, provided data showing that "a productive affiliation was feasible, but it required the Medical Staff of Moses Cone Hospital to carefully deliberate the implications of an affiliation."[77] After further discussions among those at the hospital and the medical school, the Moses Cone trustees approved the affiliation with UNC on December 21, 1966.

The affiliation of the medical school and Moses Cone Hospital was enthusiastically announced in early 1967 in the Moses Cone Hospital newsletter, with Dean Isaac Taylor and hospital director Harold Bettis saying that "they expected the program to start on a limited basis on July 1." The article elaborated:

> As presently envisioned, the program will mean the establishment of teaching services in medicine and pediatrics. Two full-time instructors from the medical school faculty will have their offices in the hospital and will function as Chiefs of the two new teaching services. A three-year program for interns and residents desiring to go into family practice is going to be offered . . .
>
> Responsibility for the recruitment of the interns and residents will be shared by the hospital and the medical school. Hospital trustees have appropriated $100,000 as sharing funds for the first year of operations of a six-year program . . . After the fourth year of operation, the program will be evaluated and a decision made as to whether or not continuation is advisable.
>
> The new affiliation is a milestone in the history of the hospital. It will mean a new type of medical care will be available in this area. According to Mr. Bettis, the hospital–medical school arrangement should facilitate the development of Moses Cone Hospital as a model medical education center "which should epitomize the manner in which a community hospital can best serve its community."
>
> The affiliation will permit the medical school to support a program of post graduate medical education which will be available to area physicians . . .

For the University, it will in the words of Dr. Taylor, "further the vital program of getting the medical school out into the state." The hospital–medical school project will be one of the first in the state. It thus will serve as a pilot study for programs yet to come.

Later, the affiliation may be extended to include other clinical services such as obstetrics-gynecology, surgery, and psychiatry, if the pilot study proves satisfactory.[78]

It was both appropriate and typical for Berryhill's role at this stage in his career that the article did not mention him, and that Dean Taylor made the announcement jointly with the hospital director. It is also of interest that the structure of the agreement between Moses Cone and the university closely followed the recommendations Cromartie had made in 1965.

William B. Herring, MD (Bowman Gray 1953), a member of the faculty in the Department of Medicine at Chapel Hill, was jointly appointed by Welt, the chair of medicine, and by Moses Cone Hospital to be the first chief of the medical teaching service at Moses Cone. He and his family moved in June 1967 to Greensboro to implement the affiliated program. Herring also became chief of the teaching services, assuming the duties of the previous part-time director of medical education.

Martha Sharpless, MD (UNC 1959), who had received her pediatric training at the Babies Hospital in New York City, was appointed by Denny, chair of pediatrics, and by Moses Cone to be the first chief of the pediatrics teaching service. She joined Herring in July, and for the next six years they were the only full-time faculty in the UNC teaching programs at Moses Cone. Sharpless soon won the respect and admiration of the pediatricians in the community because of her ready availability and skill in consulting on difficult pediatric cases. Samuel Ravenel, MD, one of the community's most eminent and long-serving pediatricians, once commented that the local pediatricians' "hymn" was "Praise the Lord but pass me Martha Sharpless."[79]

Sharpless and Herring immediately organized pediatric and medicine teaching services, and they had "a flood of fourth-year medical students eager to experience the real-life world of community hospital practice." These students came not only from UNC and nearby Bowman Gray, but also from many other states and several foreign countries.

A three-year family practice residency program was next organized. It was one of the first sixteen programs in the country approved in February 1969 by the newly constituted Residency Review Committee for Family Practice. In July 1969 the first two residents, both MD graduates from the UNC class of 1968, entered the family practice program as second-year residents and completed the program in 1971. One stayed in Greensboro and went into emergency medicine, while the other practiced family medicine in Reidsville. Herring later commented, "When I secured the approval of the family practice residency program he [Welt] chastised me for having pursued it without his approval. In that he

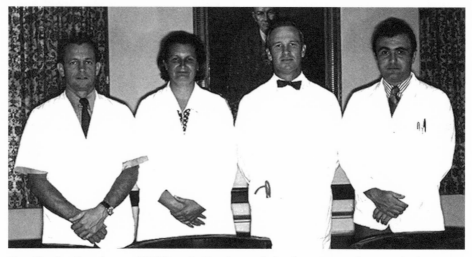

Drs. Martha Sharpless and William B. Herring with the first two residents in the family medicine program at Moses Cone, Drs. Ronald F. Joyner *(left)* and George G. Lothian *(right)*, 1970. *(Moses Cone Memorial Hospital Library)*

was correct, but if I had sought his approval it would not have been granted, and Moses Cone would not have had one of the first approved programs in the country."[80]

Three-year programs in internal medicine and pediatrics were the next to be organized and approved. They had their first graduates in 1974. By 2005 there were thirty-one full-time faculty members at Moses Cone. The hospital had approved residencies in family medicine, internal medicine, and pediatrics (the latter operated jointly with the pediatrics residency at Chapel Hill), as well as in hospital pharmacy. Some fifty primary care residents were in training at Moses Cone by 2005. Many medical students on rotation also received part of their clinical experience at Moses Cone.

An appreciation of the impact of this affiliation on the medical community in Greensboro comes from a physician practicing there at the time. He observed that from 1964, when he began to practice urology, until 1974, no new primary care physicians joined the medical community—at a time when a steady stream of new specialists were setting up practices. As residents completed the affiliated residency in family practice, however, a number of new primary care physicians joined the medical community.[81]

Herring made a more detailed estimate of the contribution of the affiliated program to the community, the state, and the nation. In 1988 there were "45 physicians practicing in Greensboro or its immediate vicinity who had all or part of their residency training at Moses Cone Hospital since 1969." Most of these were in primary care, but some went elsewhere for further training and returned to practice as specialists. In addition, ten physicians who had had medical student rotations at Moses Cone obtained their residency training elsewhere and returned to practice in Greensboro. Finally, Herring estimated that "over 1,500 physicians now practicing in the United States received clinical training at the Moses Cone Hospital, either as medical students or as house officers, for periods ranging from one month to four years."[82]

A key argument used in selling the community medicine program to the legislature was that the location of residency training is more likely to influence the location of a future physician's practice than is the medical school he or she attended. The positive results of physician recruitment in the Greensboro area following the affiliation of Moses Cone with the medical school confirmed the validity of that argument.

Affiliation Agreement with Charlotte Memorial Hospital

The community of Charlotte had long been interested in medical education. The college physicians on the campus of nearby Davidson College founded the North Carolina Medical College as a basic sciences preparatory school in 1887. After evolving into a full MD-granting medical school, the college moved in 1907 to Charlotte, on North Church Street in the Fourth Ward, in a building with a 360-seat amphitheater; physiological, pathological, and bacteriological laboratories; a library; and a dissecting hall. Five Charlotte hospitals were used for clinical instruction. Lacking the resources to meet the modern standards of the Flexner Report of 1910, however, the college closed its Charlotte school and merged with the Medical College of Virginia in Richmond, where its students transferred in 1914.[83]

The loss of the medical school only strengthened the determination of leaders in Charlotte to reap the benefits of medical education for their community. To their credit, when an MD-granting state medical school was being considered in the 1920s, the Charlotte delegation said it was more important for North Carolina to have a state medical school than to insist that it be located in Charlotte.[84] This effort to have a hospital and expanded medical school at Chapel Hill failed, however, as a result of the controversy following the proposal by President William P. Few of Trinity College (a Methodist college soon to become Duke University) for a joint Carolina-Duke medical school, as noted earlier.

When the expansion of the medical school at Chapel Hill was again being considered in the mid-1940s, Charlotte mounted a major drive to have the UNC medical school and teaching hospital located there. After the 1946 Sanger Report and the subsequent recommendation of the Medical Care Commission both supported expanding the existing medical school and building a teaching hospital at Chapel Hill, the *Charlotte Observer* published the bitter denunciation of the decision noted previously.

The medical and hospital leaders in Charlotte then turned their energies to strengthening the intern and residency programs at Charlotte Memorial Hospital. This hospital had been formed in 1940 by a city-county board that consolidated various small hospitals and is now known as the Carolinas Medical Center.[85]

Charlotte Memorial's internship program began in 1942. In the late 1950s and early 1960s the hospital had residents rotating from Montreal General Hospital due to the fact that James Alexander, MD, then chief of staff, had trained there.

David Citron, MD, a graduate of the two-year UNC medical school and then a self-described "naïve fourth-year student at Washington University" in St. Louis, later related that he decided to apply in 1944 for an internship at Charlotte Memorial Hospital. The imposing new hospital building impressed him, and he thought it would provide "a rich exposure to common medical problems [with] supervision by physicians of local renown." He wrote to Berryhill, whose

> response to my request for a letter of recommendation was prompt and laconic: No, he would not write such a letter. The teaching program at Charlotte had not yet proved its worth. I should, instead, remain in St. Louis for graduate training in internal medicine at Barnes Hospital. He would be delighted to write a letter to the departmental chairman. Having never had the temerity to question his judgment on a matter relating to medical education—or almost anything else, for that matter—I accepted his wise counsel.[86]

Citron called upon Berryhill again in the late 1950s, this time as a practicing physician trying to assist in recruiting interns for Charlotte Memorial Hospital. He told Berryhill that Charlotte now had a large number of well-educated physicians—many graduates of the UNC program—who eagerly wished to participate in training interns. He asked Berryhill's help "in attracting some of 'his' graduates for training in Charlotte." Citron related that Berryhill replied, "without hesitation and with his customary, unemotional forthrightness . . . 'No, David, I can't do that. Charlotte Memorial has a bad reputation to overcome.' And he was right. My request was premature if not foolish; and as Glenn Wilson recently reminded me, 'Dr. Berryhill suffered fools poorly.'"[87]

By 1961 Charlotte Memorial Hospital had no interns, and about two-thirds of its fifteen residents were foreign medical graduates. In 1962 the hospital lost accreditation of its internship, and the American Medical Association Council on Medical Education put three of the five residencies on probation. With the help of Dean Wilburt Davison of the Duke School of Medicine, the internship approval was extended for one year, but the pressure was on to develop quality programs or get out of house staff training all together.

At this time the hospital board, the physician staff, and the hospital administration reaffirmed a major commitment to medical education. With financial assistance from the Duke Endowment, the hospital in 1962 recruited Bryant Galusha, MD, a Charlotte pediatrician, as a full-time director of medical education. He and the new hospital director, John Rankin, were able to change the hospital staff bylaws so that donation of time to the teaching programs was a requirement for medical staff membership.

Once high educational standards were assured, Berryhill was receptive to requests for help. Galusha remembers that Berryhill, in typical fashion, still insisted, "Prove to me that you are serious and worthy of the support and we will support you."[88]

A meeting of Dean Berryhill and Charles H. Burnett, MD (founding chair of the UNC Department of Medicine), with representatives of the hospital and medical staff at Charlotte Memorial in May 1963 led to an agreement that senior residents from the internal medicine program at Chapel Hill would spend six to twelve months of their third year in the Charlotte program. Because the Charlotte program had previously only been approved for two years, this provided a full internal medicine program. At the same time members of the Department of Medicine faculty started monthly visits to Charlotte for rounds and conferences. Some five years later the Charlotte program was approved as a full three-year program.

With all these changes, the intern positions were filled, the residency programs were taken off probation, the existing three-year surgery residency was awarded full four-year approval, and a new residency in general practice (now family medicine) was added.[89] In 1967 Marvin McCall, MD (UNC 1956), a Charlotte internist, became the first full-time UNC faculty member at Charlotte Memorial, and in 1968 James C. Parke, Jr., MD (UNC 1954), became the first full-time faculty member in pediatrics. Pinckney Rankin, MD (Pennsylvania 1952), was appointed as a part-time UNC faculty member in obstetrics and gynecology in 1969, with Bobby Rimer, MD (UNC 1957), following him as a full-time faculty

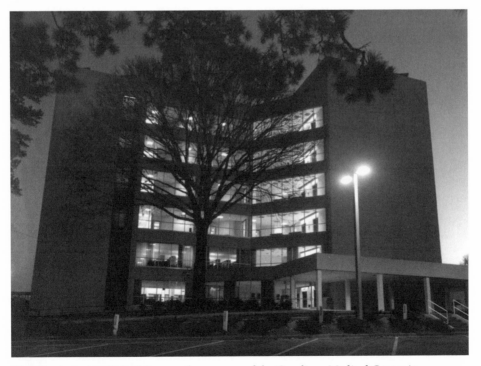

The Charlotte AHEC Building on the campus of the Carolinas Medical Center in Charlotte. *(NC AHEC Program)*

member in 1973. Clinical clerkships for UNC medical students were initially started in internal medicine, and clerkships in obstretics and gynecology and pediatrics were added later.

Today the Carolinas Medical Center has more than 200 residents and some 140 full-time faculty members. The State Health Coordinating Council has designated it the state's fifth academic medical center. It has ten fully approved residency programs including emergency medicine, family medicine, general surgery, internal medicine, obstetrics and gynecology, orthopedic surgery, and pediatrics as well as several advanced fellowship programs. Charlotte is now one of the premier sites for rotations by medical and other health sciences students from UNC.

Affiliation Agreement with the New Hanover
Memorial Hospital in Wilmington

When the announcement of the founding of the Division of Research and Education in Community Medicine was made in 1966, Lockert Mason, MD, a surgeon and the director of medical education at James Walker Memorial Hospital in Wilmington, wrote Dean Taylor to express interest in an affiliation with the medical school. Berryhill responded that negotiations for affiliations were ongoing with two hospitals in the state, but the limited resources of the Division prevented considerations of other affiliations at that time. Nonetheless, Huntley and Lyle visited Wilmington to express the Division's interest in an affiliation even though it was not then possible.

In June 1967 James Walker Memorial Hospital and the Community Hospital in Wilmington ceased operations and moved to the newly completed New Hanover Memorial Hospital (NHMH). The three-year general surgery residency program, approved in 1965 at James Walker, was transferred to NHMH, and Mason became the director of medical education for the new hospital.[90]

The affiliation of New Hanover and the medical school started informally as a different type of program from those in the other affiliations. Beginning in 1968 the airplanes of the new Medical Air Operations program were utilized once weekly to provide an interchange between the two institutions' faculty, practicing physicians, medical students, and residents. These exchanges, and the resulting affiliation agreement, were described in the Division's advisory committee report for 1970:

> Since October 1968, pediatric sub-specialists with residents have departed once a week from the University Medical Center to serve in the New Hanover Memorial Hospital in Wilmington. These pediatricians with sub-specialties in cardiology, hematology, and allergy will have approximately 300 contacts with patients this year. Without this service . . . the nearest medical center for this type of treatment is 300 miles round trip. A pediatrician from Wilmington acts as a sponsor for the visiting group. This provides an opportunity for

the local pediatrician to update his sub-specialty training; thus the program serves as continuing education for the practicing physician and provides a direct link with the university for local physicians. The aircraft, which transports the pediatricians to Wilmington, immediately returns to Chapel Hill carrying surgeons, on in some cases house staff. Since September of this year, two obstetricians have been coming to the Medical Center once a month. The surgeons spend a full day at North Carolina Memorial Hospital teaching medical students and familiarizing themselves with specialized surgical procedures. Both groups are returned by air to their respective homes at the end of the day.

[As a result] an affiliation agreement has recently been signed with this [New Hanover] hospital after two years of developmental activities coordinated through the Director of Medical Education. With the use of state funds, partial salaries for faculty positions have been made available to this hospital. Each of these physicians will head a separate teaching service for medical students and residents in the specialties of medicine, obstetrics and gynecology, and surgery.[91]

By 1971 New Hanover Hospital had approved residency programs in surgery, obstetrics and gynecology, and medicine. The impact of the medical school affiliation at Wilmington was evident almost immediately. Wilson, in a letter to Dean Taylor in support of the medical school's request to the 1971 General Assembly for expanded funding for community medicine efforts, stated, "Two physicians who will complete their training at Chapel Hill in the spring of 1971 will establish an office in Wilmington this summer. A major factor in their decision to locate in Wilmington was related to the medical school's affiliation and educational program with the New Hanover Memorial Hospital."[92]

The New Hanover Regional Medical Center now has some thirty-one full-time faculty and fully accredited residency programs in family medicine, general surgery, internal medicine, and obstetrics and gynecology. Wilmington continues to be a major site for UNC medical student rotations.

Other Affiliation Agreements

The UNC medical student class size almost tripled during the late 1960s and 1970s, and pressure increased to have affiliations for clinical training sites of third- and fourth-year medical students. Other formal affiliations were developed both before and after the NC AHEC Program was implemented, but by then Berryhill was no longer leading the Division.

STEPPING DOWN AGAIN

In August 1969 Berryhill had a conference with Dean Taylor during which he informed Taylor of his decision to resign as director of the Division. This was followed two weeks later by a letter confirming his desire to resign as soon as a successor or acting director could be appointed, but no later than December 1, 1969. Although he wished "to be relieved of the responsibilities of Director as soon as possible," he indicated that at the same time "I am so convinced that the future of this medical school—in a large measure—depends upon the continued development and strengthening of University affiliated–community hospitals educational relations, it might be tragic if a 'crash' decision were made, without careful and thoughtful appraisal of the able younger men who should be considered for this post."[93]

Berryhill related that he had turned down an offer in April 1967 "to accept the directorship of the Regional Medical Program for the State of Virginia with faculty appointments at the University of Virginia School of Medicine and the Medical College of Virginia." He also stated that he had considered resigning in 1968 but had delayed the decision "since I felt the most important contribution I could make to the activities of this Division was to exert every effort possible to get a State appropriation to insure a more stable and continuing financial basis for its future. Since these efforts, with the understanding and support of some members of the Advisory Budget Commission and, subsequently, of leaders of the 1969 General Assembly, have been successful, I feel free now to implement the above intent."

Berryhill reiterated the reasons for his resignation, which he had discussed with Taylor during their meeting, but added, "I should like to continue as an active staff member of this Division until the mandatory retirement point for me, June 30, 1971, should my successor as Director wish me to do so."

Taylor replied two weeks later accepting Berryhill's resignation effective October 1, 1969.[94] He said that Robert Smith, MD, had agreed to become acting director of the Division while a search for a permanent director was pursued. Taylor added, "Dr. Smith will be given consideration for the post, but it is one of such importance that I want to consider persons from as large a list as possible in order to be as certain as we can that the best person comes to the position." He indicated that he expected "to settle the matter prior to July 1, 1970."

Taylor stated that Berryhill, in accordance with his wishes, would "continue your work in the School as a member of the division with the title of Dean Emeritus and Sarah Graham Kenan Professor of Medicine, devoting the major portion of your time to further development of our affiliations with the Moses H. Cone Memorial Hospital and the Charlotte Memorial Hospital." He stated that both he and Smith approved of this arrangement. Taylor added, "You understand that your appointment is on an annual basis, renewable annually until June 30, 1971, subject to nomination by the department chairman and approval by the University administrative officers and by the Board of trustees."

Taylor added, "You are to be congratulated on your achievements in establishing the Division of Education and Research in Community Medical Care. I know very well the difficulties, financial and otherwise, which you have faced, and which justify special pride in the accomplishments. Of special note is the procurement of substantial state support for the Division through the Advisory Budget Commission and the 1969 General Assembly."

Berryhill resigned as director of the Division for Research and Education in Community Medicine in 1969. He remained a full-time participant in the Division until 1971, after which he served in a half-time capacity from 1971 to 1973. He then remained as a consultant to the Division from 1973 to 1975. One-time payments were made for specific consulting activities, as noted in the following January 1973 letter from Glenn Wilson, associate dean for community health services, to Dean Fordham:

> This is to request that the Division of Education and Research in Community Medical Care be granted authority to continue the services of W. Reece Berryhill, MD. We request that effective July 1, 1973, Dr. Berryhill be retained by the Division as a consultant and receive one-time payments based upon his contribution . . . As you know, Dr. Berryhill has played a central role in the development of the affiliated agreements between the medical school and the community hospitals over the past several years. The award of the federal contract for the development of an Area Health Education System in North Carolina makes his knowledge and understanding of the School and the individuals in the State of increasing importance. Dr. Berryhill continues to play a vital role in the development of the AHEC system and it will be of utmost importance that we continue to have his services available as the program develops.

In a May 1974 letter, Dean Fordham thanked Berryhill for his "great assistance to the School during this past year, your first year in 'full retirement.'" The requests for one-time payments for his consultations show him to have been involved with a number of projects, such as working with affiliated hospitals about residencies and student rotations; consulting on development of statewide policy guidelines for the AHEC Program; and consulting with participants for the statewide AHEC meeting on GME (graduate medical education) in February 1975.[95]

Robert Smith, a British physician who had recently joined the UNC faculty, became the acting director of the Division in 1969 following Berryhill's resignation. He served until July 1970, when he became the founding chair of the newly created Department of Family Medicine at UNC, a position he held until he left in 1975 to become chair of family medicine at Cincinnati.

The Coming of the North Carolina Area Health Education Centers Program

Dean Taylor recruited Glenn Wilson, MA, to UNC in 1970 as director of the Division, associate dean, and professor of medical economics. Wilson had

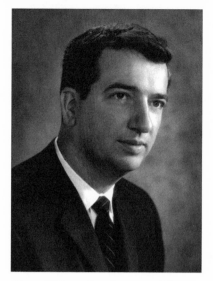

Glenn Wilson, first director of the
North Carolina AHEC Program.
(Med. Illustrations, NCC)

served as director of medical care research for a
large insurance company (1956–1962), executive
director of the Community Health Foundation in
Cleveland (1963–1969), and executive vice president
of the Kaiser Community Health Foundation in
Cleveland (1969–1970).[96]

Glenn Wilson is appropriately recognized as the
architect and implementer of the highly successful
NC AHEC Program because of his unique experiences with health care organizations elsewhere, his
many contacts with those in Washington engaged
in preparing legislation for health care manpower,
and his ability to work with community hospital
administrators and with local and state political
leaders. Wilson served as director of the NC AHEC
Program from its origin in 1972 until 1978, when
Dean Fordham appointed him chair of the Department of Community Medicine and Hospital Ad-
ministration (which later became the Department of Social Medicine). Eugene
Mayer, MD, MPH, who had been one of Wilson's early recruits to the Division
and had served as deputy director of the program, succeeded Wilson as the director of the NC AHEC Program in 1978.

Berryhill, writing in the mid-1970s, was highly complimentary of Wilson's
impact on the Division and the AHEC Program:

> The tremendous contributions in health education and health care made by
> this Division from 1970 to the present have been due in large part to Mr. Wil-
> son's previous experience in these areas for the medical and health sciences
> and his capacity to attract able associates to the Division. He had had wide
> experience [in medical care] . . . Mr. Wilson attracted a very able staff that
> worked conscientiously and imaginatively in assisting the implementation
> of joint efforts of the medical and health-science schools in these endeavors
> with community hospitals.

In an address to the Robert A. Ross Obstetrical and Gynecological Society in
1974, Berryhill elaborated on Wilson's personal qualities and his commitment to
the concept that made the affiliations and AHEC work so well:

> The major developments have evolved since 1970 when my able successor,
> Glenn Wilson, joined the faculty as associate dean, Community Health
> Services, and as director of the Division of Education and Research in Com-
> munity Medical Care. Those of you who have worked with him realize his
> extraordinary qualities of understanding, of imagination, and of sound
> leadership based on many years of experience in the fields of medical care

and medical education. Importantly also he has stood firmly on the fundamental concept and principle that the university and the community are joint partners.[97]

Wilson's seminal contributions to medical education and health care in North Carolina in his role as the founding director of the NC AHEC Program was recognized by the Program with the establishment of the Glenn Wilson Award for Public Service. It recognizes Wilson's success in assembling a team to write the initial federal AHEC grant, the largest ever received by UNC at the time; his development of the university-community partnerships necessary for its success; his leadership in obtaining permanent state funding in 1974 for facilities and programs in the nine AHECs; and his career-long commitment to access to quality health care for all. The Glenn Wilson Award is given annually to an individual who has been a leader in improving access to quality health care for the citizens of the state and who has participated in teaching health sciences students directly or through his or her organization.

Although Berryhill and Wilson differed significantly in age and background, they shared a common commitment to improve the health of the people of the state. Wilson later described his relationship with Berryhill:

> When I arrived in Chapel Hill in 1970, knowing very little about the State and its health care problems, he traveled with me, introduced me and said that what I was doing was a good idea. Without his great credibility and his saying "I'm involved" it might have taken years for AHEC to evolve; in fact without his reputation and good will among physicians in the State it might have failed. His Presbyterian sense of integrity and his commitment to the people of North Carolina made it work. He took an extraordinary chance . . . and gave me his endorsement. I respected him totally; and although we were close friends I could never address him by his first name.[98]

From the perspective of three decades later, Wilson's evaluation of the contribution of Berryhill and the Division from 1966 to the early 1970s in preparing the way for the NC AHEC is justified. It is also clear that the NC AHEC Program we have in the early part of the twenty-first century would not exist had it not been for Dean Taylor's recruitment of Glenn Wilson to UNC in 1970. Wilson brought practical experience in dealing with various health care organizations; many contacts in Washington and on the national scene; boundless energy; and the ability to work in a collegial way with those who have made AHEC work in communities across North Carolina.

The Carnegie Commission Report

While North Carolina was striving in the 1960s to find methods to improve the number and distribution of physicians and other health professionals throughout the state and to improve the quality of medical care at the community level, a parallel effort was going on nationally. The Carnegie Commission on Higher Education in 1970 released an important study of the nation's health care needs, along with recommendations for improvements. UNC President William C. Friday was one of some twenty prominent leaders in American higher education on this commission.[99]

Among the problems highlighted by the commission were serious shortages of health care personnel and wide geographic discrepancies in the quality of health care available to Americans. It recommended addressing the former primarily by building more health science centers (medical and other health science schools with teaching hospitals) and by significantly increasing the number of graduating physicians in the existing schools.

The commission saw an exciting challenge for universities and their medical centers in dealing with the maldistribution of health care personnel and services. It proposed addressing this problem by means of a new, geographic approach to medical education that included establishing area health education centers around the nation in locations without a health science center.

The commission suggested the establishment of three area health education centers in North Carolina—at Asheville, Charlotte, and Wilmington—to provide geographic balance in the state for the three existing academic medical centers at Chapel Hill, Durham, and Winston-Salem and the fourth developing center at Greenville.

Federal Funding for Community Medical Education through the AHEC Program

In late 1971 Congress passed the Comprehensive Health Manpower Training Act to address the health manpower problems that had become a critical national problem. One section, entitled Health Manpower Education Initiative Awards, provided funds to implement area health education centers. Implementation of the legislation was delayed as several agencies in Washington fought over control of the funds, but the problem was resolved when the authority was given to the Bureau of Health Manpower Education.[100]

When the federal government in the summer of 1972 finally requested applications for contract support for the operation of area health education centers, Dean Taylor asked Wilson to take the lead in preparing, within a very short time, the preliminary proposal and then the application from UNC. This successful process was later described:

> The [UNC] medical school was selected as one of twenty-seven out of ninety-three medical schools to apply for a grant and was one of eleven successful applicants. The award was for $8,563,734, which was the largest in terms of money and the only one that proposed covering a whole state in a single program. [It] was a particular tribute to a small group who worked on the proposal, primarily Glenn Wilson, Eugene Mayer, Faye Pickard, Glenn Pick-

ard, John Payne, John Parker, Shirley Jabbs, Mary Lee Erissman, and Ann Francis.[101]

Bryant Galusha, who worked on the grant application from his position as director of medical education at Charlotte Memorial Hospital, related that Wilson was the "mover" in the project. He described the frantic process as "great fun" and observed, "We were like a bunch of college kids." He characterized the grant-writing process as "teamwork at its finest": it involved numerous persons across the state, including those at UNC and the other medical schools, community college leaders, hospital administrators, practicing physicians, and political leaders.[102]

Medical Air Operations played an essential role during the preparation of the grant application, transporting people and drafts of the application and of affiliation agreements back and forth from Chapel Hill to the sites of the proposed AHECs and flying the final grant proposal to Washington. Cutchin remembers a particularly busy Saturday: in the morning seeing patients at the Tarboro Clinic and in the afternoon going over plans for what was to become the Area L AHEC with John Payne, who had flown in a medical school plane to Tarboro from Chapel Hill for the meeting.[103] Another participant in the hectic grant-writing process remembers one day when she flew from Chapel Hill's Horace Williams Airport to the Raleigh-Durham airport and thence to Fayetteville, Wilmington, Tarboro, and finally back home to Chapel Hill. She had departed at 6:30 A.M., and her day ended at 1:30 the next morning, when all those who had been flying around the state had completed reviewing and updating the latest draft of the grant proposal.[104]

Berryhill later speculated about some of the reasons for the success of North Carolina's application for the federal AHEC grant:

> The Area Health Education Centers program is an example of what can happen when the aspirations and felt responsibilities of a medical school coincide with national long-range planning. The history of the AHEC program is inextricably intertwined with the history of the medical school's Division of Education and Research in Community Medical Care since, in many ways, the former is the intellectual descendant of the latter . . .
>
> . . . A major factor [in the success of the grant application] undoubtedly was the fact that the basis for what was being proposed was a system that was already in operation and successfully so. A second factor was the enormous breadth of the proposal—a breadth which encompassed the medical school's expansive vision of its role in medical education at the community level throughout the state and further incorporated the conviction that methods and procedures which had been developed with the existing affiliation[s] could be adapted and applied to other areas in the state.[105]

A 1973 report entitled "A Statewide Plan for Medical Education in North Carolina," prepared by Ivan L. Bennett, MD, and a national panel of medical educators for the UNC Board of Governors, elaborated on North Carolina's success with the AHEC grant and with the initial implementation of the AHEC Program:

> Beginning in 1967, UNC–CH School of Medicine established affiliations with several community hospitals and in 1969 the General Assembly appropriated funds for the establishment of undergraduate and postgraduate educational programs in these institutions. By the time that Congress enacted the Comprehensive Health Manpower Training Act in 1971, UNC–CH had 16 full time faculty members located in 7 affiliated hospitals throughout the state and was in an excellent position, by virtue of this initial experience, to compete for federal funds appropriated to establish a system of AHECs. UNC–CH was awarded NIH Contract No. 72-4387 by the Bureau of Health Manpower in the amount of $8.5 millions over a five year period in a keen national competition. After less than a year of the contract, AHECs had been established in Charlotte . . . Wilmington . . . Raleigh . . . Asheville . . . and Planning Area L . . . These 5 AHECs will be supporting and training health personnel in 31 counties . . . Four additional AHECs are under discussion or are in the negotiation stage . . . During the past year, the AHEC programs have compiled a solid record of achievement . . . This is a most impressive demonstration of what has already been done. The potential for the future is bright.[106]

Significance of the NC AHEC Program

The significance of the accomplishments of those who established the NC AHEC Program in the 1970s can best be appreciated when one realizes that it took sixty years from the Flexner Report of 1910 to establish the outstanding academic medical centers that existed in the United States in 1970. These centers were traditionally committed to providing humane and scientifically sound care for the patients they served while helping to ensure even better care for tomorrow's patients everywhere through their commitment to education and research. Yet in the 1970s they were widely perceived as having failed to promote adequate health and medical services for those who lived outside the larger cities.

In North Carolina during the 1970s a totally new and parallel system of medical education at the community level was developed across the state. This system materialized as a result of the leadership of the founding AHEC Program director, Glenn Wilson; the solid support of former Dean Berryhill, Deans Taylor and Fordham, and UNC President Friday; and the cooperation and involvement of countless others at UNC, in the other medical schools in the state, in community hospitals and colleges, in the practicing physician community, and in the local and state political community.

Early Recognition for North Carolina's Efforts in Community Medicine

The NC AHEC Program has received numerous honors and recognitions over the years since its inception in 1972.

One of the earlier honors was bestowed at the Convocation Program of the American College of Physicians (ACP) in Dallas in April 1977, when the first Richard and Hilda Rosenthal Foundation Awards were given.[107] These awards were established in 1976 to be presented "to that scientist or scientific group whose innovative work is making a notable contribution to improve clinical care in the field of internal medicine." The first awards were given to one individual (Baruch S. Blumberg, MD, PhD, the discoverer of the Australia antigen and its relationship to post-transfusion hepatitis) and to two groups (the NC AHEC Program and the WAMI [Washington-Alaska-Montana-Idaho] Program for regional medical education).

Glenn Wilson accepted the Rosenthal Award on behalf of the program. The citation stated:

> The objective of the North Carolina Area Health Education Centers Program is to implement a better specialty and geographic distribution of all health personnel in North Carolina. This goal is being attained by decentralizing medical, dental, public health and pharmacologic education and by strengthening regional educational opportunities for nursing and allied health programs, thus creating regional professional environments that retain and attract additional health personnel.
>
> The Program is directed by the University of North Carolina School of Medicine at Chapel Hill and its faculty and involves its five health sciences schools and Duke University Medical Center, Bowman Gray School of Medicine, the emerging medical school at East Carolina University, five campuses of the University of North Carolina, 21 community hospitals, and 15 technical institutes.
>
> The Program represents the commitment of the faculties to extend beyond traditional academic objectives as partners with the community hospitals and their staffs to assume regional educational responsibility for one of our society's most pressing health care problems, the specialty and geographic distributions of all health personnel.

In an interview at the time of the announcement of the award, Wilson described the NC AHEC Program as a "creative partnership" among numerous institutions and individuals throughout the state to address the "socially important question" of how to improve the distribution of physicians and other health care personnel in the state and nation. He emphasized that the AHEC Program was built "on the principle that local people can best determine local needs and that local people and their institutions can begin to solve problems if given the opportunity." He added that the AHEC Program had demonstrated "an enormous reservoir of energy and talent that can be focused constructively on social problems. If the North Carolina AHEC program had to pay for the talent and energy of those who volunteer to participate in this statewide teaching effort, the cost would be several millions dollars more per year." He cited figures to show that the rate of the increase in numbers of active physicians in North Carolina in the first three years of the program was nearly twice the national rate for the same period.[108]

At the same convocation Berryhill received the American College of Physicians' highest honor when he was made a Master of the ACP. The citation for Berryhill's mastership documented his accomplishments in spearheading "the drive to expand the 2-year medical school at the University of North Carolina to a 4-year, degree-granting institution" that is "known nationally as an outstanding institution." It continued with praise for his accomplishments with the community medicine program:

> When Dr. Berryhill retired as dean in 1964, he became the first director of the School of Medicine's Division of Education and Research in Community Medical Care. Based on the enthusiastic statewide support he had gained as dean, he was able to establish cooperative arrangements with a number of the state's community hospitals.
>
> From these affiliations, which provided full-time faculty for the hospitals, was created the North Carolina Area Health Education Centers Program, recognized nationally as one of the most promising approaches to relating medical science and technology to community medical care.
>
> Dr. Berryhill, who is Sarah Graham Kenan Professor of Medicine Emeritus, still advises faculty and works with the Area Health Education Centers (AHEC) Program. A major accomplishment of the AHEC has been improving the professional environment in North Carolina's 100 counties by decreasing professional isolation for practitioners through varied local and regional educational activities.

An editorial in the *Greensboro Daily News* a few days after Berryhill's death in January 1979 recognized his modesty, his "stellar qualities of tenacity, humility and intelligence," his career as a dean in working for the expansion of the medical school at Chapel Hill, and his dedication to it "during its crucial years." The editorial continued, "But even after stepping down from the deanship in 1964, Dr. Berryhill went on to become director of the Division of Education and Research in Community Medical Care. Out of his work in broadening medical school affiliations with North Carolina hospitals came the North Carolina Area Health Education Centers Program (AHEC), now nationally recognized for its excellence."[109]

The NC AHEC Program later distributed walnut and brass plaques with the following inscription for display in each of the AHEC sites in North Caro-

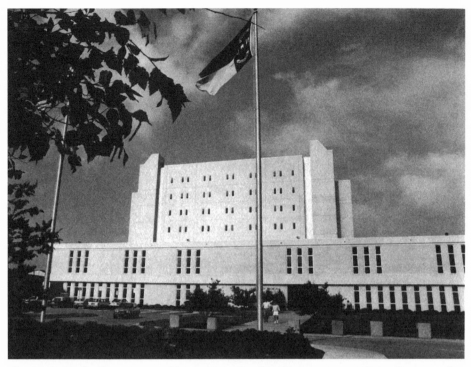

The Brody Medical Sciences Building at East Carolina University, 1982. It is adjacent to the Pitt County Memorial Hospital, which serves as the teaching hospital for the ECU School of Medicine. (Williams, *The Beginnings of the School of Medicine at East Carolina University,* 1998; courtesy of The Medical Foundation of East Carolina University)

lina: "W. Reece Berryhill, M.D. 1900–1979; Dean, U.N.C. School of Medicine, 1941–1964; In Remembrance Of His Many Contributions To University Community Relationships Which Led To The North Carolina Area Health Education Centers Program."

The NC AHEC Program Then and Now

Following the initial federal grant of $8,563,734 in October 1972, the North Carolina General Assembly in 1974 appropriated $23 million for renovation or building of facilities at the AHECs around the state as well as $4.5 million for operating expenses. This funding came after a long and bitter political fight about the need for a second state-supported medical school in the state and whether an expanded AHEC Program could achieve the same goals. The legislature in 1974 resolved the controversy by funding both the AHEC Program and a new MD-granting medical school at East Carolina University (ECU) at Greenville.[110] After having a joint ECU-UNC one-year school for several years, ECU admitted its first four-year class in 1977. In 1981 ECU graduated its first class of twenty-eight physicians and received full four-year accreditation from the Liaison Committee on Medical Education. In the intervening years the rapidly evolving ECU medical school became a strong partner in the NC AHEC Program.

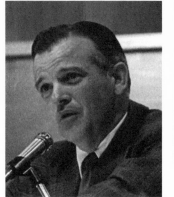

Dr. Bryant Galusha.
(NC AHEC Program)

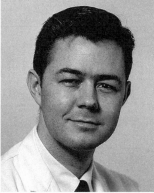

Dr. Lawrence M. Cutchin.
(Med. Illustrations, NCC)

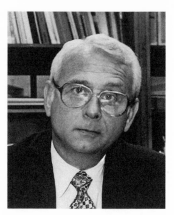

William Morrison.
(Coastal AHEC)

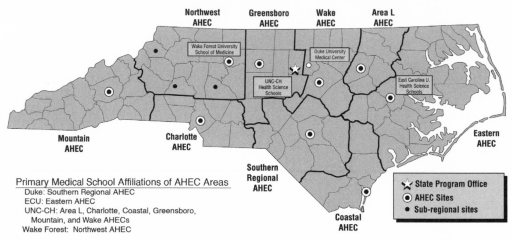

Map of the North Carolina AHEC Program. *(NC AHEC Program)*

By the fall of 1974, the NC AHEC Program could report a major change in the sources of funding for community medical education efforts in North Carolina: "Before the federal AHEC contract was received, 50 percent of the funding for these educational programs came from the individual hospital in which the program was offered, the other 50 percent was provided through state appropriations. Now [1974] funding is roughly 70 percent state, 20 percent federal, and 10 percent local."

By 2005 the total annual funding for the NC AHEC Program exceeded $160 million. Of this amount, approximately 34 percent was from local hospital support, 28 percent was from state appropriations, and 28 percent was from clinical income. The balance came from miscellaneous sources, including federal and other grants and continuing education fees.

Area L, Charlotte, and Wilmington were the first three AHEC centers in North Carolina under the first federal AHEC grant beginning in 1972. The Area

L AHEC was based in the federal and state health planning Area L and involved smaller hospitals, including Halifax Memorial Hospital in Roanoke Rapids, Nash General Hospital in Rocky Mount, Wilson Hospital, and Edgecombe Hospital, as well as the Tarboro Clinic. The first AHEC director for Area L was Lawrence Cutchin, MD. The Charlotte AHEC, based at Charlotte Memorial Hospital (now Carolinas Medical Center), was responsible for a nine-county area surrounding Charlotte. Its first AHEC director was Bryant Galusha, MD. The Coastal AHEC, based at New Hanover Hospital (now New Hanover Regional Medical Center), was responsible for the AHEC Program in Wilmington and a five-county surrounding area. Its first AHEC director was William Morrison, the administrator of New Hanover Hospital.

Moses Cone Memorial Hospital (now the Moses Cone Health System), the site of the first formal educational affiliation completed by the Division in 1967, joined the NC AHEC Program in 1974 as the Greensboro AHEC.

The 1974 report by the NC AHEC Program stated that the five established AHECs "are supporting and training health personnel for 44 counties." Four more AHECs were in development, and the report predicted that "all counties will be served by one of the nine centers" by 1975.

At the time of this writing nine Area Health Education Centers cover all 100 counties in the state: Area L AHEC, Charlotte AHEC, Coastal AHEC, Eastern AHEC, Greensboro AHEC, Mountain AHEC, Northwest AHEC, Southern Regional AHEC, and Wake AHEC. The offices of the NC AHEC Program are located on the UNC campus at Chapel Hill. Each AHEC has a primary affiliation with one of the four medical schools but works with all of them and with many other educational institutions.

In 2000–2001 the NC AHECs provided on-site primary care residency training for 165 physicians and hosted more than 1,460 months of clinical rotations by residents and more than 2,100 months of clinical clerkship rotations for medical students from the four medical schools. In other words, approximately 300 medical students and residents are at the AHECs receiving clinical training during any given month in the academic year.

In conjunction with their educational mission, the AHEC faculty and residents had a cumulative total of 454,734 outpatient visits and 184,782 inpatient visits and procedures in 2004. In addition, Duke and UNC faculty members utilized Medical Air Operations from the Horace Williams Airport to see more than 17,000 patients in specialty clinics on site at various AHEC locations in 2006.[111]

The NC AHEC Program now has some 300 faculty members with appointments in one or more of the state's four medical schools. More than 2,000 volunteer community preceptors supplement their educational efforts.

The AHEC residency training programs in North Carolina have educated more than 2,000 primary care physicians during the period from 1972 to 2005. These physicians are providing care for patients in communities throughout the state and nation. In North Carolina in 2003, some 40 percent of the nearly 2,400 family physicians in practice were trained in an AHEC-sponsored residency program.

The Final Years

The final decade of Berryhill's life brought recognition for his efforts from a number of sources. In addition to the renaming of the Basic Medical Sciences Building at Chapel Hill as Berryhill Hall in his honor in 1973, his achievements were recognized with honorary degrees from Davidson College in 1956 and from his alma mater, the University of North Carolina at Chapel Hill, in 1976. He was made Sarah Graham Kenan Professor of Medicine in 1968 and became a Master of the American College of Physicians in 1977. In spite of all the honors, he remained a reticent person who always recognized and thanked others for their contributions to the health care endeavor he championed.

Berryhill continued to have an active interest in the events in the medical school, the university, and the state until near the end of his life. After his death from complications of primary refractory anemia, secondary hemochromatosis, and emphysema,[112] Norma Berryhill wrote to Maxwell Finland, a colleague from his days at Harvard:

He lived on transfusions for three years—then the time came when the transfusions themselves could not be tolerated because of the iron buildup. His doctors were mostly old students and Harvard men, which pleased him. I was able to take care of him at home until three weeks before the end. He had gone to his office each day for a while until five weeks before the end. His last effort was the History of the Fourth Service [the Harvard Medical Unit at the Boston City Hospital] which he didn't think was up to his usual standard.

I continue to live in the country alone, though I feel Reece very near. Everyone is so dear and thoughtful.[113]

A founding father of the present UNC hospitals and medical school, Berryhill died in North Carolina Memorial Hospital on January 1, 1979, the first day of the 100th anniversary year of the beginning of medical education at Chapel Hill.

Graveside services were held for Berryhill on the afternoon of January 3, 1979, at the Old Chapel Hill Cemetery. The obituary in the *Chapel Hill Newspaper* noted that "Dr. Berryhill was credited with being the one man who could make a 60-year-old dream come true: a four-year medical school at his Alma Mater, the University of North Carolina at Chapel Hill."[114] The late Dean Isaac Manning was quoted as saying , "[Berryhill] has all the qualities of a Presbyterian deacon. He never lets a matter drop." Dr. Nathan Womack, the first chair of surgery, recalled: "A lot of people had tried to get a four-year school, but Reece was the one to hit upon a secret weapon: the alumni. The 'country boys' came through." He

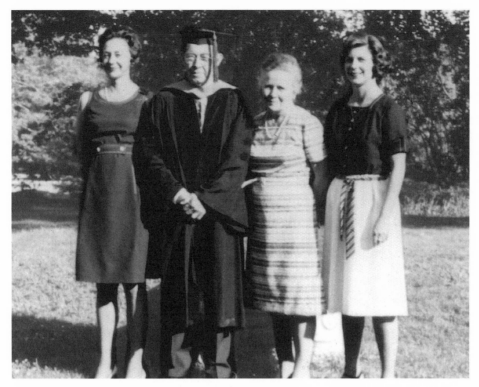

Jane, Reece, Norma, and Catherine Berryhill after Dr. Berryhill received an honorary degree from UNC, 1976. *(Berryhill Family)*

elaborated, "Many of the country boys had been [his] classmates at Chapel Hill, and many were legislators." Former Dean Isaac Taylor added, "Reece Berryhill's determined, selfless vision was the most important factor in the establishment of this great state medical school . . . Now the school itself stands as a proper monument to his great life."

A member of the two-year class of 1950 remembered Berryhill's funeral very clearly: "He would have been amazed at the enormous crowd that came in the bitter cold weather for his interment at the old Chapel Hill Cemetery across from Woollen Gym. I am sure he is still looking after the medical school from his place in heaven."[115]

Berryhill had been actively involved in the planning for the celebrations of the centennial of the beginning of medical education at UNC in 1879. Although he didn't live to participate in the events, Norma Berryhill was an active participant, and Berryhill's spirit permeated the proceedings. The centennial events in February 1979 included a scientific session at the medical school as well as an academic convocation in Memorial Hall on the university campus, with the awarding of honorary degrees by the university and an address by the director of the National Institutes of Health.

Berryhill's final contribution to the medical school he loved was the publication during the centennial celebration of the history of the first 100 years

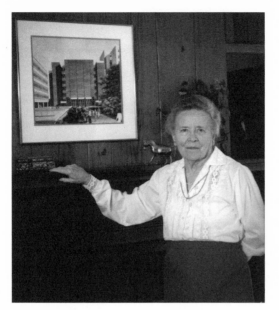

Norma Berryhill in her home in front of an architectural rendering of Berryhill Hall, 1980s. (*Berryhill Family*)

of medical education in Chapel Hill, which he had co-authored with former Dean Isaac H. Manning and professor of medicine William B. Blythe.[116]

Norma remained at their home on the farm after Berryhill's death in 1979 until about 1990, when she sold the home and property and moved to a condominium apartment in Chapel Hill. Their beautiful country homestead is now the site of several apartment and home developments, one of which is known as "Berryhill."

Norma moved in 2000 to the Carolina Meadows Retirement Community in Chatham County south of Chapel Hill after it became more and more difficult to obtain reliable help for her in the apartment. She commented in response to an inquiry by a visitor, "At 98 you aren't happy, but I am very contented here." Although her hearing and eyesight had dimmed, mentally she remained as alert as ever and enjoyed listening to audio books from the Library of Congress. She kept in close touch with activities in the community and university through frequent visitors and through attendance at occasional medical school events until she was more than 100 years old.

In March 2001 she celebrated her 99th birthday with a luncheon at the Carolina Inn for some thirty family members. The next March she celebrated her 100th birthday with another luncheon for some forty-seven of her female relatives, although she regretted that her Canadian relatives couldn't make it because they had visited earlier in the year. A month later she attended the fiftieth-anniversary banquet for the expanded medical school and hospital. At the conclusion of the formal program everyone was invited to dance. She declined a dance invitation with an enthusiastic pronouncement that "I was never much of a dancer, but tonight I am dancing in my soul!"[117]

Norma Berryhill died on July 8, 2005, at Carolina Meadows in Chapel Hill, at age 103. The obituary from the UNC news bureau commented on her unique role in the success of the expanded medical school and new hospital.

Persuading physicians to move to Chapel Hill in the 1940s and 1950s was a challenge for the Berryhills. There was only one hotel in town and few restaurants, so the responsibility for making potential and new medical faculty families feel welcome fell upon Mrs. Berryhill.

It was a task she handled with grace and dignity. She organized the Medical Student Wives Association and House Officers Wives Club to help build a sense of community among medical students, interns, residents and their spouses. She hosted dinners and teas for faculty members and their wives, readily provided meals—and often lodging—to visiting legislators or dignitaries, and always offered a casserole or dessert when a new medical-school family moved to Chapel Hill.

Perhaps most importantly, Mrs. Berryhill served as mentor, counselor and confidante to hundreds of medical students' wives. During the 1940s and 1950s, the vast majority of medical students were men, and many of them attended school on the GI Bill following their discharge from the military. They came to Chapel Hill with wives and babies and barely enough money to scrape by. While their husbands spent long hours away from home working and studying in the library, laboratory or hospital, their wives frequently turned to Mrs. Berryhill for empathy, encouragement and advice.

It was a kindness not soon forgotten. Fifty years later, now grandmothers and great-grandmothers themselves, the same women would visit Mrs. Berryhill to express their appreciation for her support.[118]

An annual lecture in honor of Norma Berryhill was started in 1985 by Dean Stuart Bondurant, with the full support of the medical school advisory committee, "as an expression of three interrelated ideas." First, the lectures are intended to provide an opportunity for faculty, and especially younger faculty, "to become acquainted with the thinking, the values, and the contributions of the

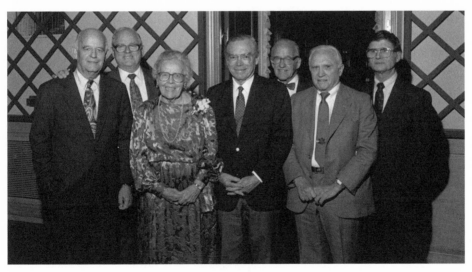

Norma Berryhill in 1991 with all of the first seven annual Norma Berryhill Lecturers except Dr. Mary Ellen Jones (1988). *Left to right:* Drs. William B. Blythe (1991), G. Philip Manire (1986), Carl W. Gottschalk (1990), Colin G. Thomas, Jr., (1989), John B. Graham (1985), and Floyd W. Denny, Jr. (1987). *(Berryhill Family)*

most senior and distinguished current members of the faculty," one of whom is selected by a faculty committee each year as the lecturer. Second, "the lecture and the subsequent reception are intended to enhance and renew the sense of community by providing a shared academic experience and social occasion to welcome new faculty members." Third, "the lectureship is named for Norma Berryhill because—both as the wife of the late Dean Reece Berryhill and independently—she has been a principal architect and engineer of the medical center. She has nurtured generations of students and faculty families and she has provided guiding wisdom to all the deans."[119] In 2000 the Medical Foundation of North Carolina published the first fifteen of these lectures.[120]

EPILOGUE

Precisely because individuals were important, American medical education did not develop in a predictable or inevitable fashion. At every point choices were made—some with good results, others with less salutary consequences. . . . [F]or those who wish to do so, opportunities to influence medical education are still present. The lesson of history is that the future is not predetermined and that individuals can make a difference.

—Kenneth M. Ludmerer, *Time to Heal*, 1999

No army is so powerful as an idea whose time has come.

—Paraphrase of Victor Hugo, *History of a Crime*, 1877

We ask only that all of us shall work together to make real a new ideal of democracy—"The equal right of every person born on earth to needed medical and hospital care whenever and wherever he battles against Disease and Death."

—North Carolina Hospital and Medical Care Commission (Poe Report), 1944–1945

W. Reece Berryhill and North Carolina's
Good Health Movement

$\mathcal{M}$*any individuals* and institutions were responsible for the remarkable transformation of health care, medical education, and biomedical research in North Carolina during the last half of the twentieth century. W. Reece Berryhill, however, was an vital player in these successes: first, as a catalyst for the Good Health Movement in the 1940s; second, as a leader from the 1940s to the early 1960s in advocating, planning, and implementing the teaching hospital and expanded medical school at Chapel Hill as part of a comprehensive university medical center with a statewide mission; and third, as an innovator in the late 1960s in establishing community medical education programs that provided the foundation for the development of the North Carolina Area Health Education Center Program.

In response to the first question posed in the Prologue, the state was fortunate in that Berryhill's upbringing, education, and career choices facilitated his future role as an innovator and leader in the bold effort to better the health of all North Carolinians.

First, Berryhill was raised at the beginning of the twentieth century in a farming community, where instant gratification was rare. He learned early that hard work and many disappointments might come between planting the seed and harvesting the crop. This experience served him well as he surveyed the three failed attempts in the first four decades of the twentieth century to establish a public MD-granting medical school for the people of his state and as he unwaveringly worked in the 1940s and 1950s to fulfill this dream.

Second, early in life Berryhill's parents and others in his community instilled in him a sense of duty and integrity, along with a deep respect for the importance of education. These traits, reinforced during his formative years as a student at the University of North Carolina, were obvious to all who had contact with him. They made it possible for him to convince others to join in his mission, even though he was neither a charismatic leader nor a powerful speaker.

Third, Berryhill's decisions to spend his undergraduate days in college at Chapel Hill and then to return there for his first two years of medical school were crucial for his ultimate success as dean and as a leader in the state's Good Health Movement. In the mid-twentieth century the political and medical leadership of the state had many ties to the university at Chapel Hill. Thus, during his six student years at Chapel Hill he had the opportunity to be educated with the state's future leaders and to meet many of their families and friends. These contacts were invaluable in his efforts to marshal support and appropriations for the hospital and medical school at Chapel Hill as part of the broader Good Health Movement and then later in his efforts to bring medical education to the communities of the state.

Finally, if Berryhill and the medical school he was to lead were not to be provincial, it was essential that he be exposed to the best in medical care, research, and education of his time. His decision to complete his medical degree at the renowned Harvard Medical School and then to finish his postgraduate education in internal medicine on the prestigious Harvard Service at Boston City Hospital provided just such an opportunity. Here he was exposed to many of the medical giants of his day, including Francis Peabody, George Minot, and Joseph Wearn, all of whom were widely respected for their dedicated care of patients, their enthusiasm for teaching, and their insatiable curiosity about patients and their illnesses. The three years he spent working as a junior faculty member at Western Reserve Medical School with Wearn further expanded his horizons as a physician and a future medical educator. These experiences in Boston and Cleveland gave him national standards with which he could plan the new medical center in Chapel Hill. Of equal importance, these national contacts were invaluable when it was time to recruit the medical school's new faculty.

Berryhill began campaigning for a full medical school at Chapel Hill unofficially after his return to Chapel Hill in 1933 as the university physician and a faculty member in the School of Medicine. He continued in earnest when he was appointed dean of the two-year medical school in 1941, shortly before the Japanese attack on Pearl Harbor and the United States' entry into World War II. His first success came when the legislature approved the teaching hospital and expanded medical school in 1947. He had the pleasure of seeing his dream realized when the North Carolina Memorial Hospital opened in Chapel Hill in 1952 and the first class of MDs graduated from the University of North Carolina at Chapel Hill in 1954.

The tall and distinguished Berryhill conveyed the image of a stern and self-disciplined physician, although he could be kindly and compassionate to students and patients alike when the occasion demanded. He was a man of few words, but when he spoke, others paid attention. Harold Roberts, a former medical student in the class of 1955 who later became a distinguished member of the medical school faculty, remembered Berryhill "as the dean who made the most lasting impression on my memory." While he never got to know him on a personal basis, "it was clear to me even as a medical student that he was effective, incisive, decisive, fair, involved, concerned, and determined. There was never any doubt in his mind about the difference between right and wrong and he was on the side of right. The uncertainties of present day political correctness, fuzzy headed thinking, and the murkiness that surrounds quality and excellence would never have occurred to Dean Berryhill. He operated on a firm basis of metaphysical principles unencumbered by trivia."[1]

Robert A. Ross, the first chair of obstetrics and gynecology, commented in 1955 on Berryhill's success in consolidating "an eminent basic science faculty" and selecting "a clinical group who had proved themselves elsewhere and who gave up tangible things to join in a new experience that would be wholly rewarding." He added, "As individuals and as a group they believed in Dr. Berryhill's word, integrity, purposefulness, and presence. None has had reason to change his belief."[2]

Many of Berryhill's efforts went on behind the scenes. This was due in part to his retiring nature, but it also reflected his astute political judgment that the campaign for the medical school should be part of a statewide Good Health Movement and not perceived just as an effort to benefit one institution. As a result, in 1950—when the hospital was being constructed and clinical faculty were being recruited—a journalist wrote: "Although he has been the moving force behind creation of the four-year school, Dr. Berryhill for the most part has gone unnoticed in the eyes of the North Carolina public. Paradoxically, he is undoubtedly one of the greatest—yet least known—men in the Old North State today."[3]

At the time of Berryhill's death in 1979, William C. Friday added: "Reece Berryhill was one of the University's noble sons. Builder of the medical school, he demanded standards of achievement and performance that insured the excellence of the school today. His concern was the good health of all citizens and his dedication was total."[4]

In response to the second question posed in the Prologue, timing was of critical importance in the success of North Carolina's efforts to improve health care for all its citizens and of the teaching hospital and expanded medical school at Chapel Hill. Berryhill himself recognized the importance of timing when he described the NC AHEC Program as "an example of what can happen when the aspirations and felt responsibilities of a medical school coincide with national long-range planning."[5]

The three unsuccessful efforts to establish a state-supported MD-granting medical school in the early twentieth century were examples of untimely endeavors. The clinical training at the UNC Medical Department in Raleigh from 1902 to 1910, which was closed following Abraham Flexner's visit, was clearly a premature effort with inadequate state funding. A state teaching hospital and medical school founded in the 1920s or 1930s would have suffered from prematurity followed by damaging or fatal malnourishment during the Depression and World War II. Furthermore, the founding of a state school in the 1920s or 1930s would have meant that one of the excellent private medical schools at Duke and Wake Forest Universities most likely would not exist in its present form. For example, if UNC had accepted President Few's proposal in the 1920s for a joint medical school, with the basic sciences on the UNC campus in Chapel Hill and the clinical program in Durham, neither Duke nor UNC would today have the complete academic medical centers that are a vital part of their university campuses. If UNC had accepted the Bowman Gray money in the 1930s for a UNC medical school and teaching hospital in Winston-Salem, it is likely that Wake Forest would still be a college in Wake County rather than Wake Forest University and School of Medicine in Winston-Salem. Furthermore, one observer speculated on the cost to the University of North Carolina of "a decision either not to expand the School or to move it to Charlotte, Raleigh, Greensboro, or Winston-Salem, all potential sites. In my opinion, we would have no School of Public Health, no School of Dentistry, perhaps no School of Nursing, and none of the many research institutes and centers which have grown from this complex. Having already lost the School of Engineering [to NC State as part of the university consolidation during the Depression years] we would have lost the opportunity to build a great multiversity."[6]

The first example of the timely confluence of state and national goals occurred in the mid-1940s, when North Carolina's and Berryhill's efforts to plan for a major postwar expansion of medical facilities in the state coincided with Congress's passage of the Federal Hospital Construction (Hill-Burton) Act in 1946 and its funding in 1947. North Carolina was better able to make opportune use of this funding than most other states because its planning for better health for its citizens had begun in 1944 while the war still raged.[7]

The second example of the timely confluence of state and national activities occurred in the field of biomedical research. The successful Manhattan Project for the atomic bomb during World War II, as well as the impressive advances in medicine such as penicillin, had convinced the public and Congress of the importance of governmental support of education and of research in medicine and the sciences. Berryhill could not have fully anticipated the massive growth of this federal mandate in the years to come. Yet his recruitment in 1946 of Kenneth M. Brinkhous from Iowa to Chapel Hill as head of the pathology department sent a clear message that the proposed expanded medical school was to be not just a production line for health care providers, but an integral part of the academic mission of the university. At the time of Brinkhous' death in 2000 he was internationally recognized for his pioneering research in coagulation; he was a member of the prestigious National Academy of Sciences; and his interdisciplinary team approach to research had provided a model for numerous such efforts on the UNC campus.

The importance of this interdisciplinary and collegial research environment at Chapel Hill was nationally recognized recently when UNC was awarded three of the first twenty-one highly competitive NIH "Roadmap" awards for interdisciplinary research. This "new initiative from the National Institutes of Health . . . encourages researchers to attack difficult problems using interdisciplinary collaboration and sophisticated computational techniques and informatics to create quick translations to patient care." Thus, while North Carolina is now tenth in the nation in population, the three Roadmap awards to UNC and one to Duke in the first round of awards ranked the state at the top in this new research initiative. In another round of awards in 2005, UNC–CH received eight Roadmap grants, more than any other institution in the nation.[8]

The wisdom of the decision more than half a century ago to have the university medical center on the university campus is only now being fully appreciated as programs such the Roadmap projects, the Carolina Center for Genome Sciences, and the UNC Lineberger Comprehensive Cancer Center thrive as organic parts of a university that is committed to exploring the universe of knowledge. This was vividly recognized recently by the director of the Cancer Center, when he wrote describing the process for the renewal of the center's five-year National Cancer Institute grant, one of the largest at UNC:

> During the last twelve months our program leaders involved virtually all 235 Cancer Center members in a stimulating exercise to plot the course of cancer discovery at UNC . . .
>
> What makes our Cancer Center and this planning process so unique is the tremendous breadth of our membership; they represent so many disciplines across societal and biomedical research. If you were to tour the UNC campus to find Cancer Center members, you would start near the Arboretum at the Department of Psychology; turn left at the Old Well to walk through Polk Place with the School of Information and Library Science on your left and the Schools of Journalism and Computer Science on your right. Then you would wind up Columbia Street past Chemistry, Biology, the Schools of Pharmacy, Nursing, Public Health and Dentistry, before turning on Manning Drive past the home of one of the greatest medical sciences faculties in the country [the School of Medicine research facilities]; and end up at the door of our clinical facilities at UNC Hospitals.[9]

The third example of the timely confluence of state and national priorities was in the Community Medicine program that Berryhill led in the late 1960s and that was the predecessor of the NC AHEC Program. The concept of the university's having a statewide obligation to its citizens dates back to UNC President Edward Kidder Graham's oft-quoted vision in 1915 of making the university's "campus co-extensive with the boundaries of the State . . . [in order] to put the University . . . in warm, sensitive touch with every problem in North Carolina life."[10] The 1946 Sanger Report reinforced this vision for the medical school by insisting that the proposed teaching hospital and expanded medical school be integrated with a network of hospitals throughout the state.[11] After Berryhill completed his service as dean in 1964, followed by a sabbatical year studying medical education in Europe and the United States, he spent the remainder of the decade establishing affiliations with community hospitals in order to bring medical education from the university to communities throughout the state. Thus, by the time the

Carnegie Commission in 1970 called for the establishment of 126 area health education centers around the country in communities not served by an academic health center, North Carolina already had the framework in place to implement such a program.[12] Although Berryhill had no direct involvement with obtaining the federal AHEC grant in 1972 or in implementing the NC AHEC Program, his patient and persistent "plowing the ground" in medical communities around the state has been widely recognized as having prepared the way for the statewide NC AHEC Program.

The success in anticipating these trends and in setting high standards for both the clinical and the research programs in the medical school was confirmed when the UNC School of Medicine was recognized as one of only four "bimodal" medical schools in the nation that were ranked by the AAMC in the top 20 percent both in numbers of graduates entering primary care and in medical research funding.[13] The alumni of the MD-granting medical school during its first half-century mirror this finding. They range from Charles Boyette, MD (UNC 1961), who was recognized nationally as Country Doctor of the Year for his thirty-nine years of service as a physician, mayor, and civic leader in his coastal community of some two thousand citizens in eastern North Carolina,[14] to Francis S. Collins, PhD (Yale), MD (UNC 1977), a Morehead Scholar who was the co-discoverer of the cystic fibrosis and neurofibromatosis genes, who headed the NIH's highly successful Human Genome Project, and who has spent vacations using his skills as an internist in developing countries.[15]

When Berryhill and others began the movement to better the health of North Carolinians in the early 1940s, the state had come from having no MD-granting medical schools in the decade after the 1910 Flexner Report to having two private MD-granting schools and one state basic science school. Yet these were not able to meet the demands for physician and other health care professionals, and the hospitals in the state were inadequate in number, distribution, and services. These deficiencies were vividly documented by the fact that North Carolina had the worst rejection rate of its young men for military service of any of the forty-eight states during World War II.

More than half a century later, at the beginning of the twenty-first century, North Carolina has four outstanding MD-granting medical schools—two private (Duke at Durham and Wake Forest at Winston-Salem) and two public (East Carolina at Greenville and UNC at Chapel Hill). Unlike some of the nation's medical schools that are free-standing or are located in different cities from the parent university, all the state's medical schools are in the same city as their university, while Duke and UNC have a university hospital on campus. Furthermore, the people of the state have at Chapel Hill one of only six of the nation's 125 medical schools with a teaching hospital and schools of dentistry, medicine, nursing, pharmacy, and public health, all located on the university campus. The state's four medical schools have educated many thousands of physicians and other health care professionals for the state and nation. Of these, more than 3,000 physicians currently practicing in North Carolina were educated at the UNC School of Medicine and/or in the residency programs of the UNC Hospitals and the AHECs.[16] Modern hospital and health care facilities provide services for patients from the coast to the mountains. These services are greatly enhanced by the presence of the statewide NC AHEC Program, the largest in the country and a model for the nation.

In the middle of the last century, the state also was in the backwater of bio-medical research, while at the beginning of the twenty-first century it is an internationally recognized leader, with its research universities, academic medical centers, a school of veterinary medicine at North Carolina State University, Nobel laureates,* and the Research Triangle Park. The latter is anchored by the thriving and impressive research endeavors of the three Triangle universities at Duke, North Carolina State, and UNC. The Park's 7,000 acres, which in the 1950s were said to be "good only for raising possums and pine trees," at the beginning of the twenty-first century are the home for more than 150 organizations and companies with an estimated annual payroll of some $2.7 billion. More than 80 percent of the Park's approximately 39,000 full-time employees work for multinational corporations.[17] The Park's tenants include the nonprofit Research Triangle Institute, the nation's second-largest independent research organization; the National Institutes of Environmental Health Sciences, the only NIH outside of Bethesda; the National Humanities Institute; and the state-supported North Carolina Biotechnology Center, which is committed to developing the biotechnology industry. The activities at the Park have spun off so many other research and manufacturing enterprises that North Carolina is now third in the nation in the number of companies in the rapidly emerging field of biotechnology.[18]

In conclusion, the statewide Good Health Movement successfully addressed the Poe Commission's challenge in the 1940s to provide "More Doctors" and "More Hospitals" for the people of the state, although this will inevitably be a continuing challenge. The third goal for "More Insurance" (that is, universal access to needed health care for all) remains unfulfilled early in the early twenty-first

*On October 8, 2007, it was announced that the 2007 Nobel Prize in Medicine goes to Mario R. Capecchi, Martin J. Evans, and Oliver Smithies "for their discoveries of principles for introducing specific gene modifications in mice by the use of embryonic stem cells." Oliver Smithies, who was born in Great Britain in 1925 and is now a US citizen, received his PhD in biochemistry in 1951 from Oxford University. He has been Excellence Professor of Pathology and Laboratory Medicine in the School of Medicine, UNC-Chapel Hill, since 1988. He joins three others from the Research Triangle Park who have received Nobel Prizes in Medicine: the late Gertrude B. Elion, 1988; the late George H. Hitchings, 1988; and the late Martin Rodbell, 1994.

century, and the situation is worsening each year. This is a failure of citizens and leaders in North Carolina and the nation to accomplish Governor Broughton's 1944 mandate: "The ultimate purpose of this program should be that no person in North Carolina shall lack adequate hospital care or medical treatment by reason of poverty or low income."[19] It is also a rejection of the Poe Commission's plea for all to support "the equal right of every person born on earth to needed medical and hospital care whenever and wherever he battles against Disease and Death."[20]

Appreciation of the leadership provided by Berryhill and many other public spirited individuals during the second half of the twentieth century to meet North Carolina's need for doctors and hospitals can provide insight and inspiration for those in the twenty-first century addressing the critical challenge of making these outstanding medical care and research advances available to all citizens.

W. Reece Berryhill: Chronology and Honors

Oct. 14, 1900	Walter Reece Berryhill born in the Steele Creek settlement of Mecklenburg County, North Carolina, the son of Samuel Reece Berryhill (1873–1930) and Minnie Eugenia Scott Berryhill (1873–1955).
1900–1916	Education in the schools of Mecklenburg County. Graduates from Dixie High School (then ten grades) in 1916. Returns to Dixie High School for a year of college preparatory work before entering the University of North Carolina at Chapel Hill.
1917–1921	UNC–Chapel Hill, AB in 1921. Di Society; Phi Beta Kappa; president of senior class.
1918	Student Army Training Corps (SATC) at UNC–Chapel Hill; stationed at Georgia Tech in Atlanta with an SATC Marine unit in summer of 1918.
1921–1922	Assistant supervisor, Baird's School, a private preparatory school in Charlotte, North Carolina.
1922–1923	Principal, Big Springs High School, Charlotte.
1923–1925	First two years of medicine at UNC–Chapel Hill; works in summers with two of the leading internists in Charlotte.
Summer 1925	Studies physical diagnosis and clinical pathology (with other students transferring from two-year schools to Harvard) at Huntington Hospital, Boston.
1925–1927	Third and fourth years of medicine at the Harvard Medical School, Boston.
1927	MD from Harvard.
1927–1929	Intern and resident on the Harvard Fourth Medical Service at Boston City Hospital.
Summer 1929	Practice of medicine with an internist at Belmont, NC.
1929–1930	Acting assistant professor of physiology at UNC School of Medicine, Chapel Hill; teaches physiology for six months while department head is on sick leave.
Aug. 2, 1930	Marries Norma May Connell of Warrenton, NC; two children, Jane Carol and Catherine Brewer.
1930–1933	At Western Reserve in Cleveland in the Department of Medicine, chaired by Charlotte native and his former Harvard attending professor, Joseph Wearn, MD. Chief resident in medicine at the Lakeside Hospital, 1930–1931, and instructor of medicine, 1931–1933. Diagnosed and treated for pulmonary tuberculosis.

1933–1941	Physician-in-chief, university infirmary, and director of student health services, UNC–Chapel Hill; assistant professor of medicine; teaches second-year course in physical diagnosis.
1937–1940	Assistant dean in charge of student affairs, School of Medicine, UNC–Chapel Hill (William de B. MacNider, MD, dean).
1940–1941	Acting dean, School of Medicine, UNC.
1941–1964	Dean, School of Medicine, UNC. Berryhill leads the effort to expand the medical school to a four-year, MD-granting school and to build the teaching hospital at Chapel Hill. He is responsible for recruiting the first clinical chairs in the medical school.
Sept. 1952	North Carolina Memorial Hospital opens; first third-year medical students start their clinical rotations.
1954	First MD graduates from the School of Medicine in Chapel Hill.
Aug. 31, 1964	Retires as dean of the UNC School of Medicine; succeeded by Isaac M. Taylor, MD.
Sept. 1964–Aug. 1965	Commonwealth Fund Traveling Fellow. Visits medical schools in Europe and the United States to study developments in the undergraduate medical curriculum, in educating family physicians, and in community medical care.
1966–1969	Director, Division of Education and Research in Community Medical Care, UNC School of Medicine. During this time he lays the foundation for the NC AHEC Program, which was funded in the early 1970s. Remains a full-time member of the Division until 1971 and then serves as part-time member until 1973 and as a consultant until 1975.
Jan. 1, 1979	Dies at North Carolina Memorial Hospital, Chapel Hill.

SELECTED HONORS AND AWARDS

Phi Beta Kappa, UNC–Chapel Hill, 1921

Alpha Omega Alpha, UNC School of Medicine, 1925

Order of the Golden Fleece, UNC–Chapel Hill, 1949

Faculty-Alumni Distinguished Service Award, UNC School of Medicine, 1955

Honorary Doctor of Science, Davidson College, 1956

O. Max Gardner Award of the University of North Carolina, 1964

Distinguished Citizens Award from the Governor of North Carolina, 1964

Sarah Graham Kenan Professor of Medicine, UNC–Chapel Hill, 1968–1979

Berryhill-Mecklenburg Medical Student Scholarship established in his honor by his friends in the Charlotte area, 1971

Basic Medical Sciences Building named Berryhill Hall, UNC School of Medicine, 1973

Honorary Doctor of Science, UNC–Chapel Hill, 1976

Master of the American College of Physicians, 1977. At the same meeting the North Carolina AHEC Program received the Richard and Hilda Rosenthal Foundation Award from the American College of Physicians

Medical Schools in North Carolina, 1850–2000

1850: No medical schools in the state. North Carolinians had to go out of state for a medical education. There were forty-two US medical schools with 17,213 MD graduates during the decade 1850–1859.

1852: Report of the North Carolina Medical Society on Medical Schools: Better to have no medical schools than to have inadequate ones with the resources available to the state at the time.

- *Edenborough Medical School at Raeford,*1867–1877. First chartered medical school in the state. Essentially an apprenticeship program with one full-time professor. Described in a 1877 report by the Medical Society as "a blight upon our profession, a burlesque upon science, and a curse to humanity."

- *Leonard School of Medicine of Shaw University at Raleigh,*1881–1914. Provided much-needed pharmacists and physicians for the black communities of the state. Closed after the Flexner Report.

- *North Carolina Medical College,*1887–1914
  - ~ 1887–1907: A basic sciences medical school at Davidson College.
  - ~ 1907–1914: A four-year, MD-granting medical school in Charlotte. After the Flexner Report, the school in Charlotte closed and merged with the Medical College of Virginia in Richmond.

- *University of North Carolina at Chapel Hill**
  - ~ 1879–1885: Basic sciences medical school at Chapel Hill.
  - ~ 1890–1952: Basic sciences medical school at Chapel Hill.
  - ~ 1902–1910: UNC Medical Department at Raleigh provided clinical years and MD degree. Closed after Flexner's visit.
  - ~ 1952–: Four-year, MD-granting medical school at Chapel Hill.

1900: One public basic sciences medical school at Chapel Hill and two private four-year, MD-granting medical schools at Charlotte and Raleigh.

- *Wake Forest College/University**
  - ~ 1902–1941: Two-year basic sciences medical school at Wake Forest.
  - ~ 1941–: Four-year, MD-granting medical school at Winston-Salem.

1910: Two private MD-granting medical schools at Charlotte and Raleigh and two basic sciences medical schools at Chapel Hill and Wake Forest.

1910: The Flexner Report: *Medical Education in the United States and Canada*

1920: Only two basic sciences medical schools at Chapel Hill and Wake Forest.

- *Duke University**
  - ~ 1930–: Four-year, MD-granting medical school at Durham.

- *East Carolina University**
  - ~ 1972–1975: A one-year medical school at Greenville with students transferring to Chapel Hill for the balance of their medical school and for the MD degree.
  - ~ 1977–: A four-year, MD-granting medical school at Greenville.

- *NC AHEC Program**
  - ~ 1972–: Now covers the entire state and involves all four medical schools.

2000: Four (two public and two private) MD-granting medical schools at Chapel Hill, Durham, Greenville, and Winston-Salem.

*Existing schools and programs are listed in boldface type.

Note: Data on US medical schools and graduates from Bowles and Dawson, *With One Voice: The Association of American Medical Colleges, 1876–2002* (Washington: AAMC; 2003), Appendix 1, 193–195.

See also: Long D. *Medicine in North Carolina: Essays in the History of Medical Science and Medical Service, 1524–1960.* Vol. 2, Part 1: Medical Schools in North Carolina, 351–552. Raleigh, NC: North Carolina Medical Society; 1972.

Medical Schools in the United States, 1900–2000

1900: 160 US medical schools with 5,214 MD graduates

1910: The Flexner Report: *Medical Education in the United States and Canada*

1920: 85 US medical schools with 3,047 MD graduates

- Pre–World War II generation included new and expanded private medical schools such as Duke, Wake Forest (Winston-Salem), and Rochester

1940: 77 US medical schools with 5,097 MD graduates

- Postwar generation included state university medical schools such as new and expanded schools in North Carolina, Alabama, Arizona, California (4), Florida, Mississippi, and Washington

1970: 101 US medical schools with 8,367 MD graduates

- 1970s generation included new community-based medical schools such as East Carolina, Northeastern Ohio, South Alabama, and South Florida, as well as expanded class size in existing schools such as UNC (Chapel Hill)

1980: 126 US medical schools with 15,113 MD graduates

2000: 125 US medical schools with 15,715 MD graduates (no two-year schools)

Note: Data on US medical schools and graduates from Bowles and Dawson, *With One Voice: The Association of American Medical Colleges, 1876–2002.* Appendix 1, 193–195. Washington, DC: AAMC; 2003.

See also: *Directory of American Medical Education, 2000–2001.* Association of American Medical Colleges, Washington, DC.

MEDICAL EDUCATION
IN THE
UNITED STATES AND CANADA

A REPORT TO
THE CARNEGIE FOUNDATION
FOR THE ADVANCEMENT OF TEACHING

BY
ABRAHAM FLEXNER

WITH AN INTRODUCTION BY
HENRY S. PRITCHETT
PRESIDENT OF THE FOUNDATION

BULLETIN NUMBER FOUR (1910)

589 FIFTH AVENUE
NEW YORK CITY

The full text of the Flexner Report is available as a free pdf file download from the web site of the Carnegie Foundation for the Advancement of Teaching at: www.carnegiefoundation. org/publications/pub.asp?key=43&subkey=977.

NORTH CAROLINA

Population, 2,142,084. Number of physicians { 1761 (Amer. Med. Direct.). Ratio, 1:1216; 1932 (Polk). " 1:1110.
Number of medical schools, 4.

CHAPEL HILL: *Population,* 1181.

(1) UNIVERSITY OF NORTH CAROLINA MEDICAL DEPARTMENT. A half-school. Established 1890. An organic part of the university.

Entrance requirement: A year of college work—not, however, strictly enforced during this, the first session in which it has been required.

Attendance: 74; 95 per cent from North Carolina.

Teaching staff: 15, of whom 10 are professors who take part in the work of the department. The instructors are trained, full-time teachers.

Resources available for maintenance: The department is provided for in the university budget. Its budget calls for $12,000. Its income in fees is $6500.

Laboratory facilities: The laboratories at Chapel Hill are in general adequate to good routine teaching of the small student body. The equipment covers pathology, bacteriology, histology, physiology, and pharmacology. Anatomy is inferior. Animals are provided for experimental work. The general scientific laboratories of the university are excellent; a small annual appropriation is available for books and periodicals. The work is intelligently planned and conducted on modern lines.

Date of visit: February, 1909.

CHARLOTTE: *Population,* 36,320.

(2) NORTH CAROLINA MEDICAL COLLEGE. Organized 1887, it has given degrees since 1893. A stock company; professorships are represented by stock and can be sold subject to the concurrence (never yet refused) of the faculty.

Entrance requirement: Nominal.

Attendance: 94, 87 per cent from North Carolina.

Teaching staff: 32, of whom 19 are professors, 13 of other grade.

Resources available for maintenance: Fees, amounting to $8345 (estimated), a large part being required to carry a building mortgage and to retire the debt.

Laboratory facilities: These comprise a poor chemical laboratory, containing one set of reagents, a wretched dissecting room, and a meager outfit for pathology, bacteriology, and histology. There is no museum, no library, and no teaching aids of any kind whatever. No post-mortems are even claimed.

Clinical facilities: The school, in virtue of a subscription, holds four weekly clinics at a colored hospital of 35 beds; other hospital connections are unimportant. Obstetrical cases are rare.

There is a poor dispensary, with a small attendance, in the school building. It occupies a fair suite of rooms.

Date of visit: February, 1909.

WAKE FOREST: *Population, 900.*

(3) WAKE FOREST COLLEGE SCHOOL OF MEDICINE. A half-school. Organized 1902. An integral part of Wake Forest College.

Entrance requirement: Two years of college work, actually enforced, but resting upon the irregular secondary school education characteristic of the section.

Attendance: 53.

Teaching staff: 6 whole-time instructors take part in the work of the department; two of them devote their entire time to medical instruction.

Resources available for maintenance: The budget is part of the college budget. Fees amount to $2225.

Laboratory facilities: The laboratories of this little school are, as far as they go, models in their way. Everything about them indicates intelligence and earnestness. The dissecting-room is clean and odorless, the bodies undergoing dissection being cared for in the most approved modern manner. Separate laboratories, properly equipped, are provided for ordinary undergraduate work in bacteriology, pathology, and histology, and the instructor has a private laboratory besides. Chemistry is taught in the well equipped college laboratory; physiology is slight; there is no pharmacology. There is a small museum; animals, charts, and books are provided.

Date of visit: February, 1909.

RALEIGH : *Population, 20,533.*

(4) LEONARD MEDICAL SCHOOL. Colored. Organized 1882. An integral part of Shaw University.

Entrance requirement: Less than four-year high school education.

Attendance: 125.

Teaching staff: 9, of whom 8 are professors, one of other grade.

Resources available for maintenance : Mainly fees and contributions, amounting to $4721, practically all of which is paid to the practitioner teachers.

Laboratory facilities : These comprise a clean and exceedingly well kept dissecting-room, a slight chemical laboratory, and a still slighter equipment for pathology.

There are no library, no museum, and no teaching accessories. It is evident that the policy of paying practitioners has absorbed the resources of a school that exists for purely philanthropic objects.

Clinical facilities: These are hardly more than nominal. The school has access to a sixteen-bed hospital, containing at the time of the visit three patients. There is no dispensary at all. About thirty thousand dollars are, however, now available ۰for building a hospital and improving laboratories.

Date of visit: February, 1909.

General Considerations

THE state of North Carolina makes a comparatively satisfactory showing in the matter of ratio between population and physicians; but this may, perhaps, in some measure be due to the fact that practitioners, unlicensed and unregistered, exist undisturbed in the remote districts. It is futile to maintain a low standard in order to prepare doctors for those parts; for the graduates, instead of scattering to them, huddle together in the small towns already amply supplied. It is admitted that all eligible locations are overcrowded. There is not the slightest danger that the necessary supply of doctors would be threatened if, for instance, the practice of medicine in the state were pitched on the plane of entrance to the state university; higher than that it probably ought not to be at this time.

The standard suggested — any real standard whatsoever, indeed — would quickly dispose of the thoroughly wretched Charlotte establishment. No clinical school would remain in the state. The two half-schools — at Wake Forest and at the state university — are capable of doing acceptable work within the limits of their present resources. Both of these schools now require college work for entrance. Is this step to be generally recommended at this time to southern universities with medical departments? Without attempting to arrive at a decision, it may be pointed out that there are two sides to the question. On the one hand, the college requirement is essential to the symmetrical development of the medical curriculum; on the other, a good medical course can be given at an actual high school level, provided that facilities and teaching are developed to a high point of efficiency. How will the university best serve the state,— by training a small number at the higher level, or by getting actual control of the state situation on a high school basis before pushing ahead to a basis just generally feasible in more highly developed sections of the country? The University of Michigan is only now requiring college work for entrance; it became a strong school of immense influence in its own community on a lower basis. Undoubtedly it is right now to go to the higher standard; perhaps it should have done so earlier. But its present efficiency and influence show— as McGill and Toronto show — that if a lower standard is felt to be a reason for better teaching and not an excuse for poor teaching, an institution unfavorably located for the initiation of the higher standard can do good work on the lower basis. In the south now is it more important to destroy commercial schools by collecting in good university institutions a sufficient body of students, or to provide high-grade teaching for a few, leaving utterly wretched teaching for the vast majority? The dilemma is worthy of very careful consideration.

A word as to the colored school at Raleigh. This is a philanthropic enterprise that has been operating for well-nigh thirty years and has nothing in the way of plant to show for it. Its income ought to have been spent within; it has gone outside, to reimburse practitioners who supposed themselves assisting in a philanthropic work. Real philanthropy would have taken a very different course. As a matter of fact, Raleigh cannot, except at great expense, maintain clinical teaching. The way to help the negro is to help the two medical schools that have a chance to become efficient,— Howard at Washington, Meharry at Nashville.

North Dakota

Population, 536,103. Number of physicians, 552. Ratio, 1:971.
Number of medical schools, 1.

GRAND FORKS: *Population, 12,602.*

STATE UNIVERSITY OF NORTH DAKOTA, COLLEGE OF MEDICINE. Organized 1905. A half-school. An organic part of the state university.

Entrance requirement: Two years of college work.

Attendance: 9.

Teaching staff: 9 professors and 7 instructors take part in the work of the department. The professor of bacteriology is State Bacteriologist.

Resources available for maintenance: The department shares in the general funds of the university. Its budget amounts to $6300; income from fees, $450.

Laboratory facilities: The laboratory of bacteriology, being at the same time the public health laboratory of the state, is well equipped and very active. Subjects given in the regular university laboratories are likewise well provided for. For the specifically medical subjects— physiology, pathology, anatomy—the provision is slighter. The students are, of course, few. A library and museum have been started.

Date of visit: May, 1909.

[*See South Dakota, "General Considerations," p. 301.*]

APPENDIX E

Recommendations of the Committee of Physicians
Presented to Governor J. Melville Broughton, January 1944

To the Governor of North Carolina
From a Committee of the Medical Profession:

One of the most important problems facing the State and the medical profession is that of providing opportunities for more adequate medical care in the post-war period for all groups of citizens. Some provision must be made for the low-income group to have adequate medical care at fees they can afford to pay and for the indigent to receive both hospital and ambulatory medical services.

In any attempt to solve this problem we are immediately faced with critical shortages of general hospital facilities and trained medical personnel of all types. In 1941 North Carolina, the 11th largest state and the 5th most rapidly growing, stood in 42nd place, tied with South Carolina, in the number of general hospital beds per thousand population and in a comparable position in the number of doctors. In addition, we have always had in this State too few trained medical personnel—nurses, dietitians, doctors of Public Health, sanitary engineers, sanitarians, medical technicians, and health educators. To quote Dean Davison of Duke University Medical School, "The South needs twice as many doctors and three times as many hospital beds" to raise medical facilities to the average for those of the country as a whole which probably will not be an adequate standard for medical needs of the State in the future.

Much progress has been made in the last few years in improving the facilities for medical care and hospitalization for patients with tuberculosis and mental diseases, although there is still a great need for additional hospital beds and additional trained personnel to care for patients with these two types of disease.

That the problem is too large and complex for any one group of individuals or institutions to satisfactorily and adequately solve seems obvious. It is a responsibility and obligation and an opportunity of the entire community, that is, the State. In spite of the magnificent contributions of the Duke Foundation, of private general hospitals throughout the State, including those of Duke University and the North Carolina Baptist Hospital of the Bowman Gray School of Medicine, and the private practitioners of Medicine toward this end, the problem is still acute. Any comprehensive plan which would insure an opportunity for complete high-standard medical services for indigent patients and for the low-income group must be coordinated with existing health and medical agencies in the State; "must have the active and guiding cooperation of the medical profession"; must provide an increase in hospital facilities, opportunities for training all types of medical personnel and opportunities and support for research into medical problems affecting the health of this section. It would require the financial and moral support of Federal, State, county and municipal agencies as well as that of private philanthropists.

As the first step in a far-reaching program of providing better medical facilities, the following proposals are presented:

1. The building of a large well-equipped general hospital, initially 500 to 700 beds, in a more or less centrally located place in the State to serve as a diagnostic and treatment center for indigent patients who might be referred by social welfare agencies or private physicians from all over the State, both for those needing hospitalization and for ambulatory patients. There should be facilities in the out-patient department adequate for examining large numbers of the latter daily. Patients certified as indigent by their county or city welfare officer would be treated free or for a small nominal registration fee. Patients referred by their physicians and financially able to pay would be charged on a fee schedule, the income to go to the hospital maintenance.

The bed capacity of the hospital should be largely reserved for ward patients, although there should be a small number of semi-private and low-cost private rooms for hospitalization of referred patients in the low-income group. More expensive private rooms should be kept at a minimum.

A system of transportation by ambulances or buses sent from the hospital on different routes throughout the State might be worked out to bring patients to the hospital. A similar plan has been successfully operated in the State of Iowa for many years.

Such a general hospital for the State would logically be placed adjoining the present buildings of the Schools of Medicine and Public Health and the Navy Hospital on the campus at the University at Chapel Hill. The present two-year Medical School, now adequately housed in a new building representing an outlay of approximately $500,000, should be expanded into a four-year

School of Medicine and the clinical teachers of the Medical School should serve as the professional medical staff of the hospital.

A hospital of the size indicated would supply adequate clinical material for teaching classes of 50 or more medical students. Past experience has shown that the best progress in Medicine is attained through the maintenance of the closest possible physical and spiritual relationship between patient, "student" (teacher, student, investigator), library, and laboratory, including the science laboratories of Chemistry, Physics, and Biology, best afforded by universities. Thus, the hospital should be integrated with the Schools of Medicine and Public Health and other facilities at the State University and would undoubtedly work in close cooperation with the State Health Department and with the other State hospitals and agencies devoted to medical care and the improvement of the general health of the State.

In effect this would establish a great North Carolina medical center which primarily would provide medical services to the indigent and train needed medical personnel of all types—doctors of medicine, doctors of public health, nurses, public health nurses, sanitary engineers, sanitarians, hospital administrators, medical technicians, dietitians, social workers, and perhaps dentists. In addition such a center would serve the practising physicians in the State on a postgraduate level enabling them to secure additional training and to keep abreast of progress in Medicine. It would be a central laboratory for research in Medicine and Public Health. The trained personnel and facilities of such an institution would be of great value in performing certain specialized services to the State tuberculosis and insane institutions. In time institutes for the study and treatment of cancer, of nutritional problems, of tropical diseases, an important problem in the post-war period, of mental diseases and many others might be added and thus enlarge the services to this State and section.

2. Obviously, one hospital could not care for all the indigent in the State who need medical attention. From time to time smaller hospitals, well equipped for diagnostic work and treatment, should be set up in different sections of the State in which there are now no hospital facilities. In certain sections existing hospitals might be enlarged. The professional direction of these additional hospital facilities should be in the hands of the medical profession in those

communities and sections of the State. A well coordinated plan could be worked out between the smaller hospitals and the larger central unit whereby the latter could supply professional consultation when requested, or obscure cases in the former presenting problems in diagnosis or treatment could be sent to the central hospital for study.

The building of small hospitals in areas where no such institutions exist and the enlargement of some of the present hospitals would not only provide vitally needed medical facilities but would tend to attract young graduates of Medicine and all other types of trained medical personnel to those areas to begin the practice of their profession. This would help greatly to improve the maldistribution of medical personnel in the State; to further encourage this movement the State might follow the plan of the Commonwealth Foundation and offer a certain number of scholarships to men and women who would agree to return to rural districts and small communities for a certain number of years.

Such a plan, well developed, operated judiciously in a coordinated undertaking with existing State health agencies under the general direction of and with the enthusiastic support of the medical profession, might eventually provide an opportunity for adequate medical services for the citizens who have not been able to afford this service. Furthermore, it might well serve as a model for other states and for the nation as a whole in improving the health and the general usefulness of our people. This tentative proposal should be a part of an overall plan sponsored by the profession of the State in cooperation with public and private agencies and individuals looking toward the eventual solution of the problem of providing complete medical care for the low-income and indigent groups of our citizens.

COMMITTEE: DR. P. P. McCAIN, *past President State Society, Chairman*
DR. JAMES W. VERNON, *President, State Society*
DR. H. B. HAYWOOD, *past President State Society*
DR. DONNELL COBB, *past President State Society*
DR. PAUL F. WHITTAKER, *President-elect State Society*
DR. WILLIAM COPPRIDGE
DR. HAMILTON McKAY
DR. W. R. BERRYHILL

APPENDIX F

Proposed Four-Year Medical School: Detail of Salaries and Wages Estimates,
Prepared by Dean W. Reece Berryhill, September 5, 1944

Proposed Four Year Medical School
Detail of Salaries & Wages Estimates
 Prepared September 5, 1944

Anatomy
1 Professor	$ 5,500
2 Asso. Prof's. @ $4,000	8,000
1 Asst. Prof.	3,400
2 Technicians @ $1,800	3,600
1 Instructor	2,500
1/2 Secretary @ $1,800	900
Total	$23,900

Biological Chemistry
1 Professor	$ 5,500
1 Asso. Prof.	4,000
1 Asst. Prof.	3,250
1 Technician	1,500
1/2 Secretary	900
Total	$15,150

Bacteriology
1 Professor	$ 5,000
1 Asso. Prof.	4,500
1 Asst. Prof.	3,600
2 Technicians @ $1,800	3,600
1/2 Secretary	800
Total	$17,500

Pathology
1 Professor	$ 7,500
1 Professor	7,000
1 Asso. Prof.	6,000
1 Asst. Prof.	4,000
3 Technicians @ $1,800	5,400
1 Secretary	1,600
	$31,500

Pharmacology
1 Professor (Kenou)	$ 6,500
1 Professor	5,500
1 Asso. Prof.	4,000
1 Fellow	1,800
1 Technician	1,800
1/2 Secretary	800
Part Time	1,500
Total	$21,900

Physiology
1 Professor	$ 6,000
2 Asso. Prof. @ $4,500.	9,000
1 Instructor	2,500
1 Fellow	1,500
2 Technician @ $1,600.	3,200
	$22,200

Medicine
1 Professor	$12,000
2 Asso. Prof. @ $7,500.	15,000
3 Asst. Prof. @ $5,000.	15,000
4 Instructors @ $3,600.	14,400
1 Fellow	1,200
Part Time	5,000
Total	$62,600

Surgery
1 Professor	$12,500
3 Asso. Prof. @ $8,000.	24,000
4 Asst. Prof. @ $6,000.	24,000
4 Instructors @ $4,000.	16,000
Part Time	5,000
Total	$81,500

Obstetrics
1 Professor	$10,000
1 Asso. Professor	7,500
1 Instructor	4,000
Part Time	2,500
Total	$24,000

Pediatrics
1 Professor	$10,000
1 Asso. Professor	7,500
1 Asst. Professor	4,000
Part Time	2,500
Total	$24,000

Psychiatry
1 Professor	$10,000
2 Asso. Prof. @ $5,000	10,000
1 Asst. Professor	3,250
Total	$23,250

Library
Librarian and Assistants	$ 7,000

Administration
1 Dean	$ 7,500
1 Assistant	1,500
2 Secretaries @ $1,800.	3,600
Total	$12,600

Medical Illustrations
1 Technician	$ 1,800

Physical Plant Opr. & Mtnce.
7 Janitors @ $936.	$ 6,552
1 Foreman	1,456
1 Animal Caretaker	1,770
1 Laborer (Grounds,etc.)	936
Total	$10,714
Total Salaries & Wages	$379,614

*Reports of the North Carolina Hospital
and Medical Care Commission (Poe Report),
October 1944 and February 1945*

Hospital and Medical
Care for All Our People

**"A Program of Great Hope, of Almost Infinite
Promise, and Yet of Great Practicability"**

EDITED BY CLARENCE POE

Reports of Chairman and Sub-Committees of

*North Carolina Hospital and
Medical Care Commission 1944-45*

(Data Revised February, 1947)

NORTH CAROLINA HOSPITAL AND MEDICAL CARE
COMMISSION AND ITS SUB-COMMITTEES, 1944-45

CLARENCE POE, Raleigh, Chairman

DR. C. V. REYNOLDS, Secretary

Hospital and Medical Care for Our Rural Population

THOS. J. PEARSALL, Chmn., Rocky Mount
DR. G. M. COOPER, Vice-Chmn., Raleigh
DR. C. HORACE HAMILTON, Raleigh, Secretary
J. B. SLACK, F.S.A., Raleigh
DR. JANE S. McKIMMON, Raleigh
HARRY B. CALDWELL, Greensboro

R. FLAKE SHAW, Greensboro
J. G. K. McCLURE, Asheville
DR. B. E. WASHBURN, Rutherfordton
DR. S. H. HOBBS, JR., Chapel Hill
M. G. MANN, Raleigh
DR. W. C. DAVISON, Durham

Hospital and Medical Care for Our Industrial and Urban Population

CHARLES A. CANNON, Chmn., Concord
CHAS. A. FINK, Vice-Chmn., Spencer
DR. I. G. GREER, Thomasville
DR. J. B. SIDBURY, Wilmington
E. T. SANDEFUR, Winston-Salem
REUBEN ROBERTSON, Canton

C. C. SPAULDING, Durham
DR. EDSON E. BLACKMAN, Charlotte
DR. C. C. CARPENTER, Winston-Salem
MISS FLORA WAKEFIELD, Raleigh
MRS. W. T. BOST, Raleigh

Special Needs of Our Negro Population

DR. E. E. BLACKMAN, Chmn., Charlotte
C. C. SPAULDING, Durham
DR. R. E. WIMBERLY, Raleigh

DR. CLYDE DONNELL, Durham
DR. N. C. NEWBOLD, Raleigh
ALEXANDER WEBB, Raleigh

Four-Year Medical School for University and Hospital Facilities

DR. P. P. McCAIN, Chmn., Sanatorium
JOSEPHUS DANIELS, Vice-Chmn., Raleigh
DR. DONNELL COBB, Goldsboro
DR. PAUL WHITAKER, Kinston
MRS. JULIUS CONE, Greensboro
DR. HUBERT B. HAYWOOD, Raleigh

JAMES A. GRAY, Winston-Salem
ALEXANDER WEBB, Raleigh
DR. W. R. BERRYHILL, Chapel Hill
DR. C. C. CARPENTER, Winston-Salem
DR. W. C. DAVISON, Durham

Mental Hygiene and Hospitalization

DR. JAMES W. VERNON, Chmn., Morganton
BISHOP CLARE PURCELL, Vice-Chmn., Charlotte
MRS. R. J. REYNOLDS, Winston-Salem
D. HIDEN RAMSEY, Asheville
JUDGE S. J. ERVIN, Morganton

PAUL BISSETTE, Wilson
JOHN W. UMSTEAD, Chapel Hill
W. G. CLARK, Tarboro
MRS. FRANCES HILL FOX, Durham
DR. MAURICE H. GREENHILL, Durham

Committee on Statistical Studies

DR. C. HORACE HAMILTON, Chairman, N. C. State College, Raleigh

Hospital and Medical Care Plans in Other States

DR. W. M. COPPRIDGE, Chmn., Durham
R. G. DEYTON, Raleigh

DR. ROSCOE D. McMILLAN, Red Springs

ii

Foreword by the Chairman

In 1944-45 I served, by appointment of Governor Broughton, as Chairman of the newly created "North Carolina Hospital and Medical Care Commission."

This commission was not only composed of 60 distinguished North Carolina men and women, representing all important classes of our citizenship, but in order to make its labors more effective, was subdivided into seven ably manned Committees as shown on the preceding page.

These sub-committees made what Dr. Carl V. Reynolds, State Health Officer, called at the time "the most comprehensive, accurate and informing review of health conditions ever made in the history of North Carolina—and probably the best ever yet made for any Southern State."

For this reason both the Medical Care Commission and the North Carolina Good Health Association have called for the republication of the veritable treasure house of information collected in these reports. In doing this it has also seemed wise to revise all data, where practicable, so as to bring it up to date. That is to say, the latest available data as of February, 1947, rather than November, 1944, is now presented herewith, in so far as possible. For this revision especial thanks are due to Dr. C. Horace Hamilton.

In effect this volume becomes a condensed but fairly complete report of all major activities of the campaign for "More Doctors, More Hospitals, More Insurance" in North Carolina from the time the Hospital and Medical Care Commission was appointed by Governor Broughton, February 28, 1944, until the officially State-sponsored Medical Care Commission took over on July 27, 1945. In this period the 60 members of the Hospital and Medical Care Commission were privileged to play an active part in four fortunately fruitful efforts:—

1. To inform and arouse our people as to existing conditions and needed remedies.
2. To secure needed State legislation.
3. To assist in the nation-wide study of hospital conditions and needed remedies by the National Committee on Hospital Care.
4. To enlist the support of all North Carolina Senators and Representatives in behalf of the Hill-Burton Act from which North Carolina should ultimately receive $17,500,000 for hospital building.

Furthermore, while resolutely determined to discover and uncover all the facts about North Carolina hospital and medical care conditions, the highlight of all our activities was not the discovery about the shockingly high 57% rejection rate of North Carolina boys in the American armies but rather the far more astonishing discovery that among draftees who had grown up in North Carolina orphanages and who had had not-too-expensive hospital and medical care plus sound but not-expensive nutrition, the rejection rate had been only 3%!

This is a beacon light to guide our people as they fare forth on a program which is indeed one of "great hope, of almost infinite promise, and yet of great practicability."

CLARENCE POE

Raleigh, March 1, 1947.

iii

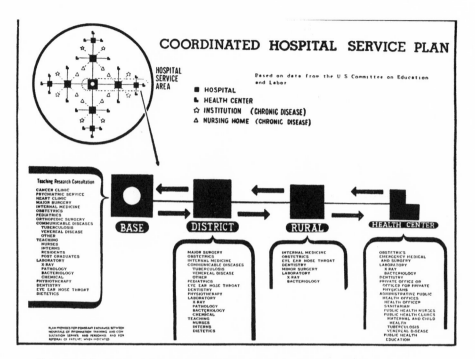

COORDINATED HOSPITAL SERVICE PLAN

Based on data from the U S Committee on Education and Labor

■ HOSPITAL
⌐ HEALTH CENTER
☆ INSTITUTION (CHRONIC DISEASE)
△ NURSING HOME (CHRONIC DISEASE)

HOSPITAL SERVICE AREA

Teaching Research Consultation
CANCER CLINIC
PSYCHIATRIC SERVICE
HEART CLINIC
MAJOR SURGERY
INTERNAL MEDICINE
OBSTETRICS
PEDIATRICS
ORTHOPEDIC SURGERY
COMMUNICABLE DISEASES
  TUBERCULOSIS
  VENEREAL DISEASE
  OTHER
TEACHING
  NURSES
  INTERNS
  RESIDENTS
  POST GRADUATES
LABORATORY
  X-RAY
  PATHOLOGY
  BACTERIOLOGY
  CHEMICAL
PHYSIOTHERAPY
DENTISTRY
EYE EAR NOSE THROAT
DIETETICS

PLAN PROVIDES FOR CONSTANT EXCHANGE BETWEEN HOSPITALS OF INFORMATION TRAINING AND CONSULTATION SERVICE SERVICE AND PERSONNEL AND FOR REFERRAL OF PATIENT WHEN INDICATED

BASE

DISTRICT
MAJOR SURGERY
OBSTETRICS
INTERNAL MEDICINE
COMMUNICABLE DISEASES
  TUBERCULOSIS
  VENEREAL DISEASE
  OTHER
PEDIATRICS
EYE EAR NOSE THROAT
DENTISTRY
PHYSIOTHERAPY
LABORATORY
  X RAY
  PATHOLOGY
  BACTERIOLOGY
  CHEMICAL
TEACHING
  NURSES
  INTERNS
DIETETICS

RURAL
INTERNAL MEDICINE
OBSTETRICS
EYE EAR NOSE THROAT
DENTISTRY
MINOR SURGERY
LABORATORY
  X RAY
  BACTERIOLOGY

HEALTH CENTER
OBSTETRICS
EMERGENCY MEDICAL
  AND SURGERY
LABORATORY
  X RAY
  BACTERIOLOGY
DENTISTRY
PRIVATE OFFICE OR
  OFFICES FOR PRIVATE
  PHYSICIANS
ADMINISTRATIVE PUBLIC
  HEALTH OFFICES
  HEALTH OFFICER
  SANITARIAN
  PUBLIC HEALTH NURSES
  PUBLIC HEALTH CLINICS
  MATERNAL AND CHILD
    HEALTH
  TUBERCULOSIS
  VENEREAL DISEASE
  PUBLIC HEALTH
  EDUCATION

Complete hospital service which is both convenient and of high quality can be provided only if there is a high degree of *coordination* of hospitals and health centers as illustrated in the above chart. *Rural hospitals and heath centers or clinics* are necessary to provide convenient medical service for minor illnesses and conditions not requiring highly specialized professional care. These small hospitals and health centers or clinics are also available for emergencies of all kinds.

The district or regional hospital is the focal point for coordinating hospital service for several rural hospitals and health centers covering either several counties or possibly a smaller but densely populated urban area. These district hospitals are large enough to provide highly specialized surgery and medical care for major or serious illness. Small hospitals and health centers refer complicated cases to district hospitals and depend upon such hospitals also for advanced laboratory and diagnostic work and for consultation.

The teaching hospitals not only serve as teaching centers for the training of students, nurses, internes, and resident physicians, but also provide facilities and personnel for post-graduate medical education, clinics and consultation services for hospitals and doctors in the small community along with specialized diagnostic research and therapeutic services.

iv

I

Our Supreme Health Needs are: 1)More Doctors, 2)More Hospitals, 3)More Insurance

(Preliminary Report to Governor Broughton and to the People of North Carolina. Adopted October 11, 1944.)

In the office of Governor J. M. Broughton on October 11, 1944, the "State Hospital and Medical Care Commission," appointed by him the preceding February, met to hear reports from State Chairman Clarence Poe and six sub-committee chairmen: Dr. P. P. McCain, "Four-Year Medical School"; Charles A. Cannon, "Hospital and Medical Needs of Urban and Industrial Population"; Thomas J. Pearsall, "Hospital and Medical Care of Our Rural Population"; Dr. E. E. Blackman, "Special Needs of Our Negro Population"; Dr. W. M. Coppridge, "Hospital and Medical Programs in Other States"; Dr. James W. Vernon, "Mental Hygiene and Hospitalization."

After discussion of all reports, the full Hospital and Medical Care Commission adopted the following preliminary report and appeal to the people of the State.

To the People of North Carolina:

On January 31, 1944, at a meeting of the Trustees of the University of North Carolina, Governor J. M. Broughton presented with strong approval a report from a committee of distinguished physicians (this committee including the president, president-elect and three past-presidents of the North Carolina Medical Society) appealing for a great forward step in the life and progress of North Carolina.

These distinguished leaders of the state's medical profession pointed out that North Carolina is now the 11th most populous state in the Union but is 42nd in number of hospital beds per 1000 population (only 6 states lower in rank) and 45th in number of doctors per 1000 population (only 3 states lower in rank) and joined Governor Broughton in recommending two far-reaching remedies as follows:

> *1. The Expansion of the Two-Year Medical School at the University into a Standard Four-Year Medical School with a Central Hospital of 600 beds or more;*
>
> *2. A Hospital and Medical Care Program for the entire state with this noble objective as expressed by Governor Brough-ton: "The ultimate purpose of this program should be that no person in North Carolina shall lack adequate hospital care or medical treatment by reason of poverty or low income."*

By unanimous action the trustees of the Consolidated University approved this twofold program. Almost immediately thereafter Governor Broughton named a "State Hospital and Medical Care Commission" which has been busy ever since investigating conditions, scrutinizing defects, and weighing suggested remedies. Subcommittees were named as follows:

Hospital and Medical Care for Our Rural Population
Hospital and Medical Care for Our Industrial and Urban Population
Special Needs of Our Negro Population
Hospital and Medical Care Plans in Other States
Four-Year Medical School for University and Hospital Facilities

After nearly eight months of investigation and study the State Hospital and Medical Care Commission now presents to the people of the state the following findings and recommendations:

1. Our basic and permanent aim should never be at any time less lofty and comprehensive than the Governor's declaration approved by the 100-man Board of Trustees of the Greater University: "The ultimate purpose of this program should be that no person in North Carolina shall lack adequate hospital care or medical treatment by reason of poverty or low income."

2. In order both to remedy the most urgent needs of today and work toward the larger program of tomorrow, three things are supremely needed:

2

B. *MORE HOSPITALS*
C. *MORE INSURANCE*

These are the three mutually indispensable legs of our three-legged stool. We cannot have enough doctors without more hospitals . . . nor enough hospitals without greater popular ability to pay for hospital service . . . and such ability to pay on the part of the poorer half of our population is impossible without insurance.

3. In each area we must be especially diligent to serve where need is direst and most challenging. This direst need is:

> Among economic groups, *the poor*
> Among occupational groups, *tenant farmers*
> Among races, *the Negro*
> In the two major geographical areas of the state, *Eastern North Carolina (and our mountain counties)*
> Inside family groups, *mothers in childbirth and infants in the first months of existence.*

Supporting Data: North Carolina ranks 41st (only 7 states lower) in maternal deaths per 1000 live births . . . and ranks 39th (only 9 states lower) in number of infant deaths per 1000 live births. Minimum approved number of hospital beds is 4 per 1000 population, but in Eastern North Carolina and Western North Carolina number of beds per 1000 population is only:

	Whites	*Colored*
Eastern Counties	1.59	.92
Western Counties	2.43	2.38

Minimum approved number of doctors is 1 for each 1000 people, but Rural North Carolina (1940) has only 1 doctor for each 3,613 people.

4. Our program is not one of communism. It is not one of "Socialized Medicine." It will not destroy the fine relationship of doctor and patient. To "Socialized Medicine" as commonly understood it has, as someone has said, the same relation that vaccination has to smallpox—*"it prevents you from getting the real thing."*

5. The masses of the people are determined to find some way to work steadily toward the goal set forth by Governor Broughton. To fail to help them may leave them to leadership dangerously unsound. Our desire is to help constructively—to co-operate for larger things with existing physicians, hospitals and other medical agencies. Our purpose indeed is "not to destroy but to fulfill."

6. We fully realize that such a program cannot be achieved overnight or at one session of our General Assembly. We do most confidently ask, however, that a realization of this fact shall not be used to prevent the state from doing less than the utmost it is possible to do.

3

For what we now face is the need not for a normal two-year gain in a program already well advanced but the imperative need for a great advance in a highly important program 20 years overdue.

7. The poor of the state have indeed heard gladly of this program. Men and women of wealth, we rejoice to say, have been equally quick to proffer their support. Just as North Carolina in 1900-1920 spent larger sums than ever before for Better Schools but found it a good investment for all classes, and again in 1920-40 greatly increased its expenditures for Better Roads with similar benefits to rich and poor alike, so we may now greatly increase our expenditures for Better Health and find all classes of North Carolinians bettered as a result.

So much for three basic health needs of our people and the spirit in which your State Hospital and Medical Care Commission has sought to find ways and means of meeting these needs. As a result of long study by your Commission and its various Subcommittees, we now recommend the following measures for approval by our people and their forthcoming General Assembly:

A. TO MEET THE NEED FOR MORE DOCTORS, BETTER DISTRIBUTED

North Carolina is faced with an imperative need both for more doctors and a better distribution of doctors. While an accepted formula is that there should be 1 doctor for each 1000 population, North Carolina has only 1 doctor for each 1,554 people . . . rural North Carolina has only 1 doctor for each 3,613 people . . . and there is only 1 colored physician for each 6,916 colored people. To remedy this situation we recommend:

A State Supported Four-Year Medical School. The Commission gives its unqualified endorsement to the proposal that the present two-year medical school at the University of North Carolina be expanded into a standard four-year medical school with a central hospital of 600 beds. North Carolina students trained in North Carolina will likely remain in North Carolina to follow their chosen profession.

Loan Funds for Medical Students. The Commission recommends that a loan fund be established by the State Legislature, particularly for promising youth, male or female, white or non-white, who wish to become physicians in North Carolina, with extra inducements provided for those who will agree to practice medicine at least 4 years in rural areas. Ability rather than wealth or social status should be the principal test for admission to the medical schools of the state.

Medical Training for Negro Youth. This Commission recognizes the high moral duty of the state to provide greatly improved opportunities for enabling capable Negro youths to become physicians serving their race, and we recommend a continuing study of various methods of achieving this end, including suggested North Carolina co-operation with adjoining states in establishing a Regional Medical School for Negroes, North Carolina to take the lead in this matter with as prompt action as possible to follow reasonably adequate time for study and investigation.

4

B. To Meet the Need for More Hospital Facilities

1. The Commission recommends that the state provide a total of $5,000,000 to be expended, as called for under prescribed regulations, for building and assisting counties and communities to build and to enlarge hospital and health centers wherever and whenever they are needed in the state. This is based on an eventual need of 6,000 additional hospital beds.

2. It is recommended that grants be made for the construction of new hospitals only in areas not adequately served by existing hospital facilities, and only for the purpose of supplementing or expanding the facilities of existing pubicly owned hospitals or those operated on a non-profit basis.

3. It is further recommended that no grant shall exceed 50 per cent of the cost of construction and equipment of a new hospital or the expansion of an existing hospital; and that within such limitation the proportion of the grant to the total cost be based on economic conditions within the areas to be served, the financial ability of the local governmental unit which will own or operate such facility, and on the availability of funds from other sources.

4. Such a state-wide program to meet the urgent hospital needs of our people should include (in addition to the Central Hospital at the Four-Year Medical School):

(a) *A small number of District Hospitals* of approximately 100 beds. These hospitals would be complete in every sense of the word, and would serve both rural and urban people.

(b) *A large number of County or Rural Hospitals* of approximately 60 beds (including improvement or enlargement of existing facilities, particularly those that are already publicly owned or operated on a non-profit basis).

(c) *Health Centers* in small rural communities (available to all qualified physicians in the area) to provide simple diagnostic and laboratory services, facilities for minor operations, dental services, obstetrical service, etc., with a small number of beds for cases not requiring services of a larger hospital. Such Health Centers should also be used by the public health service in carrying on its preventive and educational work.

(d) To provide for the more adequate care of low-income persons in hospitals, we recommend that the state appropriate $1 per day for each indigent patient treated. The Duke Endowment now provides $1 and this together with $1 from the state would provide $2 per day—counties, municipalities, etc., making up the remainder of the costs.

(e) It is recommended that the Legislature provide for a permanent State Hospital and Medical Care Council of adequately qualified persons which should adopt policies designed to maintain the highest standards of service, efficiency, economy and professional excellence in the hospital building program, the medical student loan fund, and the general administration of the state hospital and medical care program, strict provision being made to safeguard the program from

5

political interference. To encourage continuing community pride, initiative, and support, any hospital receiving state-aid should remain under the professional, administrative and financial control of its own board of trustees elected locally from representative citizens in the community.

(f) Appropriations for public health work should be increased until the state has an entirely adequate program for the prevention of disease, thus reducing needed hospital and medical care to the lowest practicable minimum.

(g) We endorse the proposal for a general examination of school children to discover remediable physical defects, such defects to be remedied at public expense in cases where parents are financially unable to pay for such treatment.

C. To Meet the Need for More Insurance

The Commission recommends that the state encourage in every practicable way the development of group medical care plans which make it possible for people to insure themselves against expensive illness, expensive treatment by specialists, and extended hospitalization. The Blue Cross plan of hospital and surgical service, with some modifications, can meet the needs of that part of the state's population able to pay all their medical care costs. It is recommended that these Blue Cross organizations be asked to expand their services to include the general practitioner and prescribed drugs. This is particularly important for rural people who depend so heavily on the general physician. *The importance of insurance for hospital and medical care in a general program such as ours can hardly be overestimated. Every citizen needs to realize that it is just as important to have insurance against sickness-disasters as against fire-disasters.*

Conclusion

In conclusion we would say that no claim is made that this is a complete or perfect program. The wisdom of the General Assembly must fill in many gaps. The physicians, press and people of the state who have so generously proffered their interest and support—all are asked to help in remedying defects and improving details. We ask only that all of us shall work together to make real a new ideal of democracy—*"The equal right of every person born on earth to needed medical and hospital care whenever and wherever he battles against Disease and Death."* And to this end we would say:

1. The family that can pay its way will do so—yet the burden on even these families should be eased through health-and-hospital insurance.

2. The family that can partly pay its way will pay this part (likewise helped by insurance to the fullest possible degree); government and philanthropic aid being provided for the remainder.

3. The family that poverty, illness, or other misfortune has left honestly incapable of paying anything for its fight against disease will nevertheless be helped to an equal chance with the rest of us as it makes the same grim battle against ever-

6

menacing Death which we must all make and see our loved ones make sooner or later.

Signed on behalf of the State Hospital and Medical Care Commission,

CLARENCE POE, *Chairman*
CARL V. REYNOLDS, M.D., *Secretary*

P. P. McCAIN, M.D., *Chairman, Four-Year Medical School for University and Hospital Facilities*
THOMAS J. PEARSALL, *Chairman, Hospital and Medical Care for Our Rural Population*
CHARLES A. CANNON, *Chairman, Hospital and Medical Care for Our Industrial and Urban Population*
E. E. BLACKMAN, M.D., *Chairman, Special Needs of Our Negro Population*
JAMES W. VERNON, M.D., *Chairman, Mental Hygiene and Hospitalization*
W. M. COPPRIDGE, M.D., *Chairman, Hospital and Medical Care Programs in Other States*
C. HORACE HAMILTON, *Chairman, Statistical Data and Publications*

7

II

"A Program of Great Hope, of Almost Infinite Promise, and of Great Practicability"

(Chairman's Final Report to Governor Cherry and the General Assembly of 1945. Presented February 10, 1945.)

"A program of great hope, of almost infinite promise, and yet of great practicability!" With these opening words the Chairman of the North Carolina Hospital and Medical Care Commission forwarded to the Governor and General Assembly on February 10, 1945 1) his own final report and 2) reports of ten committees. Especially emphasized were 3) seven paragraphs summarizing the most remarkable declarations of various committee chairman, and 4) a genuinely amazing demonstration of what good hospital and medical care had accomplished in North Carolina orphanages—and might accomplish for all our people.

GENTLEMEN:—

A message of great hope, of almost infinite promise, and yet of great practicability.

Such I submit must be a summary of ten reports on general health conditions and hospital and medical care in North Carolina which I now have the honor to transmit to you.

Along with the report of the full Commission as adopted October 11, 1944, I now submit nine detailed reports from subcommittees appointed February 28, 1944, ably officered, on which both physicians and laymen have served with equal efficiency (with first the chairman and then the vice-chairman of each committee listed) as follows:

1. Hospital and Medical Care for Our Rural Population—THOS. J. PEARSALL, DR. G. M. COOPER.

2. Hospital and Medical Care for Our Industrial and Urban Population—CHARLES A. CANNON, CHARLES A. FINK.

3. Special Needs of Our Negro Population—DR. E. E. BLACKMAN, C. C. SPAULDING.

4. Four-Year Medical School for University and Hospital Facilities—DR. P. P. MCCAIN, JOSEPHUS DANIELS.

5. Mental Hygiene and Hospitalization—DR. JAMES W. VERNON, BISHOP CLARE PURCELL.

6. Hospital and Medical Care Plans in Other States—DR. W. M. COPPRIDGE, R. G. DEYTON.

7. A Schoolchild Health Program—DR. GEORGE M. COOPER, CLYDE A. ERWIN.

8. An Enlarged Public Health Program for North Carolina—DR. CARL V. REYNOLDS.

9. A Statistical and Graphic Summary of North Carolina Hospital and Medical Care Needs—DR. C. HORACE HAMILTON.

It is the opinion of such experts as State Health Officer Dr. Carl V. Reynolds that we here present the most comprehensive analysis and review ever yet undertaken of the medical and hospital needs of all our North Carolina people—urban and rural, white and black—and that such data will be invaluable in formulating all policies for better health conditions in North Carolina for years to come.

10

Ideals With Practicability

"Hitch your wagon to a star," said Emerson—meaning that practical men should yet have ideals.

"Hitch your star to a wagon," says Dr. Arthur E. Morgan—meaning that in order to be a working success, every ideal must be tied to earth and to everyday practicability.

Both these fine principles have been kept in mind by all 50 members of your Hospital and Medical Care Commission. Every member has ideals—but every member has also shown capacity for translating his ideals into practical achievement. And we have brought you a program which is intended to meet the hard tests of practicability which North Carolina Governors and Legislatures have always mixed with their idealism.

Four Pertinent Questions Asked

From the time the North Carolina Hospital and Medical Care Commission was organized in February, 1944, to report tentatively to Governor Broughton in October and finally to Governor Cherry and the General Assembly of 1945, we have sought to anticipate the four main questions you would expect your Commission to answer:

1. *What are present hospital and medical care conditions in North Carolina? Is a change, a great change, seriously needed?*
2. *If this is established as a fact, has a practicable program for making the change been developed?*
3. *Are the costs reasonable when compared with the results to be achieved?*
4. *Can you not only cite statistical proofs and thoroughly competent judgment, but is there some specific example right here in North Carolina where the proposed program has been translated into human-interest, flesh-and-blood Tar Heel terms, and if so, with what result?*

Three Questions Answered

Answering at once the first three questions, permit us to say—

1. *As to the need for change and improvement,* our committees have found that among the 48 states of the Union North Carolina is—

—45th in number of doctors per 1,000 population
—42nd in number of hospital beds per 1,000 population

And mainly as a result, we believe, of these two conditions as cause and effect our committees also report that North Carolina is—

—With respect to *infants*—39th in percentage of infants dying under one year of age (only 9 of the 48 states making a worse showing)

11

—With respect to *women*—41st in percentage of mothers dying in childbirth (only 7 of the 48 states making a worse showing)

—With respect to *men*—48th in percentage of army rejections for physical defects by latest available data (no state with a poorer showing)

(Precise percentage of rejections: April, 1942-March, 1943, *48.1%;* February-August, 1943, *56.8%.*)

Doctors Approve Program

2. *As for the practicability of the program* advocated by your Hospital and Medical Care Commission, we need only say that the best judges should be our North Carolina doctors themselves . . . and that of 65 county medical societies that have exhaustively examined the complete program since it was announced October, 1944, the vote (as reported to Secretary R. D. McMillan) has been:

Approving the program in entirety.. 55

Approving in part.. 8

Disapproving the program 2

Costs Low Compared to Benefits

3. *As to costs,* in view of the hundreds of millions North Carolina has spent for roads and schools, the $5,000,000 the Legislature is asked to appropriate for a statewide Hospital Building Fund is astonishingly small. Both the Federal government and our own North Carolina counties, cities and towns will almost surely supplement heavily all the aid the State may provide for hospital building. For the indigent sick in hospitals the 3½ million people of North Carolina combined are now asked to provide only as much ($1 a day) as one deceased North Carolinian (James B. Duke) gives them constantly through his will. All other costs in the proposed program we believe are equally reasonable.

Question Number 4 Brings Great Hope

As proud North Carolinians, let us say to your Excellency, Governor Cherry, and the honored members of our House and Senate, it has been no pleasure to your Commission to recite the proof that North Carolina so desperately needs *"More Doctors, More Hospitals, More Insurance."*

When, however, we come to your fourth question, "Can you cite us an example where this proposed program has been translated into human-interest, flesh-and-blood Tar Heel terms . . . and if so, with what results?" then a great sunrise of hope and inspiration breaks upon the whole scene.

One of the most honored members of your Commission, Dr. I. G. Greer, as spokesman for the numerically largest religious denomination in North Carolina and its oldest social service agency, the Baptist Orphanage at Thomasville, N. C., reveals what can be done not only with our average North Carolina stock, but even with young North Carolinians who have been more-than-normally handicapped by

12

poverty—our orphans. First, let us repeat our earlier figures—48.1 and 50.8—as the percentage of army rejections of North Carolina draftees . . . and then let's listen to this officially signed report by Mr. I. G. Greer, superintendent of the Thomasville Baptist Orphanage, who wrote us February 9, 1945:

> *"Sometime ago you asked me to verify a statement I made to you regarding boys in service who grew up here in the Orphanage. At the time I think I told you we had 284 boys in uniform and that only 3 had failed to pass the physical examination. We know now that we have 318 in the service, and only 3 have failed to pass the physical examination—less than 1%."*

"Nor do our Baptist Orphanages differ from other North Carolina orphanages in this respect. From the superintendents of four other white orphanages I have just received data, making a total showing for boys of draft age who have been in these institutions as follows:

	Accepted for Service	Rejected
Baptist Orphanages (Mills and Kennedy)	*318*	*3*
Methodist Orphanage, Raleigh	*150*	*1*
Children's Home (Methodist), Winston-Salem	*225*	*2*
Barium Springs Orphanage (Presbyterian)	*220*	*5*
Oxford Orphanage	*225*	*5*
Totals	*1,138*	*16*

"This shows 1.4% army rejections, and with 1,873 children now in these orphanages there have been only 7 deaths in five years.

"Practically every child who enters our orphanages comes to us undernourished and in need of some kind of medical attention. This combined North Carolina orphanage record of 98.6% army-acceptance shows what might be done for both the children and older people all over North Carolina through improved medical and hospital care if the General Assembly approved such a program of 'More Doctors, More Hospitals, More Insurance' as the State's Hospital and Medical Care Commission is now advocating. If at any time you can use this statement in helping advance this much needed legislation, you have my permission."

The boys in our North Carolina orphanages are not coddled. They are not given luxuries. They are given sound nutrition and the reasonably adequate medical and hospital care from school age on as advocated by Governor Cherry and your Commission—and what do we find? Whereas the State's latest reported percentage of army rejections is 56.8 (and when the writer's youngest son went to Fort Bragg with 52 boys from your capital city, he was one of only 18 accepted) a not-expensive program of hospital and medical care provided for North Carolina orphanage boys of draft age brings an army acceptance of 98.6%!

NORTH CAROLINA CAN BECOME FAMOUS FOR LOW DEATH RATE

Deliberately as a result of a year-long study of all the data, good and bad, I would say this:

13

North Carolina has an almost ideal climate—seldom zero in winter or 100 in summer—and we have a remarkably sturdy middle-class population, free alike from dissipations of the idle rich and the physical deterioration of poverty-cursed slums. For these reasons of fine climate, fine physical stock, and freedom from extreme wealth and blighting poverty, our death rate has been amazingly low in spite of the absence of proper hospital and medical care.

With proper medical examination and treatment for all school children and proper hospital and medical care for all our older people, I believe that North Carolina can become nationally and even internationally famous for having the lowest death rate of any state of equal population in the American Union—with all that this would mean in increased efficiency, happiness and pride for all North Carolinians!

It is to such an inspiring opportunity for carrying North Carolina forward through adequate legislation in 1945 and 1947 that your North Carolina Hospital and Medical Care Commission presents its case!

SEVEN HIGHLIGHTS OF TEN REPORTS

Just one more question I can hear His Excellency, the Governor, and busy members of the House and Senate asking as follows:

"Every one of your Commission Reports deserve detailed study, but in every article some one statement or paragraph stands out above all else. From all your Commission Reports suppose you had to pick out seven or eight paragraphs which you think every legislator should resolve to read, re-read and remember, no matter what else he might read or miss reading, what paragraphs would you select?"

This is perhaps the hardest of all four questions to answer but here would be my selections:

I. FARMERS NEED MORE DOCTORS, MORE HOSPITALS

It is upon our farm people that the lack of doctors and lack of hospitals falls most heavily. It is heavy in cost of medical service . . . in inability to get medical attention . . . in unnecessarily prolonged illnesses . . . in unnecessary deaths. In 34 North Carolina counties—all rural counties of course—there is now not a single hospital bed for anybody, white or black! In the matter of doctor shortage we note—

> —*The American standard is................1 for each 1,000 people*
> —*Urban North Carolina, 1940, had 1 for each   613 people*
> —*Rural North Carolina, 1940, had 1 for each 3,613 people*
> —*Rural North Carolina, 1944, had 1 for each 5,174 people*

II. INDUSTRIAL WORKERS NEED THE PROGRAM

The most praiseworthy "hospital insurance" plan, in effect in various North Carolina industries, has increased the demand for hospital care where the insured workers live . . . and should be expanded to cover not only industrial employees

14

but other citizens. As a physician in a presumably typical Piedmont industrial small town testifies: "The share-croppers of Eastern Carolina are not the only people who urgently need better care. The factory workers and Negroes of this section are in need, too. Except during rare periods of prosperity, only about one-half of the people of this community are able to pay the modest fees we charge."

III. School Children Need Examination and Treatment

The need to examine and correct the defects of all school children—at private expense where possible and at public expense where necessary—as emphasized by Governor Cherry, is plain and urgent. After Pearl Harbor the State had compulsory examinations of all boys in the two upper grades and the percentage of those showing some defects was amazing—

> *—85% had dental defects*
> *—16% defective in vision*
> *—16% were underweight*
> *—14% had diseased tonsils, etc.*

A majority of the children examined in pre-school clinics each year are also found to have some defect.

A strict system of annual inspection of every school child enrolled in the schools of every county must be provided under the leadership of the State Board of Health co-operating with city and county health departments.

IV. Negroes Need Doctors, Hospitals, Insurance

The Negro death rate in North Carolina in 1940 was 146% that of the white death rate—an appalling difference . . . The State's Negro population in 1940 was 983,574 (and now probably exceeds 1,000,000) but the State has only 129 active Negro physicians—or 1 for each 7,783 Negro people . . . and only 7,760 hospital beds, or 1.7 hospital beds for each 1,000 Negroes—less than half the American standard . . . A regional Negro Medical School should be established . . . Hospital associations should be encouraged to extend the Blue Cross program to Negroes.

V. Why a Four-Year Medical School Is Needed

Average number of physicians who die or retire in North Carolina each year— 50. Average need for new physicians in order to maintain present ratio approximates—100 each year. Average number of medical students graduated from North Carolina medical schools each year who are residents of North Carolina: about 65 (Duke, 20; Wake Forest, 45). The State thus needs 50% more new North Carolina doctors each year than these two excellent schools have provided.

VI. A Statewide Psychiatric Program Is Needed

Mental disorder is more prevalent than tuberculosis and poliomyelitis, and its total cost to the State is as great as all other diseases combined, yet little attention

15

average physician's practice is devoted to the diagnosis and treatment of disorders at least partly psychiatric in nature . . . By using the psychiatric unit of the proposed Four-Year Medical School as a "receiving hospital" and establishing one other such "receiving hospital" in the State, we can decrease the number of patients in hospitals for the insane, prevent many patients from becoming permanent wards of the State, and ultimately make a vast financial saving for the State . . . Every county hospital should also have a small number of beds (5 to 10) for psychiatric patients . . . Unless psychiatric care permeates through the entire state system of hospital care in this way, North Carolina will be sorely neglecting one of its largest problems.

VII. Types of Hospital and Health Centers Needed

A large Central Hospital of approximately 600 beds . . . A small number of District Hospitals of approximately 100 beds . . . Small Rural Hospitals of approximately 60 beds . . . Some counties with less than 12,500 population might find it practical to build small 20- or 30-bed hospitals . . . There should also be "Health Centers" in small rural communities, including diagnostic and laboratory services, facilities for minor operations, obstetrical service, and a small number of beds for cases not requiring the specialized services of a larger hospital, these health centers also to be used by the public health service in carrying on its work.

In Conclusion

In conclusion, I wish to express my thanks to all the members of the Hospital and Medical Care Commission who have labored with me in finding and interpreting the facts and in seeking to present a sound and reasonable program—"To the Good Health of All North Carolina." To my constant co-laborer, President Paul F. Whitaker of the State Medical Society, the State owes more than it will ever know. And finally the thanks of all the people are due to the two Governors under whom we have labored—to Ex-Governor J. M. Broughton who acted with characteristically prompt and adequate statesmanship when the State Medical Society appealed for State action . . . and to Governor R. Gregg Cherry who not only cheered us by immediate and vigorous endorsement of our efforts the day after your Commission was appointed but enriched and rounded out our program by his statesmanlike insistence that any campaign for "Better Health in North Carolina" must begin with the boys and girls in our public schools and must equally safeguard the health and future of the child of the rich and the child of the poor.

Respectfully submitted,

Clarence Poe

Chairman.

Raleigh, N. C.
February 10, 1945.

16

Governor R. Gregg Cherry's Message to the General Assembly, February 1945;
Members of the North Carolina Medical Care Commission appointed
by Governor Cherry in 1945

Governor Cherry's Six Point Program For Hospital and Medical Care

(Extract from special message to the Joint Session of the
General Assembly, February 27, 1945)

Mr. President, Mr. Speaker and Members of the General Assembly of North Carolina:

In my Inaugural Address, reference was made to the Report of a Commission filed with my predecessor, the then Governor, recommending further steps to be taken in medical care and public health in North Carolina. Through the courtesy of Dr. Clarence Poe, the Chairman of the Commission making such Report, every member of the General Assembly has been furnished with a clothbound book entitled: "TO THE GOOD HEALTH OF NORTH CAROLINA," which book contains a copy of the Report, together with a collection of pamphlets and statements from interested and capable persons supporting the findings of the distinguished group of North Carolina citizens who served on the Commission and made the Report. . . . Since such information has been furnished to you in a clear and convenient form, this is no occasion for me to re-state the conclusions and findings of the Report and the reasons therefor, except as may be incident to my recommendations to you as hereinafter set out in this message. . . .

After innumerable conference, I have decided to recommend to you for your favorable action, the general principles of the Medical Care Program as embodied in a Bill introduced in the Senate and House last night and which is now before you for consideration. In brief outline, the subject matter of the Bill before you, the fundamental outlines and general principles of which, I strongly recommend to you for favorable consideration, involves and sets forth the following:

FIRST:

The establishment of a "North Carolina Medical Care Commission," by the present General Assembly, and in order to effectuate the same, I further recommend that you appropriate and make available the sum of Fifty Thousand ($50,000.00) Dollars for each year of the biennium for the operating expenses of the Commission and the performance of such other duties as may be required of the Commission under the terms of the pending act.

SECOND:

That you adopt the principle of State contributions for the hospitalization of indigent patients and that the Commission shall be authorized to promulgate rules and regulations for determining the indigency of persons hospitalized and the basis upon which hospitals and health centers shall qualify to receive contributions for indigent patients and the Commission is authorized and empowered to contribute not exceeding one dollar ($1.00) per day for each indigent patient hospitalized in each hospital approved by it. To effectuate this provision, I recommend that you appropriate the sum of Five Hundred Thousand ($500,000.00) for each year of the biennium; provided, however, that this appropriation shall not be available until all provisions of the General Appropriations Bill of 1945, including those relating to the emergency salary for public school teachers and State employees shall have been completely provided for. Frankly, this means that there is only a bare possibility that this appropriation will be available for the purposes mentioned.

THIRD:

That you authorize and direct the Commission to be created under the pending Act to make surveys of each County in the State to determine the need for some kind of State aid for construction and enlargement of local hospitals, and make a report of their findings and recommendations to the Governor, who shall transmit the same to the next regular session of the General Assembly for such action as it may deem necessary.

FOURTH:

That you authorize and direct the Commission to be created under the pending Act, and in accordance with rules which the Commission may promulgate, to make loans to worthy students in need of financial assistance who may wish to become physicians and who are accepted for enrollment in any standard four-year medical school in North Carolina. In order to effectuate this provision, I further recommend that you appropriate and make available for the fiscal year ending June 30, 1946, the sum of Fifty Thousand ($50,000) Dollars.

FIFTH:

That you adopt the principle and declare the policy of expanding the two-year medical school of the University of North Carolina into a standard four-year medical school, together with necessary hospital facilities, homes for nurses, internes and resident physicians as may be required for the expansion of such Medical School. It is not contemplated that any construction of buildings or acquisition of equipment to effectuate the declared policy of expansion of such medical school can be performed during the war period or prior to the next regular session of the General Assembly and therefore no appropriation is requested to carry out the capital investment of the proposed expansion of such Medical School.

SIXTH:

That you authorize and direct the Commission to be created by the pending act to make careful investigation of the necessity and methods of providing medical training for Negro students, and make a report of their findings and recommendations to the Governor, who shall transmit the same to the next regular session of the General Assembly for such action as it may deem necessary. It is also recommended that loans to Negro medical students be authorized by the Commsision from the loan fund hereinbefore mentioned, subject to such rules and regulations as may be set up by the Commission to be created under the pending act.

* * *

Many desirable services, richly deserved by our people, must be postponed for the duration of the war. . . . In like manner, much of the proposals of the Hospital and Medical Care Commission must be postponed to some future date.

But Senators and Lady and Gentlemen of the House, a most comprehensive plan of hospitalization and medical care has been laid before you and is contained in the report (of the Hospital and Medical Care Commission) now on your desks. The bill before you and now under consideration endorses the principles and partially effectuates the plan outlined in such report. I personally favor and sincerely believe that improvement in medical care in North Carolina is sure to come and that it is definitely on the way. Just when the capstone will be finally laid for a comprehensive and adequate plan of medical care in North

Carolina is a matter for future legislators—but we here today and in the succeeding days of this General Assembly, ought to lay the cornerstone and the broad foundation upon which we can build such program as our people seek to obtain and ought to have.

The people of our State at decisive times in our history have made the great decision to build a more enlightened and productive State. In our poverty we built a great school system; in spite of debts and deficits we built a great public highway system. In these days, we shall not be afraid to lay the foundations for proper medical and hospital care needed by our poorer and less fortunate fellow citizens. The voices of the sick, the suffering and even the dying cry out to us at this time for help. These voices which we hear, and voices too long unheard, come to us across the plains and hills of every part of our State. It is my belief that we should answer their calls and minister to their needs by laying the foundation of a balanced and humane program for more adequate medical care for the people of this Commonwealth.

As members of this General Assembly, you have the responsibility and privilege of making another decisive decision in the history of our State. I ask you to believe with me that "Better Schools, Better Roads and Better Health" constitute the three main high roads for the advancement of North Carolina. I have confidence that you, in this Hour of Destiny, will make the decision embracing a program for the future happiness and welfare of North Carolina.

MEDICAL CARE COMMISSION

Following the 1945 Legislature's action, the Governor appointed the following Medical Care Commission to carry forward the hospital and medical care program:

James H. Clark, Chairman, Elizabethtown
Dr. Clarence Poe, Vice-Chairman, Raleigh
J. W. Bean, Spencer
Paul B. Bissette, Wilson
Franklin J. Blythe, Charlotte
Dr. William M. Coppridge, Durham
Don S. Elias, Asheville
Sample B. Forbus, Durham
Dr. Fred Hale, Raleigh
Dr. Fred C. Hubbard, North Wilkesboro
B. Everett Jordan, Saxapahaw
Dr. W. S. Rankin, Charlotte
Dr. Carl V. Reynolds, Raleigh
Mrs. Elizabeth Dillard Reynolds, Winston-Salem
William M. Rich, Durham
William B. Rodman, Washington
Dr. C. E. Rozzelle, Asheboro
Flora Wakefield, Raleigh
Dr. Paul F. Whitaker, Kinston
Dr. Ellen B. Winston, Raleigh

Report to the North Carolina Medical Care Commission
by the National Committee for the Medical School Survey
(Sanger Report), July 1946

NORTH CAROLINA MEDICAL CARE COMMISSION

NATIONAL COMMITTEE FOR MEDICAL SCHOOL SURVEY

July 1, 1946

To: The Chairman and Members of the North Carolina Medical Care Commission.

Appointed by the North Carolina Medical Care Commission in accordance with the provision of an Act of the General Assembly (H. B. No. 594) of the State of North Carolina, the National Committee for the Medical School Survey has conducted a study of those factors pertaining to the need for and locatio of a four-year school of medicine as a unit of the University of North Caroli and related considerations. On the basis of that study, it is the recommenda tion of the Committee, amplified in more detail in the body of this report:

I.   That the Trustees of the University of North Carolina establish a four-year school of medicine situated on the campus of the University at Chapel Hill; provided:

a.   That a hospital and health center program to provide greatly enlarged facilities be carried forward and that a practicable plan for financing medical and hospital care be established;

b.   That such a school of medicine be an integrated part of a State University medical center which will include:

1.   Appropriate facilities for the basic medical sciences, for research, and an adequate general, teaching hospital;

2.   A school of nursing;

3.   A program for the preparation of essential personnel in fields ancillary to rendering medical and hospital care;

4.   The present School of Public Health for the training of personnel in that special field;

5.   The present School of Pharmacy;

6.   An active program for graduate and postgraduate education for physicians and allied medical personnel both at the medical center and in the State as a whole;

7.   Arrangements to provide hospitals throughout the State with clinical consultations, roentgenologic, pathologic, and other services as may be desired by them;

8.   A competent administrator at the medical center to coordina all the activities of the center and integrate these on a State-wide basis as needed, and desired, in order to insure the utmost effectiveness in providing a better health program for North Carolina;

c. That such a school of medicine and associated services of the medical center, responsive to the will of the people, be integrated effectively and continuously with a State-wide network of hospitals and health centers in so far as these volunteer to cooperate; merely to expand the two-year medical school at Chapel Hill in order to graduate a greater number of physicians is not regarded as sufficient justification for such expansion;

d. That full utilization be made of the facilities of the voluntary, non-profit hospitals of the State; that these institutions remain autonomous units, expected to operate with high standards of service as required to provide proper medical care to the people of the State;

e. That, as far as possible, the activities of the four-year school of medicine be coordinated with those of the privately-endowed medical schools of the State to afford maximum service within North Carolina;

II. That the planning of the medical school development proceed as may be convenient; that, however, the construction and operation of the expanded medical school appropriately be timed with the development of the program for the construction of hospitals and health centers, in order to insure a properly coordinated advancement of the total State-wide health-service project of North Carolina; further it is thought that the exact sequence of elements involved in this project cannot be committed to blueprints at this time on the basis of information available to the Committee;

III. That the State of North Carolina consider education on an inter-state or regional basis in dentistry both for white and Negro students; in medicine for Negro students and in public health nursing for Negro students as discussed subsequently in this report;

IV. That the University of North Carolina develop a philosophy of medical education, research, and medical care which will make it a service facility for the whole State.

SUPPLEMENTAL STATEMENTS

The National Committee for the Medical School Survey presents the following in support of the above recommendations:

I. THE FOUR-YEAR SCHOOL OF MEDICINE OF THE UNIVERSITY OF NORTH CAROLINA AT CHAPEL HILL.

a. Expansion of the present University of North Carolina two-year School of Medicine to a four-year school.

There are several important reasons for expanding the present two-year School of Medicine to one with the full four-year curriculum:

1. The four-year course in a single location offers the only completely satisfactory method of providing the best medical training. Inevitably, a two-year school is at a serious disadvantage in competing with those providing the complete required course of instruction. Newer ideas in medical education unquestionably will demand marked reduction of the departmentalization which has become all too prominent. Teaching will, more and more, be conducted on vertical rather than horizontal planes, with instructors of the basic sciences now taught chiefly in the first two years contributing largely to so-called clinical teaching of the last two years, and vice versa. Such a reorientation would be impossible for a two-year school, unless by agreement its curriculum is coordinated and integrated with that of a four-year school.

2. A State-financed and State-controlled medical school has the advantage of being able to carry out over a long period of time policies which have been determined as representing the best considered needs of the entire State. Such long-term policies on the part of private institutions could not be predicted with certainty.

3. A four-year school operated under State control would be the ideal type of institution to provide the apical and focal point for the proposed State-wide medical program, fully integrated with it. The success of the program is dependent in large measure upon a system of medical education, under-graduate, graduate and postgraduate, which is geared to the needs of the whole plan.

4. The projected school may be expected to have a certain effect toward providing more doctors for North Carolina. This effect is likely to be disappointingly small, however, if the entire plan proposed by the Governor's Commission is not implemented fully. The four-year medical school alone, even under State control is only a part, even though an important one, of the complex mosaic required to make adequate medical care available to the people in all parts of the State.

In weighing the question of recommending immediate establishment of the four-year school, the North Carolina Medical Care
Commission should consider the probable great difficulty of
obtaining suitable faculty under present conditions, as well
as the very high building cost prevailing at this time.

b. The expanded school of medicine should be located on the
University campus at Chapel Hill.

A number of powerful arguments favor location of the proposed
four-year school on the campus of the University of North
Carolina at Chapel Hill.

1. Progress in medicine is dependent upon close association with
the basic sciences which serve as its foundation. Dr. Alan
Gregg, Director of the Division for the Medical Sciences of
The Rockefeller Foundation, has stated, "The growing fringe,
the advancing frontier, of medical science may safely be
assumed to be dependent upon contact with the natural
sciences--indeed contact is too weak a word--coalescence would
better describe the relationship." Such a coalescence may be
anticipated reasonably only if the medical school is
situated in close physical relationship to other university
departments, such as physics, chemistry, biology, psychology
and anthropology.

2. Advancement in medicine also depends upon the integration of
social and economic factors which have a powerful influence
upon problems related to the distribution of medical
services to the people. Close association with university
activities in social sciences and the humanities will undoubtedly be essential in providing faculty and students
with modern concepts of these questions and in developing
the proposed State-wide medical care program.

3. A university atmosphere provides cultural advantages for
students and faculty and their families. The outstanding
position of the University of North Carolina in the field of
higher education would be an important inducement which
definitely would aid in bringing desirable personnel to the
medical school.

4. Administrative difficulties and expense to the University
would unquestionably be reduced by locating the medical
school at Chapel Hill.

5. A major objective of the broad program presented to the
people of North Carolina is to train more doctors for
practice in rural areas. Again using the words of Dr. Gregg,
North Carolina "for a long time will need doctors accustomed
to and contented with life in the smaller towns. Large
cities set before medical students the attractions of city
practices, of early specializing, of migration to the still
larger cities and of something nearer to commercialism than

can survive the test of rural practice." Chapel Hill offers
the small community atmosphere conducive to training men
for rural practice.

6. Medical schools in cities are likely to develop difficult
problems of relationships with the local medical profession.
On this point Dr. Gregg comments, "I know of no university
medical school in a large city which, within my memory, has
not had at least one serious quarrel between the university
and the powerful and privileged professional leaders in the
city. Unless your university medical leaders are resigned to
offering teaching positions in return for support and
collaboration of clinicians with few other claims to attention,
they may well prepare themselves for a decade of pressures and
political maneuvers. Usually if appointments are made quid
pro quo and at a distance from the university, the character
of the school depends on forces only slightly under university
control."

7. A university hospital constructed in Chapel Hill will admit
patients from all sections of the State on a basis of equality.
Such a condition would be much less likely to prevail if the
hospital were in a larger community which might reasonably
expect more favorable consideration for its own citizens in
return for such contributions as that particular city or
county had made to the site, building or maintenance of the
hospital.

8. The organized medical profession of North Carolina has
expressed itself in favor of the Chapel Hill location, and
has promised full cooperation in the development of the
school so situated.

9. Various schools and departments of the University will be
essential in providing necessary instruction for public
health workers, dentists, nurses, medical social workers,
dietitians, nutritionists, various types of technicians, and
so forth.

10. Strong arguments might be made for locating the medical
school in a large metropolitan center if one existed in
North Carolina. There are no very large cities in the
State. Therefore, it is better to take advantage of the
University environment. The available locations other than
Chapel Hill would supply relatively limited material from
within their own communities. In fact there is no possible
medical school location in the whole State which would not
require sending students for short periods to other
communities for supplemental instruction in order to secure
maximal educational results.

The Chapel Hill location involves certain disadvantages for which necessary compensation must be made. There will be a shortage of patients for teaching in obstetrics, traumatic surgery and certain other fields. Part-time specialists so useful in certain aspects of training will be less readily available than would be the case in a larger community. Health and social agencies will more nearly represent patterns to be found in rural areas, and even though this may be considered advantageous in developing rural practitioners, students should be familiarized with more complex organizations.

Medical school authorities must arrange opportunities for students to make up for such deficiencies as occur by providing affiliations with hospitals and various institutions in other parts of the State. Such arrangement may constitute a helpful factor in integrating outlying hospitals with the medical center at Chapel Hill.

c. The expanded University of North Carolina School of Medicine should develop harmonious working relationships with the other two medical schools in North Carolina in providing the best possible medical care for the people of the State.

The only type of rivalry that should be permitted to develop between the schools should take the form of eagerness on the part of each to cooperate with the others more fully and to serve better the people of North Carolina. Because of its official character the University of North Carolina School should be expected to assume leadership in organizing a coordinating committee to plan and develop a State-wide program. Such a committee might well consist of:

> Deans of the three medical schools
> State Health Commissioner
> Chairman of the N. C. Medical Care Commission
> Representative of the State Medical Society
> Representative of the State Dental Society
> Representative of the State Nurses' Association
> Representative of the State Pharmaceutical Association
> Representative of the State Hospital Association

and it should have an advisory rather than an administrative function.

Plans will be required:

1. To assist the North Carolina Medical Care Commission in its allocation of loans for students to be trained for rural practice.

2. To plan teaching programs so that all medical teachers within the State may be utilized to best advantage. In the past there have already been examples of excellent cooperation between the schools in utilizing certain faculty members on a joint basis. Such arrangements should be encouraged in the future whenever possible.

3. To plan intern and resident training, with the fullest possible utilization of such opportunities as can be developed in hospitals other than the University hospitals in various population centers of the State.

4. To plan postgraduate instruction, not only at the medical school but on the periphery of the districts of which the medical schools form the centers.

5. To improve laboratory service throughout the State.

6. To provide consultation service whenever necessary and practicable.

7. To assist in coordinating the State-wide medical care program.

8. To integrate medical care with public health and with health education activities so that there is a minimum of overlapping and duplication and with the objective of providing complete coverage of the State.

X. A PHILOSOPHY WILL BE DEVELOPED.

a. Progress in health is North Carolina's next step.

North Carolina has developed its industry, agriculture, systems
of public education and roads, and has made general economic
progress during the past few decades. Now the attention of its
people has concentrated upon the field of health; for it has
been recognized in recent years that North Carolina has been
backward in medical care and hospitalization for the sick. The
lack of these health services has been pronounced in the rural
areas of the State and among the low income families of all races.

b. The University of North Carolina will lead the way.

Progress in other fields has been due in no small measure to the
enlightened leadership of units of the Greater University of
North Carolina. It is only natural, therefore, that the people
of the State should assume that an expanded School of Medicine
of that University would provide the leadership and guidance
required in the development of a broad health program.

c. Development of the good health movement.

The North Carolina Hospital and Medical Care Commission, appointed
by the Governor in 1944, made its theme, "More doctors, more
hospitals, more insurance", familiar to all the people. The
1945 session of the General Assembly enacted House Bill 594 into
law and thereby provided for the implementation of certain
sections of that Commission's report while authorizing further
studies which would lead to the formulation of a detailed program
for improved health facilities. The Act created a permanent
North Carolina Medical Care Commission and gave it the
responsibility for developing that program.

d. Work of the National Committee for the Medical School Survey.

1. The new North Carolina Medical Care Commission was directed
by the law to survey the cities of the State to determine the
preferred location for the expanded medical school and the
medical center which the Board of Trustees of the University
was authorized and empowered to erect under certain conditions.
At the same time, the Act provided for the appointment by the
Commission of a committee of experts in medical education
and related fields who would make an independent survey and
advise the Commission as to the best site for the medical
school and medical center. When appointed, that group of
experts became known as the National Committee for the
Medical School Survey. Its first meeting was held in Raleigh
on January 7, 1946 and there have been three subsequent
sessions. The National Committee has studied the data which
pertain to the health of the people of North Carolina.

The seven members have considered the many factors involved in demonstrating the need for another medical school in this State. They have surveyed the potential sites for the proposed four-year medical school and medical center. They have reached a decision concerning these important matters.

2. Although some difference of opinion existed among the members of the National Committee with regard to certain features of the medical care program recommended by the 1944 report of the North Carolina Hospital and Medical Care Commission, the opinion supporting the recommendation of the National Committee as embodied in the present report was over-whelming. It is apparent to the members of the National Committee that the mere expansion of the present two-year medical school will contribute little to the medical resources of the State. It is for that reason that the present report has recommended expansion to a four-year medical school only with the provision that that school be integrated with all the health facilities in North Carolina in a manner which will insure improvement in medical, public health, and hospital service throughout the State.

3. In the supplemental statements, the members of the National Committee have outlined the principles which are believed to be essential in the formulation of the comprehensive health program which has been envisioned for North Carolina. Methodology has been discussed in only a general way. It is believed that maximum effectiveness can be realized only through flexibility in developing those harmonious working relationships between the many individuals, organizations, and institutions which are essential to success. The members of the National Committee have been impressed by the fine spirit of cooperation exhibited by the representatives of the various interests and agencies in the State.

4. The very first of the supplemental statements suggested the creation of a coordinating committee which would serve to smooth the rocky road of progress in a new field. The importance of such a body cannot be overemphasized. The need of subcommittees of comparable type may be recognized as the program develops.

****

Through their elected representatives in the General Assembly, the people of North Carolina have placed their trust in the North Carolina Medical Care Commission and the University of North Carolina in their search for the road to good health for all. In response to popular demands, the University, through the four-year School of Medicine and the medical center, will develop ultimately a philosophy of medical education, research, and medical care which will make it a service facility for the whole State.

Respectfully submitted:

_____ Chairman
William T. Sanger, Ph.D., President
Medical College of Virginia
Richmond, Virginia

_____
Eugene L. Bishop, M.D., Director of Health
Tennessee Valley Authority
Chattanooga, Tennessee

_____
Graham L. Davis, Hospital Director
W. K. Kellogg Foundation
Battle Creek, Michigan

_____
John A. Ferrell, M.D., Medical Director
The John and Mary R. Markle Foundation
New York, New York

_____
Victor Johnson, M.D., Secretary
Council on Medical Education and Hospitals
American Medical Association
Chicago, Illinois

_____
Hugh R. Leavell, M.D.
The Rockefeller Foundation
New York, New York

_____
Samuel Proger, M.D., Medical Director
The Joseph H. Pratt Diagnostic Hospital
Boston, Massachusetts

Ex-Officio: _____ Secretary
Clement C. Clay, M.D., Executive Secretary
North Carolina Medical Care Commission
Raleigh, North Carolina

Minority Report of the National Committee for the Medical School Survey, July 1946

MINORITY REPORT

STATEMENT BY GRAHAM L. DAVIS, AND VICTOR JOHNSON, M. D.

The health program for North Carolina, outlined in this report, may be defined in terms of finances, facilities, and personnel. All of the committee members agree that until there is a change in present methods of financing medical service and hospital care and hospitals and health centers are greatly enlarged and improved, it would be a hopeless task to attempt to increase materially the number of physicians, dentists, nurses, dietitians, technicians, public health engineers, and other workers in the health field. Under these circumstances the creation of another medical center, primarily to educate physicians, becomes of secondary importance. This statement is by the members of the committee who are not convinced another four-year school of medicine will ever be needed in North Carolina. There is no evidence to support the conclusion that another school as such would add a single physician to the number now practicing in the State.

North Carolina has two schools of medicine that rank with the best in the nation. Authorities agree that the education resources of one good medical center, which would include a school of medicine, can supply the health personnel needs for about three million people. North Carolina has a population of 3,700,000, but its medical schools are regional and national in character, which is to their credit. Medical service has reached such high standards in this nation because of the absence of provincialism in medical education to any large extent. A medical school limited in its service to one state, either by policy or law, tends to stagnate. Several of the state university schools do draw the major portion of their students from their respective states, but fortunately many of these physicians go to other states for graduate and postgraduate education and to practice. The argument is that North Carolina needs a school narrowed in its functioning to the production of physicians and other health personnel almost entirely for North Carolina. North Carolina would be better off without such a school.

What attracts a physician to a given community is its cultural and social advantages and an opportunity to make a decent living by practicing medicine the way he has been taught to practice. The principal reason that many areas in North Carolina do not attract a sufficient number of physicians and other health personnel to meet community needs is economic. The income per capita is low. The reason that other states have doubled the number of physicians in proportion to population is because these states have doubled the income per capita. Another medical school will not solve that problem. It can only be solved by pooling the resources of the state on the insurance principle or by taxation or by a combination of the two methods, with perhaps some assistance from the Federal government. The preferred method is a voluntary prepayment plan with some assistance from the taxpayer with the care of the people in the lower income brackets and the indigent.

Another major difficulty to be overcome, if the public is to get the health services it needs, is the lack of facilities. Health departments are usually housed in jails or in the basement of the county courthouse and hospitals in rural communities are frequently old houses or similarly inadequate structures. The offices of physicians and dentists are frequently makeshift and inadequate. All these facilities belong together in a community health center. In this way the community would be more efficiently and economically served.

After North Carolina has provided the facilities and an adequate method of financing their operation, it will be time to worry about education of personnel to staff these facilities. Any other approach to the over-all problem would be putting the cart before the horse. As a practical matter, North Carolina need not worry about health personnel. On a competitive basis, the nation's existing medical schools, including the two in North Carolina, will provide it with all the physicians, dentists, nurses, public health officers and other health personnel it needs. The reason most of the graduates of North Carolina medical schools go elsewhere to practice is because the opportunities are greater.

The shortage of physicians, dentists, nurses, dietitians and technicians in recent years was largely caused by the war. This shortage and the war-time maldistribution of physicians are not justification for the establishment of more mediocre medical schools. The nation needs better, rather than more medical schools. Construction and operation of a good medical school and teaching hospital at the University of North Carolina would cost the taxpayers a lot of money, which could be used to better advantage in other ways.

A town so small and so located that it does not support even a small community hospital at present certainly is not the place for a medical center with a large teaching hospital, particularly when a medical school in a medium size city is only 12 miles away. No medical school and teaching hospital exists on this continent in a town as small as Chapel Hill. The medical schools in the smaller communities are frequently not the best and they are all seriously handicapped for clinical material for teaching purposes in certain departments, such as pediatrics and obstetrics. These are two of the strongest departments in the best schools.

A 600-bed teaching hospital in Chapel Hill would be filled to capacity if constructed now and, because of the shortage of beds and general prosperity, would continue to be filled for a number of years, provided the taxpayer takes over responsibility for the payment of hospital bills and medical care when prosperity runs out. What will happen eventually, if the North Carolina Medical Care Commission carries out the mandate of the General Assembly, is that the standards of service and adequacy of facilities in other communities will be built up to the point where it will not be necessary for patients to go to a university teaching hospital to get the medical care and hospital service they need.

People should not be required to travel long distances to get these services and they are not going to do it indefinitely. Under these circumstances it would not be in the public interest to artificially stimulate a flow of patients to Chapel Hill to keep a medical school alive.

The comprehensive educational and service program recommended in this report has not been attempted in all its details anywhere in the world. Several medical schools have made progress with certain of its phases. Medical science, medical service, and medical education are advancing so rapidly that the application of existing knowledge to the maximum needs of the people lags behind. Under these circumstances the two medical schools in North Carolina cannot be criticized to any considerable extent for failure to have such a program now in effect. The medical schools play an important part, but numerous other institutions and agencies, both official and voluntary, including the State itself, have definite responsibilities that have not as yet been assumed.

These schools are public trusts, they are owned and controlled by the two strongest churches in the State, they are responsive to the needs of the people, and they have a long record of effective service. They have never failed to produce when their responsibility was clearly defined. To assume they would fail to meet this challenge to greater service does not sound reasonable.

Respectfully submitted:

/s/   Victor Johnson, M. D., Secretary
Council on Medical Education and Hospitals
American Medical Association
Chicago, Illinois

Graham L. Davis, Director
Division of Hospitals
W. K. Kellogg Foundation
Battle Creek, Michigan

July 12, 1946

W. R. Berryhill, "The Location of a Medical School:
Considerations in Favor of Locating a Medical School on a University Campus,"
Proceedings of the Annual Congress on Medical Education
and Licensure, Chicago, February 6 and 7, 1950*

THE LOCATION OF A MEDICAL SCHOOL: CONSIDERATIONS IN FAVOR OF LOCATING A MEDICAL SCHOOL ON A UNIVERSITY CAMPUS

W. R. BERRYHILL, M.D.
Dean, University of North Carolina School of Medicine
Chapel Hill, N. C.

The majority of medical schools in this country have developed in population centers, in most part for the practical reason that access to the wards and clinics of existing hospitals and utilization of the outstanding practitioners of the area provided the only, or certainly the most economical, means of financing the undertaking. Because of economic and transportation difficulties existing at the time it was easier to bring students to a concentration of charity patients than the reverse.

Before the development of the scientific era in medicine there was little if any appreciation of the importance of the close affiliation of the medical school with a university or of the need for faculties having a primary interest in teaching and research, with the result that often when a university sponsored a medical school in the same large city the two might be miles apart in location and still further apart in educational policies, relations and standards. Many of the older medical schools at the time of their founding had at best only a speaking acquaintance and not too cordial at that with the university whose name they bore and under whose aegis they functioned.

So firm was the belief that a medical school could not successfully perform its function away from a large concentration of population that some universities located in smaller communities developed their medical schools in large cities at varying distances from the campus of the parent institution. A few universities, however, placed by historical accident in small towns had the temerity to develop a medical school and a university hospital on their own campuses either because it was recognized that medicine belonged in the uni-

*Reprinted with the permission of the American Medical Association.

versity or because no completely satisfactory arrangements could be worked out in larger cities within the state.

Through the years each arrangement has had advantages and disadvantages. Each school has attempted to work out its difficulties and to solve its problems by capitalizing on or supplementing the local conditions. In each type of organization there have developed some great schools.

If medicine is in truth a learned profession and not a trade and if it has finally become, after a long and somewhat devious course, a university discipline, then it is logical to believe that a school of medicine whenever possible should be an integral part of a university, physically and spiritually.

I assume that today most of us who are concerned with medical education would agree that the university campus is the ideal location for a medical school provided adequate funds are available (a) to insure modern physical facilities for laboratories—teaching and research, hospital clinics and wards, (b) to secure a faculty of a high order of excellence, (c) provided patients sufficient in number and in variety of types of illness can be assured for a sound teaching program, and (d) provided the faculty and administration, in addition to scientific and clinical accomplishments, have an awareness of the mission of a modern medical school and of its importance in the total life of the community.

For a university fortunately located in a large city there should be no problem, but the question arises whether these requirements can be successfully and adequately met on a university campus located at a distance from a large population center and whether the educational advantages of close university association outweigh the disadvantages of a smaller concentration of population. This problem is of more than academic interest. In fact, it becomes one of serious concern in view of its importance in determining the location and hence the future adequateness and effectiveness of new or expanded medical schools now being planned as a part of several state universities. It may be of importance also in view of the possible eventual necessity of decentralization of large urban facilities as a result of the world situation which now faces us.

I have been asked to present one point of view on the basis of the decision made by the Administration and Board of Trustees of the University of North Carolina after a comprehensive study. During the past five years several excellent surveys dealing with this problem have been made in Missouri, Florida, Mississippi, and North Carolina, and since I have neither original nor profound thoughts to add to these studies it may be helpful to restate as a summary some of the more important considerations, elementary perhaps, but it is well to remember that elementary principles are so often fundamental and just as often overlooked or disregarded.

EDUCATIONAL ADVANTAGES IN THE TRAINING OF THE MODERN DOCTOR IN A UNIVERSITY ENVIRONMENT

It is axiomatic that progress in medicine is dependent on close association with the basic sciences which serve as its foundation. This has perhaps been best stated by Dr. Alan Gregg in the report on the University of Missouri Survey of Medical Education, "the growing fringe, the advancing frontier, of medical science may safely be assumed to be dependent upon contact with the natural sciences—indeed contact is too weak a word —coalescence would better describe the relationship" [1] and "the physics and chemistry of today become the physiology and pathology of tomorrow and the clinical medicine of the day following." [2] A scientific environment which would permit and encourage such a coalescence cannot be provided easily or adequately away from close physical relationship with the total scientific resources of a university and its departments of physics, chemistry, biology, psychology, mathematics, and anthropology, and certainly not without staggering cost and duplication which no institution can afford at the present time.

In medicine today, to quote from Dr. Vernon Lippard's Florida survey, "Departmental barriers and the barriers between students and faculty are being broken down and it is not unusual to find a medical student, a graduate student in chemistry, biology, or physics, a physiologist, and a surgeon studying a common problem." [3] This helpful and hopeful trend can certainly be furthered more efficiently and economically when the school of medicine is in the university.

1. The Board of Curators Report on the University of Missouri Survey of Medical Education, 1945, p. 12.
2. Ibid., p. 25.
3. Education for the Health Services in the State of Florida. State Board of Education and State Board of Control, 1949, p. 13.

In his *The University at the Crossroads,* Dr. Henry Sigerist comments, "we still need, more than ever, a scientific physician well trained in laboratory and clinic. But we need more: we need a social physician who, conscious of developments, conscious of the social functions of medicine, considers himself in the service of society." [4] Intimate contact with the humanities and the social science departments in a modern university, therefore, is likewise vitally important to the advancement of medicine and has been too long neglected in the training of the present day physician. An understanding of the importance of the social and economic factors which influence the distribution of medical care to the people and a recognition that "the progress of medicine is dependent also on the prevailing attitudes of society toward disease and health, toward our economic and material resources, prevalent interpretations of the role of government and the structure of our society" [5] are perhaps as important to the welfare and success of the future doctor as his understanding of the sciences. He is the person whose obligation and opportunity it becomes to aid medicine in its adjustment to its changing environment and responsibilities. In this perhaps of all times "free and easy access to the humanities and the social studies which a modern university affords" [6] should be available to the medical student during his professional training and to the medical faculty as well.

There are definite educational advantages in the close interrelationships between the medical school and the other professional schools of the university with public health, dentistry, and pharmacy in the medical area and professional schools in the non-medical area—the graduate school and the schools of engineering, law, agriculture, business and public administration, social work, library science, and education. The importance of cooperative research and graduate training programs between the graduate school departments of the natural and physical sciences and the medical school should be emphasized. The relationships with other professional schools "are of practical significance in the development of special curricula within the university for emergent

---

4. Sigerist, H. E., The University at the Crossroads. Schuman (New York, 1946).
5. The Board of Curators Report on the University of Missouri Survey of Medical Education, 1945, p. 12.
6. Ibid., p. 12.

fields auxiliary to medicine, for such vocations as laboratory technology, dietetics, medical record library service, physical therapy, occupational therapy, hospital administration, medical social worker, and clinical psychologists." [7] A corps of professionally minded people in various fields who are able to work together on projects in the university are thus more likely to form a basis for future cooperation in attacking problems—medical, social, and economic—outside the university that affect the welfare of the community.

Two other advantages should be mentioned here: (1) the easy accessibility to the resources of a large university library is invaluable to the medical school, both educationally and administratively; (2) a close working arrangement with an active extension service, maintained as a part of the educational program of most state universities, provides important support for the medical school in its postgraduate program. By utilizing an existing university organization the medical school is enabled more effectively and more economically to extend its postgraduate training, both extramural and intramural, and its services throughout the state.

THE ADMINISTRATIVE ADVANTAGES

There are advantages from the standpoint of the over-all university administration in having the medical school and hospital on the university campus. The centralization of administration, of accounting, of purchasing and of maintenance and servicing organizations lessens duplication of departments and staff and lowers the cost of servicing, maintenance, and administrative supervision, and promotes economy of operation throughout. In the opinion of Dr. Alan Gregg again, "all administration of the university officers is weakened and retarded by separating the medical faculty from the rest of the university." [8]

University standards are more easily maintained and the medical school enjoys more freedom from 'pressure groups'—medical and other—when it remains physically a part of the parent institution. A prominent medical educator recently stated, "I know of no medical school in a large city which, within my memory, has not had at least one serious quarrel between the uni-

7. Ibid., p. 14.
8. Ibid., p. 25.

versity and the powerful and privileged professional leaders in the city. Unless your university medical leaders are resigned to offering teaching positions in return for support and collaboration of clinicians with few other claims to attention, they may well prepare themselves for a decade of pressures and political maneuvers. Usually if appointments are made *quid pro quo* and at a distance from the university the character of the school depends on forces only slightly under its control." [9]

The location of the medical school on a university campus in a small community demands in large measure a full time faculty, at least in the geographical sense. From the standpoint of developing a sound educational and research program this is advantageous and furthermore, such an arrangement promotes a closely knit organization and an *esprit de corps* perhaps more difficult to achieve under other arrangements.

With emphasis on teaching and research and with an adequate salary scale from the university, supplemented from a limited consulting practice with a definite ceiling on total income, a university environment becomes an added inducement in attracting and holding a competent faculty.

Another asset to the clinical teaching when the medical school is on the campus is the utilization of the student health service of the university. As pointed out by Dr. Lippard, "increasing interest in the prevention of disease and periodic health examinations make auxiliary facilities of this type highly desirable for instruction of medical students who, in the large city hospital, are so overwhelmed with seriously ill patients that they often lose sight of healthy people and the main illnesses which will make up a large proportion of their practices." [10]

The medical school must control an adequate supply of clinical material for a satisfactory educational program both for undergraduates and for graduates. While for the most part it is possible to have such control if the medical school is separated from the university, either in the same large city area or in a different city, nevertheless, all too often the teaching services in

---

9. Ibid., p. 25.
10. Education · for the Health Services in the State of Florida, State Board of Education and State Board of Control, 1949, p. 20.

hospitals under such an arrangement do not have the security or the freedom inherent in a hospital owned by the university and located on its campus.

DISADVANTAGES

While strong educational and administrative arguments can be advanced for the university campus location it should be recognized that when the university is in a small town there are two disadvantages or handicaps, to overcome for which provisions must be made:

1. There is the problem of providing an adequate supply of clinical material with a sufficient variety of disease states to insure a well rounded teaching program. To many doctors and medical educators accustomed to teaching hospitals and clinics in large population centers, it would seem very difficult, if not impossible, to secure abundant clinical material in a small town. Many think in terms of an older concept that the students have to be taken to the patients. Before twentieth century roads and modern transportation facilities were developed this was a more forceful argument than in 1950. Fortunately, most universities in small towns are now located amidst a network of good roads. Nearly everybody today has access to automobile transportation, and presently air transport of patients to and from medical centers will still further simplify and facilitate free and easy mobility of our population. Actually patients from rural areas or towns can now travel thirty to fifty miles to a hospital in a small university town about as easily and as quickly and with less physical and emotional fatigue than they can go from one end of a large metropolitan area to another. From the Florida Survey the following statement is pertinent: "among those not intimately acquainted with medical education, there is a tendency to relate excellence of instruction to the number of patients a student sees or the number of physicians on the faculty rather than how carefully the patients are studied or how much time and interest members of the faculty devote to teaching and research. It is our opinion that a large population and a large number of part time instructors are not essential to the development of a good educational program."

"The experience of medical schools in small communities has not indicated that they are handicapped seriously by lack of patients. If adequate facilities are provided and a superior faculty assembled, people find their way to the medical center in numbers and with a variety of illnesses more than sufficient to supply material for clinical observation." [11] The experiences in this country at the Universities of Iowa, Virginia, Michigan, Wisconsin, Duke and Bowman Gray, and at the Mayo Clinic at Rochester, Minn., have over the years borne out the truth of this statement.

It should be kept in mind also that with the spread of prepaid hospital and medical care insurance all teaching institutions must in the future look for a broadened economic basis from which to draw teaching material if they are to continue even their present sized classes. Experiments are under way in some institutions in using private patients for undergraduate teaching, and indications are that such an arrangement can be successful. This practice will almost certainly become commonplace in the near future as the indigent patient of the medical school days of twenty-five to fifty years ago is replaced by the part-pay or full-pay patient.

The argument has been advanced that the clinical material available for a teaching hospital in a small town is likely to be limited in certain fields, particularly in obstetrics, pediatrics and acute traumatic surgery. In certain locations in the past, in the early days of the operation of the university hospital, this has been true. But this handicap is frequently a blessing in disguise because compensation can be and has been made for any shortage of clinical material through affiliation of the university hospital and medical school with special or general hospitals in neighboring centers of larger population. There are mutual advantages and opportunities in such an arrangement in that hospitals in other areas and competent part time teachers are brought into the university's sphere of influence and additional clinical facilities and material are made available for undergraduate and graduate medical training. The level of medical care in such affiliated institutions is usually elevated to the benefit of the general public, perhaps an even more important consideration than that of furnishing teaching material for the medical students.

2. A second handicap to the location of a medical school in a small center of population is the lack of

11. Ibid., p. 18.

readily available qualified part time clinical teachers in the medical and surgical specialties. We all recognize that this group of teachers are invaluable to medical schools, indeed if it were not for their services perhaps a great many of the schools would be forced to close. We recognize also that this group of able and faithful teachers perhaps never or seldom receive from the medical school the rewards or recognition, academic or financial, that they merit. At the same time it is unfortunately true that some medical schools have been forced to depend too largely on voluntary clinical instructors, over whom by the very nature of the local situation the institution exercises little control.

Few university medical schools located in small towns are not close enough to larger centers of population to avail themselves of the services of qualified part time clinical instructors. In that situation the university can exercise more freedom in its choice of part time staff members and has a larger measure of control over it. Furthermore, these men, within a radius of thirty to fifty miles, are as easily accessible to the university hospital as are some of their professional counterparts in the large metropolitan areas, who may live an equal distance from and travel through more congested traffic to the hospital for their clinic or teaching duties.

THE FACTORS INFLUENCING THE UNIVERSITY OF NORTH CAROLINA DECISION

For many years the University of North Carolina has been confronted with the problem of how and where medical education should be developed. In fact, its Board of Trustees in 1846 first approved the establishment of a department of medicine. Since 1879 the first two years of medicine have been taught on the campus at Chapel Hill.

Beginning in 1944 as a part of a statewide popular movement to improve medical care and hospital facilities within the State, predating the passage of the Federal Hospital Construction Act, the University Trustees again faced the problem of fully developing the medical school, this time as a State University Medical Center in the capacity of the focal point in a program of hospital and medical service expansion. The question of the location of the school was studied and the medical and hospital needs of the entire state surveyed by a commission of fifty prominent citizens. Subsequently a committee headed by Dr. W. T. Sanger, President of the Medical College of Virginia, reviewed the data and the majority recommended that the school be expanded on the University campus in Chapel Hill provided "that the school of medicine and associated services of the medical center—i. e., a school of nursing, a program for training essential personnel in fields ancillary to rendering medical and hospital care, the existing School of Public Health, an active program for graduate and postgraduate education for physicians and allied medical personnel, arrangements to provide hospitals with clinical and laboratory consultations— be integrated effectively and continuously with the hospitals and health centers in the area so far as these volunteer to cooperate, and that full utilization be made of the facilities of the voluntary, non-profit hospitals of the State." [12]

This philosophy of the role of the medical school as the heart of a state university medical center taking the lead with the cooperation of and active participation by the other schools in the state in integrating medical education at all levels with medical and hospital services in those hospitals which wish to become affiliated with the teaching institutions of the area, has guided the thinking and planning of the university in the development of its medical program and that of the state in its hospital building program. With this background and this concept of the function and place of its medical school in relation to the overall medical care and hospital program in North Carolina, the University Administration and Board of Trustees, and the State Legislature without a dissenting vote, accepted the report of the Survey Committee to expand the medical school on the campus of the University at Chapel Hill for the following reasons:

1. Those already enumerated as educational and administrative advantages for such a location.

2. The university already had an investment in a modern medical science building and a 100 bed hospital, both constructed in the preceding seven years, which represented a replacement value of approximately $1,750,000 to $2,000,000.

---

12. Final Report of the National Committee for the Medical Survey, North Carolina Medical Care Commission, 1946, pp. 1-2.

3. There are no large cities in North Carolina and no possible medical school location in the whole state sufficient in size to supply all the clinical material necessary from within its local environs. Furthermore, a university hospital constructed at Chapel Hill would admit patients from all sections of the state on a basis of equality. Such a condition would be much less likely to prevail if the hospital were located in a larger community which might reasonably expect more favorable consideration for its own citizens in return for such contributions as that particular city or county had made to the state.

4. In the larger cities hospital facilities were not available to the university comparable in size or suitability for teaching and research purposes to those which the State Legislature had shown a willingness to provide funds to build on the University campus. Nor could the university secure that control of any hospital in the larger cities which its trustees deemed essential to assure a sound teaching program. Many existing hospitals offered their facilities to the university "as far as practicable," but this did not seem a sufficient guarantee in perpetuity of a workable arrangement.

Probably the most important reasons for the final decision to place the medical center on the university campus lay in (a) the position of the university in the state and (b) the role envisioned for the medical school in the State Medical Care Program.

From its beginning as a provision in the first State Constitution in 1776 the University of North Carolina has been in a real sense an institution of the people of the state, yet withal singularly free from political influences and pressures. I believe it would be fair to say that the university is more than the geographical center to the people of North Carolina.

The trustees felt that the support, both in terms of legislative appropriation and endowment from private sources, would in the long run be greater if the medical school remained in Chapel Hill where traditionally for over one hundred and fifty years public and private support have been given and service and leadership expected and accepted than if it were operated as an isolated unit in a larger city of the state.

THE FACTORS INVOLVED IN SUCH A LOCATION

Construction has begun on a 400 bed hospital and outpatient clinic building, to be followed within the next few months by a 100 bed tuberculosis unit, buildings for nurses and resident staff, and an expansion of the present Medical Science Building. It is anticipated that within a year a 50 to 100 bed psychiatric wing will be added as the teaching and research unit of the state mental hospital program.

·Chapel Hill is a small community of 10,000 permanent residents and the University has a student body of 7,000. It is located in a thickly populated section of North Carolina. Within a radius of fifty miles there are approximately 900,000 people. A network of good roads, bus lines, together with railroad and air transport, provide easy accessibility from all parts of the State and from central Virginia and South Carolina as well.

Negotiations are being completed for affiliations with two general hospitals totalling approximately 800 beds within an hour's drive of the University. These are intended to provide permanent arrangements for undergraduate and graduate training and represent the beginning of a program that looks to wider affiliations for educational and service functions. Within this area also are two mental hospitals with a capacity of 4,000 patients in which the university medical school already has charge of the pathology service and which can be utilized for other teaching activities.

There are available in larger cities—within easy commuting distance—capable men for part time clinical instructors in the University Hospital.

In summary, through such an arrangement as has been outlined we believe it is possible for a medical school as an integral part of a university, even though it is located in a small community, to have all the educational advantages available in such an environment—administrative, scientific, humanistic, and cultural—and at the same time to secure maximal results in its medical training program both in its own hospital and by the utilization of the facilities and the well trained potential teaching talent in other hospitals of the region.

Printed and Published in the United States of America

Historical Table of Organization of the
University of North Carolina at Chapel Hill, 1776–1977

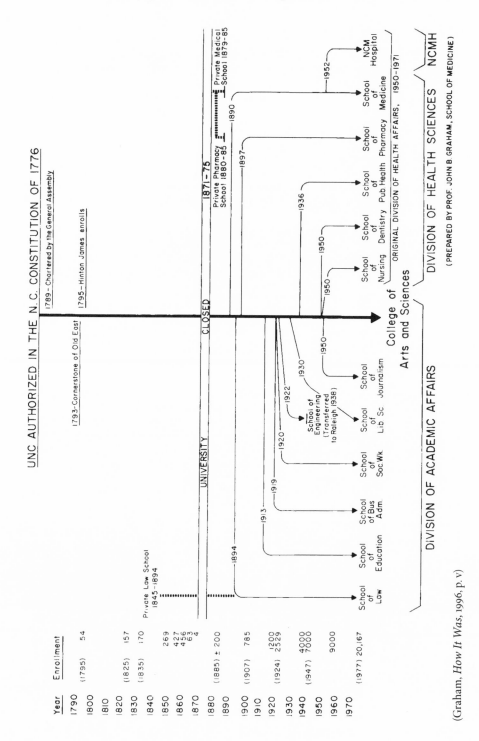

(Graham, *How It Was*, 1996, p. v)

Table of Organization of the UNC Health Care System, 2006

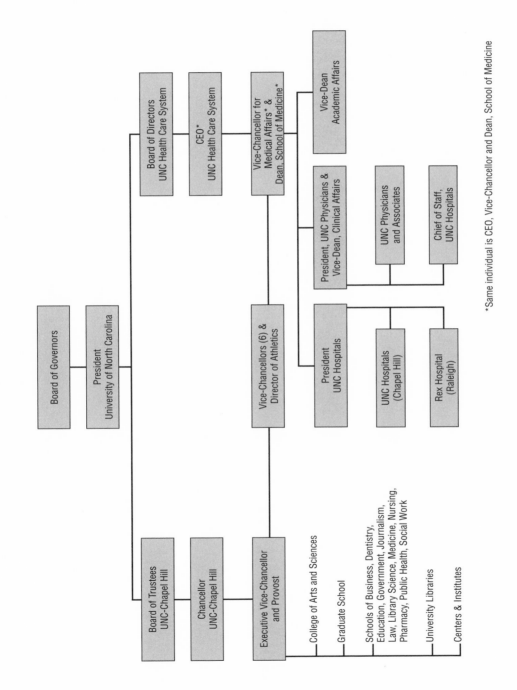

*Same individual is CEO, Vice-Chancellor and Dean, School of Medicine

University of North Carolina Campus, 1940

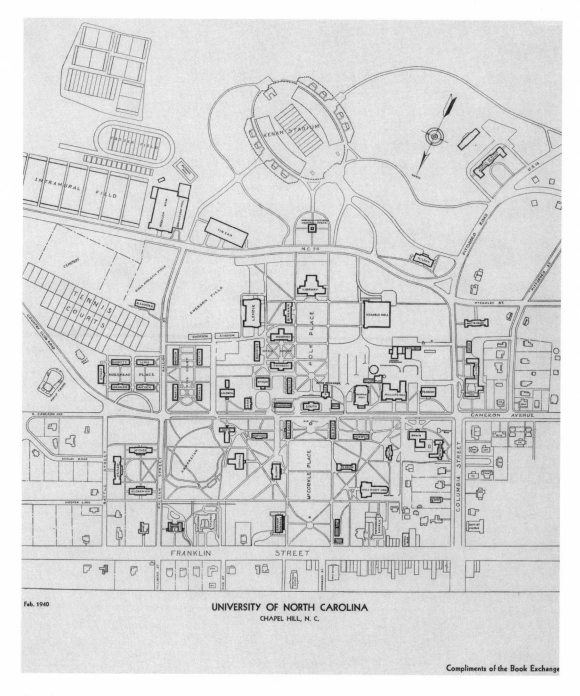

(NCC)

APPENDIX O

University of North Carolina Campus, 1954

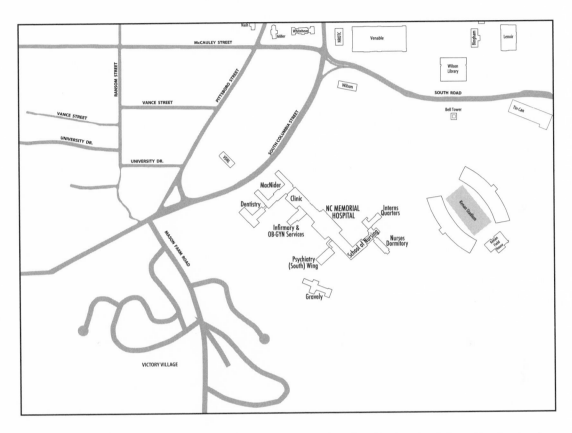

(© 2007 UNC-Chapel Hill Design Services. Based on mapping data from Engineering Information Services.)

University of North Carolina Campus, 2007

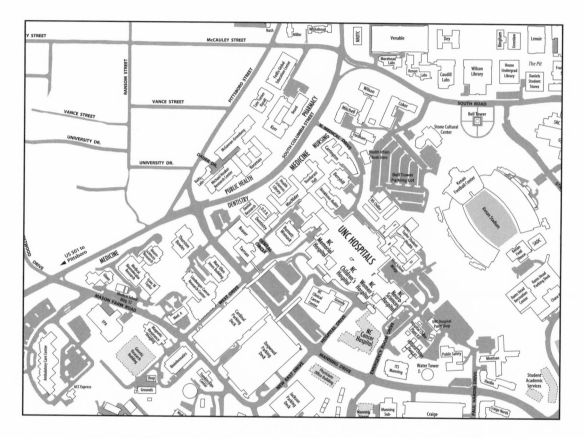

(© 2007 UNC-Chapel Hill Design Services. Based on mapping data from Engineering Information Services.)

Abbreviations

BBM	Berryhill, Blythe, and Manning, *Medical Education at Chapel Hill,* 1979
FPG	Frank Porter Graham
FWD	Floyd W. Denny, Jr.
HSL	Health Sciences Library, UNC–Chapel Hill
JMSS	J. Marion Saunders Scrapbook of Newspaper Clippings, 1944–1946
NCB	Norma Connell Berryhill
NCC	North Carolina Collection, Wilson Library, UNC–Chapel Hill
SHC	Southern Historical Collection, Wilson Library, UNC–Chapel Hill
SMEDAR	School of Medicine Annual Reports, UA, SHC
UA	University Archives, SHC
UNC–CH	University of North Carolina at Chapel Hill
WBB	William B. Blythe
WDM	William de Berniere MacNider
WDMP	William de Berniere MacNider Papers, SHC
WRB	Walter Reece Berryhill
WRBP	Walter Reece Berryhill Papers, SHC
WRBUA	Walter Reece Berryhill personnel file in UA, SHC
WWM	William W. McLendon
YY	*Yackety Yack,* UNC–Chapel Hill Student Annual, NCC

Notes

~~~~~~~

PROLOGUE: The Dean of North Carolina Medicine

1. This chapter is modeled after the first chapter, entitled "The dean of American medicine," in Flexner and Flexner, *William Henry Welch,* 1941.

2. J. Charles Daw, "Medical Sciences Teaching Laboratories, School of Medicine, University of North Carolina at Chapel Hill" (1976, revised 1985 and 1998). Unpublished documents in WRBP.

3. The dedication of Berryhill Hall was on the afternoon of Thursday, March 22, and the full-day continuing medical education program on Friday, March 23, was on the topic "The Permissive Society: Drugs, Sex, VD." See: Program for the Annual Meeting, Medical Alumni Association, UNC School of Medicine, March 22 and 23, 1973. WRBP.

4. "A Certificate in Medicine [CMED] was originally awarded to graduates of the two-year medical course [at UNC at Chapel Hill] between 1941 and 1952. Later retroactive certificates were offered to living alumni who requested them. During the 1970s when General Alumni and Medical Alumni records were being computerized . . . a retroactive certificate was listed for former students, living and dead, who were believed to have completed the one-year or two-year medical course in which they enrolled." See: Mann, ed., *Medical Education at Chapel Hill: Centennial Alumni Directory,* 1979, p. xx.

5. William T. Mallon, Association of American Medical Colleges, to WWM, April 19, 2006.

6. *YY,* 1921. NCC.

7. C. C. Fordham, in McLendon, Blythe, and Denny, *Norma Berryhill Lectures,* 2000, p. 5.

8. Dedication program, Berryhill Hall, March 22, 1973. WRBP.

9. Erle Peacock, True greatness makes others believe in greatness, *Chapel Hill Newspaper,* March 25, 1973. NCC.

10. *YY,* 1921, p. 35. NCC.

11. Henderson, The president, 1915.

12. Wilson, *The University of North Carolina,* 1957, pp. 304 ff.

13. *YY,* 1921, p. 35. NCC.

14. See Appendix B for a chronological listing of former and existing medical schools in North Carolina.

15. Wilson, *The University of North Carolina,* 1957. The best-known graduate of the UNC Medical Department at Raleigh was William de Berniere MacNider, MD, a leading pharmacologist, a widely recognized researcher in renal disease, a pioneering gerontologist, and a UNC faculty member for almost fifty years. MacNider served as dean of the medical school from 1937 to 1940, during which time Berryhill served as assistant dean for student affairs.

16. Correspondence in papers of Francis Preston Venable, 1909–1910. UA, SHC.

17. Flexner, *Medical Education in the United States and Canada,* 1910.

18. Lafferty, *The North Carolina Medical College,* 1946.

19. Long, *Medicine in North Carolina,* vol. 2, pp. 364–372.

20. BBM, pp. 29–34; Gifford, *The Evolution of a Medical Center,* 1972; Davison, *The Duke University Medical Center,* 1966.

21. BBM, pp. 46–40. Carpenter, *The Story of Medicine at Wake Forest University,* 1970, pp. 25–30.

22. BBM, pp. 58–68.

23. North Carolina Hospital and Medical Care Commission and Poe, *Hospital and Medical Care for All Our People,* 1947.

24. North Carolina Medical Care Commission, *Official Report,* 1946.

25. Chapel Hill has competition for medical school (editorial), *Durham Morning Herald,* March 24, 1946. JMSS, SHC.

26. G. M. Cooper to WDM, October 4, 1922. WDMP.

27. Berryhill, The location of a medical school, 1950; Ashby, *Frank Porter Graham,* 1980, pp. 192–206.

28. BBM, pp. 162–167.

29. Jean Swallow, Med school building carries his name: Berryhill—"Simply a great man." *Daily Tar Heel,* March 23, 1973.

CHAPTER 1: A Childhood in the Rural South

1. F. P. Venable, The university and the state: address by President Venable, *Charlotte Daily Observer,* October 14, 1900; 2:9. Venable's address was also reprinted in the *University Record:* Venable, The university and the state, 1900. NCC.

2. John Calvin, *Institutes of the Christian Religion, Book Third,* chapter 7, section 5, 1845.

3. Genealogical information from family papers shared with the authors by Norma and Walter Reece Berryhill's daughters, Jane Berryhill Neblett and Catherine Berryhill Williams.

4. Mecklenburg County came into existence during colonial times when it was separated from Anson County in 1762. The county is located in south central North Carolina along the South Carolina border and was named for the home of Princess Charlotte of Mecklenburg-Strelitz, a region in northeast Germany. She became the wife of King George III of England in 1762. The town of Charlotte was established in 1768 and was named for Queen Charlotte of England; it has been known since as the Queen City.

5. Historical Committee of 1976, *The History of Steele Creek Presbyterian Church,* 1978. See also: Web site for listing of graves in the Steele Creek Presbyterian Church Cemetery. This lists over sixty Berryhills, including a William Berryhill who died on October 28, 1799, "age 60 [and a] Revolutionary War Soldier," http://members.aol.com/wmbigham/bigham/sccem. html

6. Berryhill, Robert Alexander Ross, 1966. Reprinted in: Hendricks, Cefalo, and Easterling, *Obstetrics & Gynecology,* 2000, pp. 221–225.

7. Tar Heel of the Week: Walter Reece Berryhill, *Raleigh News and Observer,* February 24, 1960.

8. Sam Summerlin, Tar Heel of the Week: Walter Reece Berryhill, *Raleigh News and Observer,* February 26, 1950.

9. Historical Committee of 1976, *The History of Steele Creek Presbyterian Church,* 1978.

10. Historical Committee of 1976, *The History of Steele Creek Presbyterian Church,* 1978.

11. Orr, *Charles Brantley Aycock,* 1961.

12. Powell, *North Carolina through Four Centuries,* 1989.

13. Cochran, *Catalogue of Public Schools,* 1907. NCC.

14. Scott's 1810 poem is a fictional account of an epic struggle between two clans in sixteenth-century Scotland, while Jane Porter's historical novel (also published in 1810) concerns the struggles of William Wallace (Braveheart) and Robert the Bruce, King of Scotland, around 1300 to achieve Scottish independence from the English.

15. Program temporarily loaned to the authors by Norma and Reece Berryhill's daughters.

16. Transcript from University of North Carolina, Chapel Hill, for Walter Reece Berryhill, 1917–1921; 1923–1925.

17. NCB to WBB.

18. Wilson, *The University of North Carolina,* 1957, p. 207.

19. The daughters of Norma and Reece Berryhill loaned this essay and the paper that is described in the following paragraphs to the authors.

20. For a discussion of this historical controversy see: Powell, *North Carolina through Four Centuries,* 1989, pp. 176–177.

21. The quotes are from Berryhill's handwritten copy. For a short biographical sketch of Grady and a more complete text of the address see: Grady, The New South, 1907. For the circumstances of the address see: Ayers, *The Promise of the New South,* 1992, p. 21.

22. John B. Graham and George D. Penick to the authors.

23. Catherine Berryhill Williams to WWM, December 11, 2006.

24. Ayers, The first occupation, 2005.

25. Among Northerners who questioned Reconstruction policies was William Henry Welch, MD, a pathologist and bacteriologist who was born in Connecticut and who would become one of America's outstanding medical leaders as the first dean of the Johns Hopkins Medical School. In 1876 at age twenty-six he embarked for Europe on what his biographer called "a voyage of exploration that was in its results perhaps the most important ever taken by an American doctor." In Germany Welch was exposed to the leading medical education and science of his day and brought back these lessons when he designed the Johns Hopkins Medical School, which opened in 1893. He was very impressed with what had happened in Strasbourg, which had been annexed by Germany in 1870 following its victory over France in the Franco-Prussian War. He noted that Germany had sent their most promising young men to the university there so that its medical school in a few years was second only to Berlin's. In a letter from Strasbourg Welch commented to his sister, "One can not help contrasting with our unsatisfactory policy of reconstruction in the South, the strong and skillful manner in which the German empire is transforming a region hostile to them for centuries into a friendly one and so acquiring one of their fairest provinces." Flexner, *William Henry Welch,* 1941, p. 78.

26. Gerald Johnson, quoted in William D. Snider, The burdens of Tar Heel history, *Greensboro News and Record,* August 16, 1981, p. G3.

27. Breeden, Disease as a factor in Southern distinctiveness, 1988.

28. F. D. Roosevelt, http://www.sreb.org/main/Publications/Roosevelt/1938intro.asp (accessed October 15, 2002).

29. See: Henry Louis Mencken, 1880–1956, in Wilson and Ferris, *Encyclopedia of Southern Culture,* 1989.

30. Thomas, "I got these hands dirty saving a life," 1998.

31. H. G. Jones, Foreword, p. xviii, in Covington, *Favored by Fortune,* 2004.

32. Ashby, *Frank Porter Graham,* 1980, p. 9.

33. Pleasants and Burns, *Frank Porter Graham and the 1950 Senate Race,* 1990.

34. *Sketches of Charlotte,* 1902.

CHAPTER 2: Undergraduate, Teacher, and Medical Student

1. The overview of UNC's history is based on Snider, *Light on the Hill*, 1992.

2. See chapter 16, Bonds of mind and spirit, pp. 429 ff., in Woodward, *Origins of the New South*, 1951; and Snider, *Light on the Hill*, 1992, pp. 115 ff.

3. Powell, *North Carolina through Four Centuries*, 1989, pp. 470–471.

4. For Robert B. House's observations on life in Chapel Hill, see: House, *The Light That Shines*, 1964.

5. "WLB" [W. LeGette Blythe], History of the class of 1921, *YY*, 1921, pp. 35–40.

6. Harvard Medical School Application by Walter Reece Berryhill for Admission to the Junior Year, February 9, 1925. WRBP.

7. NCB to WBB.

8. W. LeGette Blythe to WBB.

9. For the story of UNC during World War I, see: Wilson, *The University of North Carolina*, 1957, chapter 21, pp. 260 ff. See also: *YY*, 1919. NCC.

10. *YY*, 1919. NCC.

11. WLB, History of the class of 1921, *YY*, 1921, pp. 35–40.

12. Kolata, *Flu*, 1999. For information on the identification of the 1918 influenza virus see also: Taubenberger, 1918 influenza, 2006.

13. Col. Victor C. Vaughan, MD, quoted in Kolata, *Flu*, 1999, p. 16.

14. Rufus Cole, MD, president of the Rockefeller Institute, quoted in Flexner and Flexner, *William Henry Welch*, 1941, pp. 376–377.

15. Wolfe, *Look Homeward, Angel*, 1929.

16. Editorial, *Journal of the American Medical Association*, 1918.

17. D. Hart, "There had passed a glory from the earth": The Spanish flu of 1918 brought down Chapel Hill leaders, as it exacted a toll on the nation and the world greater than any war. *Chapel Hill News*, November 19, 2003. Wilson, *The University of North Carolina*, 1957, pp. 275 ff.

18. WLB, History of the class of 1921, *YY*, 1921, pp. 35–40.

19. Dr. C. Alphonso Smith, quoted in Snider, *Light on the Hill*, 1992, p. 168.

20. Wilson, *The University of North Carolina*, 1957, p. 290.

21. Edward Kidder Graham, quoted in Archibald Henderson, The president, 1915.

22. Wilson, *The University of North Carolina*, 1957, pp. 295–301.

23. WLB, History of the class of 1921, *YY*, 1921, p. 38.

24. Wilson, *The University of North Carolina*, 1957, p. 305.

25. Sam Summerlin, Tar Heel of the Week: Walter Reece Berryhill, *Raleigh News and Observer*, February 26, 1950.

26. NCB to WBB.

27. *University of North Carolina Catalogue*, 1923–1924, p. 67. NCC.

28. Grant, *Alumni History*, 1924, p. 49.

29. *YY*, 1925. NCC.

30. *University of North Carolina Catalogue*, 1924–1925. NCC.

31. UNC transcript for Walter Reece Berryhill, 1917–1921, 1923–1925. WRBP.

32. *University of North Carolina Catalogue*, 1923–1924, p. 293. NCC.

33. UNC transcript for Walter Reece Berryhill, 1917–1921, 1923–1925. WRBP.

34. Manire, *The First Hundred Years*, 2002.

35. *University of North Carolina Catalogue*, 1923–1924, p. 296. NCC.

36. Manire, *The First Hundred Years*, 2002, pp. 10–11.

37. *University of North Carolina Catalogue*, 1923–1924. NCC.

38. Berryhill, W. Reece Berryhill, 1982, p. 56.

39. *YY,* 1924. NCC.

40. Jack B. Hobson to WWM, 1998.

CHAPTER 3: Harvard, UNC, and Western Reserve

1. Berryhill's UNC transcript shows that a copy was sent "To Harv. Med Sch 1/20/25" and to "Pa. Med Sch 3/13/25."

2. NCB, interviews by FWD, 1998–1999.

3. WRB records from Harvard Medical School, 1925–1929. WRBP.

4. WRB in Finland, *The Harvard Unit at Boston City Hospital,* 1982, vol. 2, part 1, p. 56.

5. NCB, interviews by FWD, 1998–1999.

6. Beecher, *Medicine at Harvard,* 1977, p. 39.

7. Beecher, *Medicine at Harvard,* 1977, p. 87.

8. Ludmerer, *Learning to Heal,* 1996.

9. "To this day, the Harvard Medical School has no hospital—unless one counts the Huntington, a hospital that exists on paper and is encompassed by the Massachusetts General complex." Beecher, *Medicine at Harvard,* 1977, p. 168.

10. Parkins, *The Harvard Medical School,* 1916. The book is now in the HSL at UNC, but is stamped in red with "Zoology" and is inscribed in front in cursive, "University of North Carolina/Dept. Zoology."

11. WRB transcript from Harvard Medical School. WRBP.

12. WRB in Finland, *The Harvard Medical Unit at Boston City Hospital,* 1982, vol. 2, part 1, pp. 55–61.

13. Beecher, *Medicine at Harvard,* 1977, pp. 302 ff., and Finland, *The Harvard Unit at Boston City Hospital,* 1982, vol. 2, part 1, pp. 12 ff.

14. Peabody, The care of the patient, 1927.

15. Peabody, *Doctor and Patient,* 1930.

16. WDM to WRB, January 28, 1931. WRBP. William Osler, MD (later Sir William Osler) (1849–1919) was appointed the first professor of medicine at the new Johns Hopkins School of Medicine in Baltimore in 1888. His book, *The Principles and Practice of Medicine,* was first published in 1892 and in subsequent editions was the leading medical textbook for several decades. After serving sixteen years at Johns Hopkins he became the Regius Professor of Medicine at Oxford University.

17. WRB in Finland, *The Harvard Unit at Boston City Hospital,* vol. 2, part 1, p. 57.

18. Worth Hale to Harry D. Clough, December 1, 1926. WRBP.

19. WRB in Finland, *The Harvard Unit at Boston City Hospital,* 1982, vol. 2, part 1, p. 57.

20. George R. Minot (1885–1950): inquiring physician, 1967.

21. WRB in Finland, *The Harvard Unit at Boston City Hospital,* 1982, vol. 2, part 1, pp. 55–61.

22. WRB in Finland, *The Harvard Unit at Boston City Hospital,* 1982, vol. 2, part 1, p. 59.

23. NCB, interview by George Johnson, MD, 1996. HSL.

24. Charles S. Mangum to Harry Woodburn Chase, August 31, 1929. WRBUA.

25. WBB, Walter Reece Berryhill, 1984. See also: NCB, interview by George Johnson, October 1996. HSL.

26. WRB to WDM, September 10, 1932.

27. Dr. Joseph T. Wearn, 91, dies; former medical school dean. *New York Times,* October 9, 1984. See also: *The Encyclopedia of Cleveland History,* http://ech.cwru.edu/ech-cgi/article.pl?id=WJT (accessed April 10, 2007).

28. NCB, interview by George Johnson, October 1996, part 3, pp. 11–12. HSL.

29. Unless otherwise noted, this section is based on interviews of NCB by George Johnson, October 1996, HSL, and by FWD in 1998–1999.

30. McLendon, Blythe, and Denny, *Norma Berryhill Lectures,* 2000, pp. 3–4.

31. WDM to WRB, September 19, 1930. WRBP.

32. WRB to WDM, September 10, 1932. WRBP.

33. WRB to WDM, March 24, 1933. WRBP.

34. WRB to WDM, August 16, 1933. WRBP. Jane Carroll Berryhill Neblett died at age seventy-two in Charlotte, NC, on March 30, 2005. She had been a teacher in Charlotte and at the Child Development Center at Presbyterian Hospital. She was survived by her mother, Norma Connell Berryhill of Carolina Meadows, Chapel Hill; her sister, Catherine Berryhill Williams of Chapel Hill; a son, John Neblett; and three grandchildren. See: *Chapel Hill News,* April 3, 2005.

35. Berryhill, W. Reece Berryhill, 1982, pp. 58–59.

36. Spies and Berryhill, The calcification of experimental intraabdominal tuberculosis, 1932.

37. WRB to WDM, February 6, 1932. WRBP. NCB, interview by George Johnson, October 1996. HSL.

38. WRB to WDM, July 10, 1932. WRBP.

39. Julian Wood Selig, Jr., MD, to WBB, July 9, 1998. WRBP.

40. WRB to Julian Selig, November 9, 1956. WRBP.

CHAPTER 4: University Physician and Medical School Faculty Member

1. NCB, interview by WWM, March 22, 2001. WRBP.

2. Papers of William de Berniere MacNider, SHC #837, and Papers of Walter Reece Berryhill, SHC #4174.

3. WDM to WRB, November 3, 1932. WRBP.

4. WRB to WDM, October 18, 1932. WRBP.

5. Wilson, *The University of North Carolina,* 1957, and Snider, *Light on the Hill,* 1992.

6. A journalist recently said that Sam Ervin, Jr., a conservative Democrat and then a representative in the state legislature (and later a US senator), "delivered in 1925 one of the more memorable speeches in legislative history. Ervin used both humor and reason to undercut the anti-evolution bill, calling it 'an attempt to limit freedom of speech.' 'I know nothing about evolution,' Ervin said. 'Neither do I care anything about it. To be very frank with you, gentlemen of this House, I don't see but one good feature in this thing, and that is that it will gratify the monkeys to know they are absolved from all responsibility for the conduct of the human race.'" Rob Christensen, N.C. cool to zeal of far right, *Raleigh News and Observer,* March 19, 2006.

7. Snider, *Light on the Hill,* 1992, p. 192.

8. Norman H. Clark, "Prohibition," http://encarta.msn.com.

9. WRB to WDM, December 16, 1931. WDMP.

10. WRB to WDM, July 9, 1932. WDMP. Robert R. Reynolds, D-NC, served in the US Senate from December 1932 until January 1945. See: www.senate.gov.

11. WRB to WDM, August 5, 1933, and August 16, 1933. WDMP.

12. Florence Sabin (1871–1953), in a speech on February 9, 1931. http://education.yahoo.com/reference/quotations/quote/56489 (accessed June 12, 2006).

13. Snider, *Light on the Hill,* 1992.

14. Snider, *Light on the Hill,* 1992, p. 209. For full text of the speech see: UNC–CH Wilson Library, call number FC378/UK3/1931/Graham.

15. William Osler (1849–1919) was the first professor of medicine and William Henry Welch (1850–1934) the first dean at the new Johns Hopkins University School of Medicine, which opened in 1893. Roscoe Pound (1870–1964) was dean of the Harvard Law School from

1916 to 1936 and wrote several important works, including *The Spirit of the Common Law* in 1921.

16. WRB, *The Location of a Medical School,* 1950 (see Appendix K).

17. Ashby, *Frank Porter Graham,* 1980, p. 95.

18. Ashby, *Frank Porter Graham,* 1980, pp. 87–88.

19. Ashby, *Frank Porter Graham,* 1980, p. 91.

20. Ashby, *Frank Porter Graham,* 1980, pp. 129–130.

21. Ashby, *Frank Porter Graham,* 1980, p. 92.

22. WDM to WRB, July 14, 1932. WRBP.

23. Frank Porter Graham, *YY,* 1938. NCC.

24. *YY,* 1932 and 1933. NCC.

25. *YY,* 1931. NCC.

26. WRB to WDM, March 24, 1933. WRBP.

27. WRB to WDM, July 9, 1932. WRBP.

28. *YY,* 1938. NCC. See also: Louis Round Wilson, The University of North Carolina under consolidation, 1931–1963: history and appraisal, unpublished typescript, 1964. NCC.

29. WRB to WDM, January 30, 1932. WRBP.

30. WDM to WRB, February 3, 1932. WRBP.

31. Gifford, *The Evolution of a Medical Center,* 1972.

32. Ashby, *Frank Porter Graham,* 1980, pp. 124 ff.

33. WRB to WDM, September 10, 1932. WRBP.

34. WDM to WRB, September 14, 1932. WRBP.

35. The correspondence between WRB and Reverend W. M. Currie is in a folder of Berryhill's letters and clippings labeled "Presbyterian Church" that was given to the authors by Norma Berryhill. It will be added to the WRB Papers in the SHC after the publication of this biography.

36. WRB to WDM, March 24, 1933. WRBP.

37. Leuchtenburg, *Franklin D. Roosevelt,* 1963, pp. 18, 29.

38. NCB, interview by George Johnson, 1996.

39. NCB, interview by George Johnson, 1996.

40. Undated [probably 1933] handwritten letter from WRB to WDM. WDMP.

41. Undated [probably 1932 or 1933] handwritten letter from WRB to WDM. WDMP.

42. WDM to WRB, January 1933. WRBP.

43. WRB to FPG, May 27, 1933. WRBP.

44. WRB to WDM, December 16, 1931. WRBP.

45. WDM to WRB, January 6, 1932. WRBP.

46. WDM to WRB, February 1, 1933. WRBP. Both Davison and Amoss were considered by President Few for the position of the first dean of the Duke medical school. After Davison was appointed, Amoss was one of his first faculty appointments. Amoss resigned in 1933 following a unanimous request from the other department chairs that he do so. This resulted in much negative state and national publicity for Duke. See: Durden, *The Launching of Duke University,* 1993. See also Campbell, *Foundations for Excellence,* 2006, p. 57.

47. WDM to WRB, May 11, 1932. WRBP.

48. WDM to WRB, January 19, 1933. WRBP.

49. WDM to WRB, February 1, 1933. WRBP.

50. WDM to WRB, May 15, 1933. WRBP.

51. Telegram from WRB to FPG, May 26, 1933, and letter from WRB to FPG, May 27, 1933. WRBUA.

52. WDM to WRB, June 7, 1933. WRBP.

53. FPG to WRB, June 27, 1933. WRBUA.

54. NCB, interview by George Johnson, 1996.

55. NCB, interview by George Johnson, 1992.

56. Catherine Berryhill Williams, interview by WWM, February 14, 2005.

57. Catherine Berryhill Williams, interview by WWM, February 14, 2005.

58. Jane Berryhill Neblett, interview by WWW, June 25, 2000.

59. Sam Summerlin, Tar Heel of the Week: Walter Reece Berryhill, *Raleigh News and Observer,* February 26, 1950.

60. William N. Hubbard, Jr., to FWD, July 9, 1997. WRBP.

61. Sam Summerlin, Tar Heel of the Week: Walter Reece Berryhill, *Raleigh News and Observer,* February 26, 1950.

62. Catherine Berryhill Williams, interview by WWM, February 27, 2001.

63. Catherine Berryhill Williams, interview by WWM, February 14, 2005.

64. Manire, Carolina: A research university, 2000, pp. 40–41.

65. Jane Berryhill Neblett, interview by WBB, June 25, 2000.

66. Handwritten note from NCB to WDM on 246 Glandon Road, Chapel Hill, North Carolina stationery, undated [?1934]. WDMP.

67. NCB to William and Sally MacNider, undated [?1934]. WDMP.

68. Sam Summerlin, Tar Heel of the Week: Walter Reece Berryhill, *Raleigh News and Observer,* February 26, 1950.

69. NCB, interview by George Johnson, 1996.

70. Catherine Berryhill Williams to WWM, December 2006.

71. Rachael E. Long, Building notes: University of North Carolina at Chapel Hill, unpublished manuscript compiled in 1984 and revised in 1993. UNC–CH Library. See also: Henderson, *The Campus of the First State University,* 1949.

72. Henderson, *The Campus of the First State University,* 1949, pp. 177–178.

73. WRB to WDM, August 16, 1933. WRBP.

74. WRB to A. B. Denison, Western Reserve University, September 1931. WRBP.

75. WRB to Dr. P. A. Leddy, New Haven, December 1932. WRBP.

76. WRB to Dean I. H. Manning, UNC, May 27, 1933. WRBP.

77. WDM to WRB, June 7, 1933. WRBP.

78. *University of North Carolina Catalogue,* 1938–1939; *University of North Carolina Catalogue,* 1941–1942, p. 10.

79. WRB to WDM, February 6. 1934. WDMP.

80. Sheldon White, interview by WWM, December 18, 1997.

81. F. A. Blount to WBB, August 13, 1998.

82. John F. Lynch to FWD, 1997.

83. Berryhill, Primary atypical pneumonia, 1943.

84. See: J. A. Ramirez, Atypical pneumonia, *Current Treatment Options in Infections Disease* 2001;(3):173–178, http://www.treatment-options.com/article_frame.cfm?PubID=ID03-2-2-01&Type=Opinion&KeyWords=atypical%20pneumonia&HitNum=4 (accessed February 17, 2005).

85. Berryhill, Spontaneous pneumothorax, 1944.

86. WRB to I. H. Manning, May 27, 1933. WRBP.

87. WRB in Finland, *The Harvard Medical Unit at Boston City Hospital,* 1982, vol. 2, pt. 1, pp. 55–61.

88. BBM, pp. 56–57.

89. *The UNC–CH Record: The General Catalogue,* 1934–1935.

90. WRB to Dr. Tom Jones, Durham, NC, April 1, 1936. WRBP.

91. WRB to Dr. P. P. McCain, May 9, 1935. WRBP.

92. In North Carolina's still segregated society in the 1930s, the white patients in Durham were treated at Watts Hospital, and the black patients were treated at Lincoln Hospital.

93. WRB to R. B. House, June 4, 1935. WRBP.

94. Medical School Advisory Committee, Recommendations for the Clinical Courses, May 4, 1936. WRBP.

95. BBM, p. 57. Watts Hospital, which opened its doors in 1895 for the care of the white citizens of Durham, had been a gift to the community from George Washington Watts. The patient services of Watts and the formerly black Lincoln Hospital were consolidated in 1976 in the new Durham County General Hospital (later Durham Regional Hospital). After renovations, the former Watts Hospital facility opened in September of 1980 as the campus for the North Carolina School of Science and Mathematics, a two-year boarding high school for highly talented students from across the state. See also: Reynolds, *Watts Hospital of Durham,* 1991.

96. BBM, p. 58.

97. WRB to WDM, May 6, 1936. WDMP.

98. WRB to WDM, May 9, 1936. WDMP.

99. WRB to R. B. House, September 30, 1936. WRBP.

100. R. B. House to WRB, December 14, 1936. WRBP.

101. WRB to Dean Mangum, May 28, 1937. WRBP.

102. *YY,* 1938. NCC.

103. *YY,* 1942. NCC.

104. William N. Hubbard, Jr., to FWD, July 9, 1997.

105. F. A. Blount to WBB, August 13, 1998.

106. William N. Hubbard, Jr., to FWD, July 9, 1997.

107. Lewis S. Thorp to WWM, November 2, 1999.

108. James H. Scatliff to WWM, December 2006.

CHAPTER 5: Dean of the Two-Year School of Medicine

1. BBM, pp. 36–37. See also: Halperin, Frank Porter Graham, Isaac Hall Manning, and the Jewish quota at the University of North Carolina Medical School, 1990.

2. BBM, p. 52.

3. WDM to Dr. Duncan R. McEachern, February 22, 1936. WDMP.

4. BBM, pp. 37–38.

5. BBM, p. 105.

6. BBM, pp. 38–39.

7. UNC Record, *The General Catalogue,* 1936–1937, pp. 242–243.

8. UNC Record, *The General Catalogue,* 1940–1941, p. 301.

9. Statement Concerning the Advisory Committee of the Medical School of the University of North Carolina, signed by MacNider and dated "6/xxx/'36." WDMP.

10. R. B. House to C. S. Mangum, W. de B. MacNider, and W. R. Berryhill. WDMP.

11. C. S. Mangum to R. B. House, March 1, 1936. WDMP.

12. Statement Concerning the Advisory Committee of the Medical School of the University of North Carolina, signed by MacNider and dated "6/xxx/'36." WDMP. The statement began, "I think this following statement should be found in my papers which are concerned with the conduct of the Medical School during the past year."

13. Memo to file concerning the negotiations with President Graham concerning the deanship of the School of Medicine, 1937. WDMP.

14. MacNider memo for the file dated May 15, 1937. WDMP.

15. WDM to FPG, May 29, 1937. WDMP.

16. FPG to WDM, May 29, 1937. WDMP.

17. G. L. Donnelly to FPG, May 28, 1937. WDMP.

18. WRB to WDM, June 28, 1937. WDMP.

19. WDM to WRB, July 3, 1937. WDMP.

20. Ehle and Kuralt, *Dr. Frank,* 1993, pp. 53–55.

21. BBM, p. 43.

22. BBM, p. 41.

23. WRB to John Mebane, July 7, 1937. WDMP.

24. Hall, The University of North Carolina, 1940. Hall's allusion to a "mad world" was in reference to the start of World War II in Europe with Hitler's invasion of Poland on September 1, 1939.

25. BBM, p. 50.

26. BBM, p. 52.

27. Mecklenburger named head of UNC medical school: trustees make natural choice, *Charlotte Observer,* September 10, 1941.

28. *YY,* 1952, pp. 188–189. NCC.

29. Minutes of the Administrative Board of the Medical School, December 4, 1941. UA.

30. Ludmerer, *Time to Heal,* 1999, pp. 125 ff.

31. BBM, p. 53.

32. Snider, *Light on the Hill,* 1992.

33. The medical school class photos from 1943 to 1945 show only a few men and one or two women students in civilian clothes, while all of the other men are in military uniform. See: Mann, *Medical Education at Chapel Hill,* 1979.

34. G. Walter Blair, Jr., to FWD, March 4, 1997.

35. Minutes of the Administrative Board of the Medical School, November 29, 1945.

36. WRB, School of Medicine Annual Report for 1945.

37. WRB, School of Medicine Annual Report for Year Ending December 31, 1946.

38. Ludmerer, *Time to Heal,* 1999, p. 131.

39. *Tar Heel Topics,* brochure published by the Admissions Office, UNC–CH, Chapel Hill, NC, Roy Armstrong, Director of Admissions, vol. 19, no. 4 (September 1946).

40. Catherine Berryhill Williams to WWM, December 2006.

41. Arthur Clark to WWM, May 18, 2005.

42. John F. Lynch to FWD, nd (probably 1997).

43. Shahane R. Taylor, Jr., to the authors, 1997.

44. Citron, Dr. Berryhill's third career, 1984.

45. C. Craven, Dean Berryhill visualized topflight medical center, *Raleigh News and Observer,* September 1, 1963.

46. John L. McCain to the authors, June 2, 1997.

47. B. S. Guyton to J. B. Bullit, July 11, 1951, and J. B. Bullit to B. S. Guyton, July 26, 1951. WRBP.

CHAPTER 6: The Poe Commission, the Sanger Report, and the Good Health Movement

1. North Carolina Hospital and Medical Care Commission and Poe, *Hospital and Medical Care for All Our People,* 1947, p. 71.

2. North Carolina Hospital and Medical Care Commission and Poe, *Hospital and Medical Care for All Our People,* 1947.

3. State's financial status reported best in history, *Greensboro Daily News,* July 31, 1946. JMSS. "Skyrocketing returns from all tax sources during the war years—and the first year of peace—have placed the state of North Carolina in the best financial condition in its history.

Governor Cherry reported today that on June 30—end of the 1945–46 fiscal year—the state's general fund had a surplus of $27,438,017 and the highway fund had a surplus of $50,821,491. The general fund surplus does not include a postwar reserve fund which was set aside by the General Assembly of 1943 and which now amounts to $20,537,701."

4. Unless otherwise noted, the material in this section is from Wilson, *The University of North Carolina,* 1957, or from BBM.

5. This study was also supported by the AMA Council on Medical Education, which had been established in 1904 with Arthur D. Bevan, MD, as chairman and N. P. Colwell, MD, as secretary. This joint sponsorship was not publicized at the time because of fears that organized medicine would appear to be trying to decrease competition by closing medical schools. Colwell did accompany Flexner on some of his visits, including those in North Carolina in February 1909. For details see: Ludmerer, *Learning to Heal,* pp. 166 ff., 1985; Flexner, *I Remember,* 1940; Bonner, *Iconoclast,* 2002; Felts, Abraham Flexner and medical education in North Carolina, 1995. In his 1940 autobiography, Abraham Flexner addressed the frequent, and often angry, criticism that he surveyed medical schools but was not a physician. When Henry Pritchett first asked Flexner to do the medical school survey, he thought Pritchett was confusing him with his brother, Simon Flexner, MD, a professor at the Johns Hopkins medical school. Pritchett replied, "I think these professional schools should be studied not from the point of view of the practitioner but from the standpoint of the educator. I know your brother, so that I am not laboring under any confusion. This is a layman's job, not a job for a medical man." Flexner added, "Time and again it has been shown that an unfettered lay mind, if courageous, imaginative, and determined to master relationships, is, in the very nature of things, best suited to undertake a general survey . . . Dr. Pritchett was right: even though I might well have been the wrong choice, the proper person to study medical education was a layman with general educational experience, not a professor in a medical school." He observed that Dr. Colwell's reports for the AMA CME "were creditable and painstaking documents, which, however, as Dr. Pritchett foresaw, had to be extremely diplomatic, because they were prepared by a committee of physicians about medical schools, the faculties of which consisted of their fellow physicians. Dr. Colwell and I made many trips together, but, whereas he was under the necessity of proceeding cautiously and tactfully, I was fortunately in position to tell the truth with utmost frankness." See: Flexner, *I Remember,* 1940.

6. Francis Venable Papers. SHC.

7. Flexner, *Medical Education in the United States and Canada,* 1910. See also: Appendix D.

8. Although the two schools in Raleigh closed fairly quietly, the reaction to the closure of the Charlotte school was "one of resentment and denial," as recently documented by a medical historian. The North Carolina Medical College "had begun in 1886 as a preparatory program for Davidson College students who planned to become physicians," but by the time it moved to Charlotte in 1907 it had become an MD-granting proprietary school: "Such schools were particular targets of the Carnegie study," and "Flexner severely criticized the Charlotte faculty as a private venture, money-making in spirit and object . . . Its teaching chairs were bought and sold by physicians who pocketed most of their students' fees." The resentment toward Flexner was outspoken in editorials in the *Charlotte Medical Journal,* edited by E. C. Register, MD, a professor of the practice of medicine at the Charlotte school. One editorial stated that Flexner's assault on the private schools was "so autocratic . . . unreasonable . . . untrue [that] his assertions would have little influence." Although the Charlotte school did close and merge with the Medical College of Virginia in 1914, the historian noted that three of the graduates and four of the faculty members served as presidents of the North Carolina Medical Society through the years. See: Felts, Abraham Flexner and medical education in North Carolina, 1995. A short history of the school published privately in 1946 by a former faculty

member was similarly critical of the Flexner report and its sponsorship by "the Rockefeller Foundation [*sic*], which had started on a campaign to eliminate all small medical schools." See: Lafferty, *The North Carolina Medical College,* 1946. The author's son, a radiologist in Charlotte, said in a letter written in 1960 to WWM, "I believe that if he were living now, he would not write what he did . . . concerning the Rockefeller Foundation [*sic*] and the Flexner report. Specialists are spreading out through the small towns of North Carolina in spite of the difficulties of four years of college and four years of medical school . . . It is my feeling from what I have heard of the North Carolina Medical College that it was not a proprietary school simply to make money for the founders. I know it did not make any fortune for [my father] or any of the others with whom I have been personally acquainted."

9. Unless otherwise noted, the main source for this section is Wilson, *The University of North Carolina,* 1957.

10. G. M. Cooper to WDM, October 4, 1922. WDMP.

11. See: Wilson, *The University of North Carolina,* 1957, pp. 562 ff. The account in BBM, 1979, differs somewhat with regard to Few's proposal and the timing. See also: Gifford, *The Evolution of a Medical Center,* 1972.

12. *Raleigh News and Observer,* December 21, 1922. Quoted in Wilson, *The University of North Carolina,* 1957, p. 564.

13. *Raleigh News and Observer,* December 22, 1922. Quoted in Wilson, *The University of North Carolina,* 1957, pp. 564–565.

14. BBM, pp. 34, 174–176.

15. Robert H. Woody, Biographical appreciation, in *The Papers and Addresses of William Preston Few, Late President of Duke University,* Duke University Press, 1951.

16. Felts, Abraham Flexner and medical education in North Carolina, 1995.

17. Report by Acting Dean Charles S. Mangum, nd, in file entitled "Administrative Board—Med. School." UA. This was undoubtedly in 1929 because the AAMC annual meeting was held in New York City on Nov. 7–9, 1929, per the AAMC Staff, June 29, 2006, and Mangum served as acting dean in 1929–1930 while Dean Manning recuperated from surgery. A note by MacNider in a folder of documents on the Hoey Commission, 1938–39, lists eight approved two-year schools—Alabama, Dartmouth, Mississippi, Missouri, North Carolina, Wake Forest, West Virginia, and Utah—as well as two unapproved schools, North Dakota and South Dakota. WDMP.

18. Carpenter, *The Story of Medicine at Wake Forest University,* 1970.

19. Ashby, *Frank Porter Graham,* 1980, p. 195.

20. Plowing up doctors, *Raleigh News and Observer,* October 1, 1935, quoted in Carpenter, *The Story of Medicine at Wake Forest University,* 1970.

21. FPG, interview with Ashby, quoted in Ashby, *Frank Porter Graham,* p. 196, 1980.

22. William T. Mallon, AAMC, to WWM, June 27, 2006: "There are no longer any LCME-accredited 2-year medical schools. University of Minnesota–Duluth was the last one, but it stopped being a separately accredited campus a few years ago [and] is now a two-year regional campus of the University of Minnesota main campus." See also: *Directory of American Medical Education,* 2000–2001, Association of Medical Colleges, Washington, DC.

23. See BBM, pp. 46–49, 1979.

24. Carpenter related that they accepted the available funds and proceeded with "faith in God and man and hard work." He did add that after the agreement was completed, "Dr. Kitchin went to New York to solicit additional support from the Rockefeller Foundation. He was thoroughly discouraged by Dr. Alan Gregg, medical director of the foundation, and was advised to use the $600,000 to strengthen the premedical departments at Wake Forest. Of course, Dr. Gregg's advice could not be followed because the Gray gift was for a four-year medical school in Winston-Salem, so Dr. Kitchin returned with no money and many words

of discouragement." See: Carpenter, *The Story of Medicine at Wake Forest University,* pp. 26–30, 1970.

25. WDM to O. M. Mull, November 3, 1938. WDMP.

26. O. M. Mull to WDM, November 4, 1938. WDMP.

27. Dr. Robert A. Lambert, associate director of medical sciences at the Rockefeller Foundation, recorded in his diary for April 29, 1940, a conversation he had had in Chapel Hill with Dean MacNider: "It is definitely settled that if and when the University can add the two clinical years to make a four-year medical school, this will be done at Chapel Hill and not at Greensboro, Charlotte, Raleigh, or any other 'commercial town.' Neither MacNider nor President Graham was ever approached by the trustees of the Bowman Gray Fund. The report, therefore, that the University was offered and refused the Gray money is not true. Had there been such an offer, however, it would have been promptly declined." From: Robert A. Lambert Officer's Diary, April 29, 1940, RG 12.1, Rockefeller Foundation, Rockefeller Archive Center, copy courtesy of Walter E. Campbell.

28. Carpenter, *The Story of Medicine at Wake Forest University,* pp. 22–27, 77, 1970, and *AAMC Directory of American Medical Education,* 2000–2001.

29. BBM, 1979, p. 49.

30. BBM, pp. 50–51.

31. School of Medicine Annual Report, 1939–1940, dated December 13, 1940. UA.

32. BBM, p. 58, and School of Medicine Annual Report, December 17, 1941. UA.

33. BBM, p. 58.

34. BBM, pp. 58 ff., 177 ff.

35. Broughton, *Public Addresses, Letters and Papers of Joseph Melville Broughton,* 1950.

36. North Carolina Hospital and Medical Care Commission and Poe, *Hospital and Medical Care for All Our People,* p. 112, 1947.

37. BBM, pp. 60 ff; Whitaker, The history of the North Carolina Medical Care Commission, 1972; and North Carolina Hospital and Medical Care Commission and Poe, *Hospital and Medical Care for All Our People,* 1947. See also: James Roland Pritchett, North Carolina Medical Care Commission, MA thesis, 1956, Davis Library, UNC–CH.

38. Poe, *My First 80 Years,* 1963.

39. James Roland Pritchett, North Carolina Medical Care Commission, MA thesis, 1956, Davis Library, UNC–CH, p. 33.

40. WRB to WWM, July 11, 1973.

41. L. P. McLendon, Highlights in history, 1944 to 1952, unpublished address at tenth anniversary of expansion of the UNC medical school, March 22, 1963.

42. Whitaker, The history of the North Carolina Medical Care Commission, 1972. In a presentation to a group during a North Carolina Farm and Home Week meeting in August of 1946, Graham reiterated the two main objectives of the six-point "North Carolina Plan" for improving the health of the citizens of the state: "1. To provide more hospitals and rural health centers, and 2. To train in North Carolina more doctors, nurses and medical technicians for those hospitals and centers. On these two pillars the program stands or falls together. The few who would undermine either pillar are striking at the foundations of the total program. Without more hospitals, rural health centers and diagnostic facilities, as far as I am concerned the heart of the program would be left out. This is and has been the position of all the advocates of the program as the record clearly shows." Quoted in an editorial in the *Durham Sun,* August 21, 1946. JMSS.

43. North Carolina Hospital and Medical Care Commission and Poe, *Hospital and Medical Care for All Our People,* 1947.

44. FPG to Louis R. Wilson, December 11, 1961. HSL.

45. Wilkerson, *History of the North Carolina Medical Care Commission,* 1992.

46. Cherry and Corbitt, *Public Addresses and Papers of Robert Gregg Cherry,* 1951.

47. Ashby, *Frank Porter Graham,* p. 202.

48. *Raleigh News and Observer,* August 24, 1946. JMSS.

49. BBM, p. 63.

50. Dr. Robert A. Lambert, associate director of medical sciences at the Rockefeller Foundation, reported during a visit to Duke University in March 1946 that "D. [Dean Davison] says North Carolina needs a thousand more physicians, but he is doubtful if a four-year school at Chapel Hill will contribute materially toward such an increase. Believes a statistical inquiry would show that most of the two-year students at U. of N.C. who go elsewhere to complete the course eventually return to the State." Lambert then notes that Fred Hanes [chair of medicine at Duke] "says that in the minds of the University of N.C. constituency, the question is not that of the need of such a school; it is simply that whatever Duke has, N.C. must have." Lambert added that in his opinion, "The strongest argument for a four-year school, is that anything less is inadequate for the teaching of modern medicine. That is, a medical school should offer the complete course, or nothing. The division between clinical and pre-clinical subjects is artificial and no longer valid." From: Robert A. Lambert Officer's Diary, March 8–10, 1946, RG 12.1, Rockefeller Foundation, Rockefeller Archive Center. Copy courtesy of Walter E. Campbell, October 2005.

51. Whitaker, The history of the North Carolina Medical Care Commission, 1972.

52. BBM, p. 73.

53. Whitaker, The history of the North Carolina Medical Care Commission, 1972.

54. Berryhill later praised James H. Clark, Sr., who died after a long illness in 1969. "A highly respected leader in the General Assembly over a number terms, chairman of the Advisory Budget Commission, university trustee, and the first chairman of the NC Medical Care Commission, Mr. Clark contributed enormously and in a lasting fashion to the development of education and the improvement of medical care in North Carolina. His wise leadership and effective support of the NC Good Health Program . . . were the determining factors in the legislative approval and implementations of these [recommendations]—including the expansion of the university medical school." In recognition of his many contributions to the university and medical school, he received the Distinguished Service Award of the School of Medicine in 1957. BBM, p. 131.

55. Wilkerson, The history of the North Carolina Medical Care Commission, 1972.

56. L. P. McLendon, Highlights in history, 1944 to 1952, unpublished address at tenth anniversary of expansion of the UNC medical school, March 22, 1963.

57. *Durham Morning Herald,* March 21, 1946. JMSS.

58. Greensboro Chamber of Commerce, Greensboro as the site of the Medical School, 1946, NCC.

59. *Durham Morning Herald,* March 24, 1946. JMSS.

60. North Carolina Medical Care Commission, *The Official Report,* 1946.

61. Data from George Sheldon, MD, Norma Berryhill Lecture, 2000.

62. North Carolina Medical Care Commission, *The Official Report,* 1946.

63. Paul F. Whitaker, quoted in North Carolina Medical Care Commission, *The Official Report,* 1946.

64. *Durham Sun,* August 5, 1946. JMSS.

65. Editorial from the *Wilson Times,* reprinted in the *Raleigh News and Observer,* August 3, 1946. JMSS.

66. *Charlotte Observer,* July 20, 1946. JMSS.

67. *Asheville Citizen,* July 23, 1946. JMSS.

68. *Raleigh News and Observer,* August 10, 1946. JMSS.

69. *Raleigh News and Observer* and *Charlotte Observer,* September 5, 1946. JMSS.

70. H. C. Cranford, Good Health promoters use music to enliven campaign, *Raleigh News and Observer,* February 16, 1947. NCC. Wooten and Broom, *Jubilee: A 50-Year Illustrated Retrospective,* 2002.

71. FPG, Address at dedication of the Medical Center, 1954. Graham elaborated later on this Good Health campaign in a 1961 letter to Louis R. Wilson: "I have found in this and other state-wide movements that the more people there were who had a sense of personal and creative part in such a movement, the more creativity and momentum the movement gathered and the more effective were the developments from the very sincerity of their own original devotion." See: FPG to Louis R. Wilson, December 11, 1961. HSL.

72. See Ashby, *Frank Porter Graham,* 1980, p. 202.

73. FPG to Louis R. Wilson, December 11, 1961, p. 21.

74. Cherry, Christmas radio message to the people of North Carolina, December 25, 1946, in Cherry and Corbitt, *Public Addresses and Papers,* 1951.

75. BBM, pp. 72–73. Ashby, *Frank Porter Graham,* 1980, p. 206.

76. L. P. McLendon, Highlights in history, 1944 to 1952, unpublished address at tenth anniversary of expansion of the UNC medical school, March 22, 1963, pp. 8–9.

77. L. P. McLendon, quoted in BBM, 1979, p. 72.

78. BBM, p. 73. According to the *News and Observer,* the Joint Appropriations Committee on March 18, 1947, unanimously approved the "$7,844,800 permanent improvement appropriation for the University, including $3,790,000 for expansion of the two-year Medical School and erection [of] a 400-bed teaching hospital at Chapel Hill." Efforts the next day to delay the medical school and teaching hospital part of the health care bill were overwhelmingly defeated. UNC med school approved, *Raleigh News and Observer,* March 19, 1947, and Medical school wins again, *Raleigh News and Observer,* March 20, 1947. NCC.

79. Annual Report by Dean Reece Berryhill to Chancellor House, for 1949. UA.

80. Dewitt E. Carroll, University rejects Cone Hospital merger: medical school will not come to Greensboro, *Greensboro Record,* December 10, 1947.

81. L. P. McLendon, Highlights in history, 1944 to 1952, unpublished address at tenth anniversary of expansion of the UNC medical school, March 22, 1963, p. 13.

82. BBM, p. 183, appendix I, Excerpts from the *Charlotte Observer* story of December 10, 1947.

83. Berryhill, The location of a medical school, 1950. See Appendix K.

84. Annual report from Dean Berryhill to Chancellor House for year ending December 1947, dated June 22, 1948. UA.

Chapter 7: Building and Recruiting

1. BBM, p. 78.

2. Berryhill later noted that Lennox P. McLendon, Sr., who passed away in 1968, had served on the board of trustees as well as being "the first president of the Medical Foundation from 1948 until his appointment to the Board of Higher Education in 1956 . . . His understanding of the problems as well as the opportunities of the School of Medicine and the other health-related professional schools, his wise guidance, and his support within the university, the Board of Trustees, the General Assembly, and as a highly respected leader in the state were truly invaluable. Often this made the difference between the success or failure of proposals or projects essential to the future of the medical school." In recognition of his services McLendon was awarded an honorary LLD degree by the university and the Faculty-Alumni Distinguished Service Award by the School of Medicine. BBM, pp. 131–132.

3. SMEDAR for 1947, dated June 22, 1948.

4. L. P. McLendon, Highlights in history, 1944 to 1952, unpublished address at tenth anniversary of expansion of the UNC medical school, March 22, 1963. NCC.

5. SMEDAR, 1939–1940, dated December 13, 1940.

6. BBM, p. 97, says this was approved in 1941 by Graham and House, while the SMEDAR for 1942–1943 says that it came into operation in the winter of 1942.

7. SMEDAR for 1942–1943, dated January 9, 1943.

8. Unless otherwise noted, the information in this section is from BBM, pp. 97–100.

9. Graham, Walter Reece Berryhill, 1984.

10. According to Henry Clark, the "main elements of that report, which related to the organization and function of the Division and the duties and responsibilities of the Administrator, later became the introductory paragraphs of the 'Code,' i.e., 'Rules, Regulations and Policies of the Division of Health Affairs.'" Clark, *Oral History,* 1999, pp. 89–90.

11. According to Clark, he agreed to the title of administrator "with some reluctance because I foresaw, as proved correct, that in the future I would frequently be thought of as the head of the hospital only. The term Vice Chancellor would have been more descriptive and would have carried more prestige." Clark, *Oral History,* 1999, p. 93.

12. Clark, *Oral History,* 1999.

13. Clark, *Oral History,* 1999, p. 214.

14. Morris, "Maternal and Child Health," in Denny et al., *From Infancy to Maturity,* 1996, pp. 521–527.

15. Clark, *Oral History,* 1999, pp. 95–96.

16. Clark, *Oral History,* 1999, p. 96.

17. See chapter 9, where Berryhill did address the challenge of the "brave new world of the Sanger Report"—*after* a firm academic and clinical base had been established in Chapel Hill at the medical school and hospital.

18. Clark, *Oral History,* 1999, p. 96.

19. Clark, *Oral History,* 1999, p. 93.

20. BBM, pp. 98–99.

21. Clark, *After 71 Years,* 1950.

22. SMEDAR, 1951, dated June 12, 1951.

23. SMEDAR, 1953–1954, dated May 17, 1954, pp. 29–30.

24. SMEDAR, 1954–1955, dated April 30, 1955, pp. 31–32.

25. Graham, Walter Reece Berryhill, 1984. Henry T. Clark, in his *Oral History,* gave his view of these developments. In 1955 and 1956 "the organizational unrest in the senior ranks in the School of Medicine overflowed and created one of the most turbulent periods in the history of the University at Chapel Hill." He reiterated the complaints of the medical faculty and the opposition of the other health sciences deans to any change. After many months of discussion and contention, the Trustees' Committee on Health Affairs ultimately made the decision in April 1956 based on the recommendations of a committee led by Acting UNC President William Friday. Although Clark opposed the organizational move of the hospital, he was pleased with the adoption of the Health Affairs Code, the addition of three new positions to the administrator's office in health affairs, and the move of the health affairs administrative office from Miller Hall to South Building, the site of the UNC–CH chancellor's offices. Clark summarized that Berryhill "had gotten the Trustees' approval of one of the School of Medicine's requests in the case of the authorized transfer of the Hospital, but he had been soundly defeated in his efforts to abolish the Division Board and to report directly to the Chancellor. Indeed, apart from authorizing the Hospital's transfer, the basic organizational and functioning of the Division of Health Affairs had been reaffirmed and the office

of the Division Administrator had been significantly strengthened, at least on paper, by the Trustees' ruling." See: Clark, *Oral History,* 1999, pp. 141–146.

26. SMEDAR, 1955–1956, dated May 1, 1956, pp. 27–28, #417.

27. Report on the Division of Health Affairs by William B. Aycock, with attached correspondence and minutes, 1956. UA.

28. Aycock's continuing contributions to the Division as chancellor from 1956 to 1964 were documented in a 1964 report by George Watts Hill, chairman of the Trustees' Committee on Health Affairs, to Governor Terry Sanford, chairman of the UNC trustees. Aycock's "grasp of the essential problems and the potentialities of this complex Division with its 1577 full-time students . . . 375 full-time and 160 part-time faculty, 1500 supporting personnel, $19,000,000 annual operating budget covering teaching, research and patient care programs, has been outstanding. His patience has been long-suffering, he has listened and then acted with precision and sound judgments . . . Your Committee believes that the Division of Health Affairs, despite its growing pains, has been developing along sound lines. Many of its programs have achieved national and international recognition. After fourteen years of operation of the enlarged Medical/Health Center, may I on behalf of your Trustees Committee express the hope that we so act that we take full advantage of the team potential of the six elements composing the Center and go forward through education, research and service for the ever increasing Good Health of all the people of North Carolina." George Watts Hill to Governor Terry Sanford, May 25, 1964. Filed with William B. Aycock's 1956 Report. UA.

29. David R. Perry to WWM, January 2, 2004: "The Health Affairs Code has been in force and effect without interruption since the mid-1950s to the present. The document underwent substantive revision in 1978 and 1997, during the chancellorships of Ferebee Taylor and Michael Hooker, to reflect primarily changes in the governance and administration of the faculty practice plans of both the School of Medicine and the School of Dentistry. In later 2003 and early 2004 the School of Medicine undertook a series of major revisions to the portion of the Health Affairs Code outlining the policies and regulations governing its faculty practice plan, the primary impetus for which was the statutory creation of the UNC Health Care System in November 1998. It is expected that the recommendation for the next substantive revision of the Health Affairs Code will be transmitted to Chancellor James Moeser in the first half of 2004."

30. Report of Survey of the University of North Carolina School of Medicine, Chapel Hill, NC, by the LCME of the AMA and the AAMC, January 21–24, 1963. UA.

31. BBM, p. 100.

32. SMEDAR, 1950–1951, dated June 12, 1951, p. 12.

33. Marie Mitchell, School of Medicine Dean's Office, to WWM, April 2007.

34. For further information on the early days of the School of Pharmacy, see: Noble, *The School of Pharmacy,* 1961.

35. School of Pharmacy Web site, http://www.pharmacy.unc.edu/about-us (accessed August 4, 2006); and Office of the Dean of the School of Pharmacy to WWM, December 2006.

36. For more of the early history of the School of Public Health, see: Korstad, *Dreaming of a Time,* 1990.

37. Rachel E. Long, *Building Notes,* University of North Carolina, Chapel Hill, 1993. pp. 478 ff. Unpublished manuscript, UNC-CH Library.

38. Clark, *Oral History,* 1999, p. 72.

39. UNC School of Public Health Web site, http://www.sph.unc.edu/ (accessed August 4, 2006); and Office of the Dean of the School of Public Health to WWM, December 2006.

40. Long, *Building Notes,* 1993.

41. School of Dentistry Web site, http://www.dent.unc.edu/ (accessed August 4, 2006); and Office of the Dean of the School of Dentistry to WWM, 2007.

42. UNC School of Nursing Web site, http://nursing.unc.edu/ (accessed August 4, 2006); and Office of the Dean of the School of Nursing to WWM, December 2006.

43. UNC–CH Department of Allied Health Sciences Web site, http://www.med.unc.edu/ahs/about.htm (accessed August 6, 2006); and Lee K. McLean to WWM, December 2006.

44. SMEDAR, 1950–1951 Annual Report, June 12, 1951, pp. 8–9.

45. BBM, 1979, pp. 34, 56, 84. Long, *Building Notes,* 1993. Diane McKenzie, HSL, to WWM, February 17, 2004.

46. Josephus Daniels, letter to editor dated June 14, 1922, published in the *Raleigh News and Observer,* June 22, 1922, and reprinted in part as BBM, Appendix B, p. 173.

47. Henry Clark later recalled, "The logical name, which carried a hallmark of quality, was The University of North Carolina Hospital, but during the Good Health Movement, which occurred just after the close of World War II, there had developed some sentiment state-wide to establish a major hospital as the capstone of a state-wide hospital system which would be a fitting memorial to all North Carolinians who had died in past wars in the service of their state and county. So 'The North Carolina Memorial Hospital' became the name." Clark, *Oral History,* p. 93, 1999. Several decades later the North Carolina Memorial Hospital and the newer hospitals on the campus were collectively renamed the UNC Hospitals.

48. BBM, 1979, pp. 88–89.

49. Curriculum vitae of Robert Randall Cadmus, MD, 1975.

50. *Raleigh News and Observer,* September 3, 1950, quoted in twenty-second anniversary issue of the *Tar Healer,* 1974.

51. BBM, 1979, p. 124.

52. Long, *Building Notes,* 1993, p. 381.

53. Personal communication, Rachel E. Long to WWM, December 17, 2003.

54. For some years a sign with this inscription stood in front of North Carolina Memorial Hospital, as shown in the photograph on page 69 of Wooten and Broom, *Jubilee,* 2002. This same statement was installed in the new hospital concourse in 2002 as part of the fiftieth-anniversary celebrations.

55. Robert R. Cadmus, Reminiscences of the hospital past, unpublished address on the occasion of the twenty-fifth anniversary of the opening of North Carolina Memorial Hospital, 1977. UA.

56. BBM, p. 99.

57. The organization of the hospital as a division in the medical school reporting to the dean remained in place until 1972. By that time it had become clear that the hospital needed more fiscal and operational flexibility than was provided within the university system if it were to survive and meet the challenges of the rapidly changing health care environment in the nation. The General Assembly made the hospital a separate unit in the University of North Carolina system, with its own board of directors, who were responsible directly to the board of governors through the university president. Nine members of the hospital board were to be appointed by the university, while the medical school dean and the UNC–CH vice chancellors for health sciences and for business and finance were to be ex officio members of the board (BBM, pp. 158–159). In 1989 the General Assembly created a new entity, UNC Hospitals, the operating units of which include the North Carolina Memorial Hospital, an adult acute care unit; the North Carolina Children's Hospital, a unit devoted to the special health care and treatment needs of children; the North Carolina Women's Hospital, a unit providing obstetrical services and the special health care and treatment needs of women; the North Carolina Neurosciences Hospital, an adult and pediatric psychiatric and neurological care and research unit; and the UNC Lineberger Comprehensive Cancer Center, a center that

coordinates the various diagnostic and therapeutic services of UNC Hospitals for patients with cancer. The clinical component of the latter will operate temporarily in the Gravely Building until construction of the North Carolina Cancer Hospital is completed in about 2009. With the further statutory reorganization of the university's medical complex in 1998, UNC Hospitals became part of the UNC Health Care System, with the hospital director becoming the hospital president, who reports through the CEO of the health system (who also serves as the medical school dean and vice chancellor for medical affairs) to the board of directors of the UNC Health Care System. The health system in turn reports through the university president to the board of governors. See: www.med.unc.edu/schoolhistory.htm, updated October 2005 (accessed August 1, 2006). See also Appendix M.

58. Publications on the history of the Auxiliary, 1952–1977, and of the history of the Department of Volunteer Services, 1952–1990, in the possession of WWM. See also: Wooten and Broom, *Jubilee,* 2002.

59. SMEDAR, 1947–1948, dated June 22, 1948.

60. SMEDAR, 1948–1949, dated June 18, 1949.

61. BBM, p. 79.

62. BBM, pp. 78–84.

63. Hendricks, Cefalo, and Easterling, *Obstetrics & Gynecology,* 2000, pp. 20–21, 45–49, 120–122.

64. BBM, p. 84.

65. SMEDAR, 1943–1944, dated January 26, 1944.

66. Jay Jenkins, UNC–CH Division of Health Affairs, *Charlotte Observer,* July 21–26, 1958. Reprinted in *UNC–CH Alumni Review* 1958;66(7):172–176.

67. See "The Full-Time System," pp. 207–213, in Ludmerer, *Learning to Heal,* 1996.

68. Knudtzon and Crandell, *From Quonset Hut to Number One,* p. 371.

69. Clark, *Oral History,* 1999.

70. SMEDAR, 1950–1951, dated June 12, 1951.

71. Jay Jenkins, UNC–CH Division of Health Affairs, *Charlotte Observer,* July 21–26, 1958. Reprinted in *UNC–CH Alumni Review* 1958;66(7):172–176. Since the 1950s the total annual salary compensation for clinical faculty at the UNC (and later the ECU) School of Medicine has been authorized and constrained by salary ceilings set each year by the board of governors of the UNC system. To adapt to the rapidly changing nature of physician compensation in the US health care system, more comprehensive clinical faculty compensation plans were adopted in 1996 and revised in 2001. The plan for UNC now includes an "academic base salary" based on the academic rank, an annually "negotiated" component that goes up or down depending on the faculty member's productivity and the financial condition of his or her appointing department, and an optional "performance bonus" for individual faculty members who demonstrate particularly outstanding performance. Such compensation plans were commonplace in most US medical schools by the early 2000s, and the UNC–CH plan is viewed as a successful adaptation to the turbulent economics of contemporary medical practice in the United States. (David R. Perry, executive associate dean, UNC School of Medicine, to WWM, January 2, 2004.)

72. In 1978 the Private Patient Service (PPS) became the Medical Faculty Practice Plan (MFFP), and then in 1990 it was reorganized to become UNC Physicians and Associates (UNC P&A). UNC P&A was governed by a board composed of clinical chairs and elected faculty representatives and was directed by an administrator with the title of executive director, who reported to the dean. In the reorganization of the medical endeavor in 1998 to form the UNC Health Care System, UNC P&A became a part of the health system, and the director is now the chief operating officer (COO) of UNC P&A and executive vice president of clinical services in the health system, reporting to the dean and CEO of the health system.

Since its origin, the faculty practice plan has had faculty oversight, with an advisory committee composed of clinical chairs and elected medical faculty members. Charles G. Foskey, former executive director of UNC P&A, to WWM, January 5, 2004. See Appendix M.

73. SMEDAR for year ending December 31, 1944, dated March 6, 1945.

74. See: http://www.medicalfoundationofnc.org/whoweare.shtml (accessed August 2, 2006).

75. SMEDAR, 1949–1950, dated May 22, 1950. BBM, pp. 113–116.

76. L. P. McLendon, Highlights in history, 1944 to 1952, unpublished address at tenth anniversary of expansion of the UNC medical school, March 22, 1963. NCC.

77. BBM, p. 114.

78. Jane M. McNeer, Medical Foundation of North Carolina, to WWM, February 23, 2004.

79. As of March 31, 2006, the Medical Foundation of North Carolina, Inc., held $155.6 million in invested accounts, a significant portion of which is endowed funds. More than $24.8 million in private gifts was raised in fiscal year 2006, with an additional $32 million raised in research grants from corporations or foundations. Private gifts from all sources to UNC medicine totaled just over $57 million in FY 2006. Stephanie C. Stadler, Medical Foundation of North Carolina, to WWM, August 4, 2006.

80. Graham, *How It Was*, 1996, p. 34, 47.

81. John Graham asserted that Governor Gregg Cherry held up the money waiting for the time when the state could "get a dollar's worth of building for a dollar," in the mistaken belief that the postwar inflation of building costs would soon be coming down. Graham, *How It Was*, 1996, p. 37.

82. SMEDAR, 1947–1948, dated June 22, 1948 , and BBM, pp. 78 ff.

83. Clark, *Oral History*, 1999, p. 94.

84. *Greensboro Daily News,* October 20, 1949, quoted in *The Tar Healer,* North Carolina Memorial Hospital twenty-second anniversary issue, October 1974.

85. Long, *Building Notes,* 1993.

86. BBM, p. 84.

87. *Greensboro Daily News,* April 19, 1951, quoted in *The Tar Healer,* North Carolina Memorial Hospital twenty-second anniversary issue, October 1974.

88. Roland Giduz, *Durham Morning Herald,* July 15, 1950, quoted in *The Tar Healer,* North Carolina Memorial Hospital twenty-second anniversary issue, October 1974.

89. Giduz, "Who's Gonna Cover 'Em Up?," 1958.

90. *New York Times,* September 17, 1950, quoted in *The Tar Healer,* North Carolina Memorial Hospital twenty-second anniversary issue, October 1974.

91. BBM, p. 121. See also: Denny, *From Infancy to Maturity,* 1996, pp. 482–484.

92. SMEDAR, 1961–1962. UA.

93. Jack Masur, Report of the National Advisory Committee on Long Range Planning of the Division of Health Affairs, University of North Carolina, Chapel Hill, NC, April 1958. Papers of Henry T. Clark, SHC.

94. Arthur N. Tuttle, Development of Medical Center, *North Carolina Architect,* September/October 1969. Copy in Papers of Henry T. Clark, SHC.

95. SMEDAR, 1963–1964, p. 3.

96. Wilson, *Historical Sketches,* 1976, p. 272; BBM, pp. 121 ff.; and Clark, *Oral History,* 1999, pp. 169 ff. In the half century since the hospital opened in 1952, multiple renovations and additions have expanded the hospital complex to four hospitals now known collectively as UNC Hospitals—the renovated and enlarged North Carolina Memorial Hospital for adult patients; the North Carolina Neurosciences Hospital, which opened in 1996; and the North Carolina Children's and North Carolina Women's Hospitals, occupied in 2002. These four hospitals are now joined by a concourse for patients and visitors named for Eric Munson, the dynamic

and visionary hospital president for a quarter of a century during the time of the planning, financing, and construction of the new hospitals. (See: W. W. McLendon, Munson transformed UNC Hospitals, *Chapel Hill News,* February 10, 2004.) The UNC Hospitals in 2003 had a total of 688 licensed and opened beds, with many specialized inpatient and outpatient units. The hospitals in 2003 occupied almost two million square feet of space on the campus and at several off-site locations in the area. In addition, the 130,000-square-foot Ambulatory Care Center (occupied in 1992) on the medical campus is owned by the university, but it is leased by the hospital for outpatient facilities (personal communication, Nancy Parker to WWM, February 4, 2004). During FY 2003, UNC Hospitals had 5,066 full-time-equivalent staff, 983 attending physicians, and 550 house staff members. There were 30,212 discharges (not including newborns), 24,445 surgical cases, 258 transplant cases, and 2,919 births. There were 519,129 ambulatory patient visits, and the emergency department had 41,829 visits. The hospitals' operating budget for fiscal year 2003 was $582 million, which included a state appropriation of $37.8 million for indigent care. UNC Hospitals Financial Statement for June 30, 2003, and UNC Hospitals "Useful Facts" Card for FY 2003.

97. Long, *Building Notes,* 1993.

98. Long, *Building Notes,* 1993.

99. In the early 2000s the MSRB was closed for renovations and additions to convert it to office and classroom use for the eight divisions of the Department of Allied Health Sciences, the dean's office, and the alumni affairs office. It was rededicated in April of 2006 as Bondurant Hall in honor of Stuart Bondurant, MD, dean from 1979 to 1994 and interim dean in 1996–1997.

100. SMEDAR, 1947–1948, dated June 22, 1948.

101. SMEDAR, 1949–1950 Annual Report, dated May 22, 1950.

102. One of the authors (WWM) and his new bride in 1952 rented a one-room efficiency apartment in Victory Village for $15 a month, including free coal for the potbellied stove that provided heat in the winter.

103. Graham, *How It Was,* 1996, pp. 33–34.

104. Frederick A. "Ted" Blount, MD, to WBB, August 13, 1998.

105. Frederick A. "Ted" Blount, MD, to WBB, August 13, 1998.

106. Long, *Building Notes,* 1993.

107. Berryhill, Medical progress at Chapel Hill, 1953, p. 9.

108. Long, *Building Notes,* 1993.

109. Manire, Carolina: a research university, 2000, p. 49.

110. Benji Cauthren, Common good: Highland Woods, *Chapel Hill News,* February 13, 2004.

111. BBM, pp. 85–86.

112. BBM, pp. 85–86.

113. Graham, Walter Reece Berryhill, 1984.

114. Denny, Growth and development of pediatrics, 2000.

115. Manire, Carolina: a research university, 2000.

116. SMEDAR, 1950–1951, p. 11.

117. McDevitt, *History of the Nathan A. Womack Surgical Society,* 1995.

118. Nathan Womack, Annual Report, 1953, quoted in Kagarise, *Legends and Legacies,* 1997, p. 36.

119. Erle E. Peacock, Jr., quoted in Kagarise, *Legends and Legacies,* 1997, p. 36. For original article see: Peacock, Nathan Womack, 1989.

120. Robert Zeppa, quoted in McDevitt, *History of the Nathan A. Womack Surgical Society,* 1995, p. 3.

121. Gottschalk, Carolina's Contributors to Nephrology, 2000.

122. Denny, Growth and development of pediatrics, 2000.

123. William B. Wood to WWM, December 2003.

124. Gottschalk, Carolina's Contributors to Nephrology, 2000.

125. Denny, Growth and development of pediatrics, 2000.

126. Burnett, Department of Medicine Annual Report for 1956–57 with Summary Report for 1951–57, pp. 42–44.

127. BBM, p. 86.

128. SMEDAR, 1952–1953, p. 89 (Psychiatry).

129. Web sites for UNC Department of Psychiatry and the George Ham Society (accessed August 8, 2006): http://www.psychiatry.unc.edu/ and http://www.psychiatry.unc.edu/ devalum/hamsociety.htm. Today the Psychiatry Department, which is housed in the Neurosciences Hospital completed in 1997, has one of the largest graduate education programs in the nation, with some sixty residents and fellows each year. It now receives more than $33 million a year in NIH research funding, ranking it number 4 in the nation among psychiatry departments. *Connections: A Newsletter for UNC Health Care System People* 68 (March 2, 2004).

130. Denny, Growth and development of pediatrics, 2000, p. 70. Mary Fleming Davidson (daughter of William L. Fleming) to WWM, January 23, 2004.

131. SMEDAR, 1952–1953, dated June 6, 1953.

132. SMEDAR, 1952–1953, p. 14.

133. Denny, Growth and development of pediatrics, 2000.

134. BBM, pp. 87, 130.

135. Seaman, *Ernest Harvey Wood,* 1975.

136. Richard Clark, Department of Radiology, to WWM, February 9, 2004.

137. SMEDAR, 1952–1953, p. 68.

138. Judson J. Van Wyk, in Denny, *From Infancy to Maturity,* 1996, pp. 40–41.

139. Per Gifford, *The Evolution of a Medical Center,* 1972, p. 67: "Bayard F. Carter, Professor of Obstetrics and Gynecology at the University of Virginia, agreed to head up that department beginning in 1931. Until his arrival Durham obstetrician Robert A. Ross would serve as acting head" of ob-gyn at Duke Hospital, which opened in July of 1930.

140. Berryhill, Robert Alexander Ross, 1966.

141. Charles Flowers, quoted in Hendricks, *Obstetrics & Gynecology at UNC,* p. 12.

142. Hugh Shingleton, quoted in Hendricks, *Obstetrics & Gynecology at UNC,* pp. 18–19.

143. Denny, Growth and development of pediatrics, 2000.

144. Hendricks, *Obstetrics & Gynecology at UNC,* pp. 3–7.

145. Hendricks, *Obstetrics & Gynecology at UNC,* pp. 22–24.

146. Colin G. Thomas, quoted in Kagarise and Thomas, *Legends and Legacies,* pp. 45–46.

147. David Hawkins to WWM, August 30, 2005.

148. Harrie R. Chamberlin to FWD, March 24, 1997.

149. SMEDAR, 1951–1952, dated April 17, 1952, p. 1.

CHAPTER 8: Dean of the Four-Year School of Medicine

1. L. P. McLendon, Highlights in history, 1944 to 1952, unpublished address at tenth anniversary of expansion of the UNC medical school, March 22, 1963. NCC. See also BBM, pp. 119–120, for tenth-anniversary celebration.

2. Berryhill, Medical progress at Chapel Hill, 1953.

3. To serve the people [editorial], *Bulletin of the School of Medicine,* 1953.

4. BBM, pp. 91–92.

5. Rachel E. Long to WWM, 2001 and December 2003. Lute Barrett and Anne W. McLendon, both early hospital employees, to WWM, 2000.

6. Office of Medical Center Public Affairs, UNC Hospitals: 40 Years of Caring, September 2, 1992.

7. Rachel Long, quoted in Clark, Gray, and Cadmus et al., The complete story, p. 131.

8. Wilson, *The University of North Carolina,* 1957, p. 119.

9. Wallace M. Womble, quoted in Clark, Gray, and Cadmus et al., The complete story, 1953, p. 54.

10. Robert R. Cadmus to R. B. House, August 8, 1952, quoted in Caring—The North Carolina Memorial Hospital: The First 25 Years, 1977. Unpublished brochure.

11. Robert R. Cadmus, quoted in Clark, Gray, and Cadmus et al., The complete story, 1953, p. 35.

12. Office of Medical Center Public Affairs, brochure, "UNC Hospitals: 40 Years of Caring," September 2, 1992.

13. Thomas Hughes to WWM, January 26, 2002; Joni Perry, Director of Medical Information Management, UNC Hospitals, to WWM, 2004 and 2006; UNC Hospital today admits first patient, *Durham Sun,* September 2, 1952.

14. Thomas Barnett to Karen McCall, 2002.

15. Kagarise and Thomas, *Legends and Legacies,* 1997.

16. Berryhill, Medical progress at Chapel Hill, 1953.

17. Berryhill, Medical progress at Chapel Hill, 1953.

18. Clark, Gray, and Cadmus et al., The complete story, 1953.

19. BBM, 1979, pp. 92–94.

20. SMEDAR, 1952–1953, p. 6.

21. Clark, Gray, and Cadmus et al., The complete story, 1953, p. 39.

22. George T. Wolff to WWM, March 25, 1999.

23. Office of Medical Center Public Affairs, brochure, "UNC Hospitals: 40 Years of Caring," September 2, 1992.

24. SMEDAR, 1952–1953, p. 17.

25. BBM, 1979, p. 91.

26. Clark, Gray, and Cadmus et al., The complete story, 1953, p. 39.

27. J. Maryon Saunders, Chapel Hill Letter, 1953, NCC.

28. UNC Medical Center Edition, RNO, April 19, 1953, NCC.

29. Graham, A challenge to the medical schools and the medical profession, 1954.

30. Population data from US Census Bureau 2000 figures, as quoted in www.rtpnet.org/rtp/ (accessed January 3, 2005).

31. The size of the Chapel Hill community in 1952 was also indicated by the hospital's initial four-digit telephone number: 9031.

32. *Chapel Hill Weekly,* August 22, 1952, quoted in Office of Medical Center Public Affairs, 22 years of service, 1974.

33. Joseph P. Greer, quoted in Clark, Gray, and Cadmus et al., The complete story, 1953.

34. North Carolina Memorial Hospital, Information for Physicians, 1953. NCC.

35. Robert R. Cadmus to North Carolina Memorial Hospital Staff, February 18, 1953.

36. Cadmus, quoted in Clark, Gray, and Cadmus et al., The complete story, 1953, p. 37.

37. BBM, pp. 112–113.

38. Gloria Nassif Blythe, first Chief Technologist of the Clinical Chemistry Laboratory, North Carolina Memorial Hospital, to WWM, May 2005.

39. William B. Aycock, interview by WWM, September 3, 1997.

40. Jay Jenkins, UNC Division of Health Affairs, *Charlotte Observer,* July 1958, reprinted in *UNC Alumni Review,* August 1958;46(7):172–176. NCC.

41. BBM, p. 113.

42. Robert R. Cadmus to Henry T. Clark, April 21, 1956. UA.

43. BBM, p. 99.

44. Robert R. Cadmus personnel file, 1960–1961. UA.

45. Robert R. Cadmus and Rachael E. Long, The potential for graduate medical education at the Moses H. Cone Hospital, 1966, unpublished report in Greensboro Historical Medical Library at the Moses H. Cone Memorial Hospital, Greensboro, NC.

46. Robert R. Cadmus to Dean Isaac Taylor, May 30, 1966. Robert R. Cadmus personnel file. UA.

47. W. R. Berryhill to Chancellor W. B. Aycock, February 11, 1962. Robert R. Cadmus personnel file #693. UA.

48. BBM, p. 146.

49. BBM, #7, pp. 148, 158 ff.

50. William W. McLendon, Munson transformed UNC Hospitals, *Chapel Hill News*, February 10, 2004.

51. Berryhill, Medical progress at Chapel Hill, 1953.

52. BBM, pp. 95–96.

53. Malcolm Fleishman to WWM, January 9, 2001.

54. Warren, Some modern health care problems, 1954.

55. SMEDAR, 1954–1955, p. 9.

56. BBM, p. 96.

57. Edward S. Williams, Jr., to WWM, January 8, 2005.

58. Broom, What a milestone, 2004.

59. BBM, pp. 104, 153.

60. BBM, pp. 103–105. See also: SMEDAR, 1963–1964, p. 5.

61. Noel B. McDevitt to FWD, September 2, 1997.

62. John H. Bradley, Jr., to WWM, November 2001.

63. SMEDAR, 1953–1954, pp. 1, 29–30.

64. Graham, Walter Reece Berryhill, 1984.

65. SMEDAR, 1953–1954, p. 9.

66. Dunlap, Dr. Berryhill, 1984.

67. William E. Easterling, Jr., to WWM, November 24, 2004.

68. Graham, Walter Reece Berryhill, 1984.

69. Graham, Walter Reece Berryhill, 1984.

70. Thomas W. Farmer to FWD, 1997.

71. BBM, pp. 105–107.

72. SMEDAR, 1953–1954, p. 10.

73. BBM, pp. 107–110.

74. SMEDAR, 1953–1954, p. 9.

75. BBM, p. 112.

76. The position of joint fiscal officer was created in 2004 as part of the leadership team of the UNC Health Care System. Charles Ayscue to WWM, August 21, 2006.

77. BBM, p. 155, and p. 190.

78. SMEDAR, 1951–1952.

79. SMEDAR, 1963–1964, p. 5.

80. BBM, pp. 101 ff. and 187 ff.

81. Denny, Growth and development of pediatrics, 2000, pp. 63 ff.

82. BBM, pp. 129 ff.

83. SMEDAR, 1954–1955, p. 8.

84. This trend of increasing numbers of graduate students in School of Medicine departments continued, so that in 2005–2006 there were 746 graduate students in eight departments and three curriculums offering master's and/or doctoral degrees. In addition, there

were 384 postdoctoral fellows in research positions in the basic and clinical sciences departments and centers. The latter number does not include clinical fellows. Dede Corvinus, Office of Research, School of Medicine, to WWM, August 21, 2006.

85. Quoted from Vannevar Bush's 1945 Report to the President in Manire, Carolina: A research university, 2000, pp. 44–45. For the original report, see: United States Office of Scientific Research and Development and Bush, *Science, the Endless Frontier*, 1945.

86. Manire, Carolina: A research university, 2000, pp. 45–46.

87. Berryhill, The location of a medical school, 1950.

88. Joe W. Grisham related in his 1998 Norma Berryhill Lecture that Richard H. Whitehead overcame the deficiencies in research support in the School of Medicine at Chapel Hill in the early years by doing research in the summer months at Johns Hopkins from 1891 to 1900 and at Chicago from 1901 to 1905, both in the laboratories of Lewellys Barker, MD (who returned to Johns Hopkins in 1905 to succeed Osler as professor of medicine). "From his summertime research, Whitehead amassed a respectable research bibliography, including a neuroanatomy textbook and several articles published in highly regarded journals . . . Whitehead's performance as teacher-scientist set a high-water mark of excellence for faculty at UNC–CH Medical School that still maintains a century later." See: Grisham, From morbid anatomy to pathogenomics, 2000, p. 286.

89. Manire, Carolina: A research university, 2000, pp. 48–49.

90. Graham, *How It Was*, 1996, pp. 136–137, 216.

91. BBM, photo p. 187.

92. Web sites of the Markle Foundation and the Rockefeller Archive, where the papers of the foundation are now housed: http://www.markle.org/about_markle/foundation_history/index.php and http://archive.rockefeller.edu/collections/nonrockorgs/markle.php (accessed August 21, 2006).

93. See: Gottschalk, Carolina's contributions to nephrology, 2000, pp. 131–147; and Gottschalk, Micropuncture study, 1959 and 1997; the 1997 article is the 1959 paper reprinted as a classic article with a commentary.

94. SMEDAR, 1950–1951.

95. Richard M. Peters to FWD, May 1997.

96. SMEDAR, 1953–1954.

97. Langdell, Effect of antihemophilic factor, 1953.

98. Graham, Canine hemophilia, 1949; Brinkhous, Hemophilia in the female dog, 1950.

99. SMEDAR, 1951–1952.

100. Manire, Carolina: A research university, 2000, p. 51.

101. In contrast to other clinical studies that are epidemiological in nature or that retrospectively or prospectively study natural history and/or treatments in large groups of patients, the clinical research carried out in this unit is "defined as studies where the investigator and the patient are in the 'same room at the same time.'" See: Web site for the UNC General Clinical Research Center, http://gcrc.med.unc.edu/home.html (accessed May 1, 2007).

102. BBM, pp. 118–119. Four decades after its origin, the General Clinical Research Center is still funded by an NIH grant of more than $5 million per year. It is located in recently renovated space on the entire third floor of the bed tower near the center of the medical center. It has ten inpatient beds, outpatient examination rooms, supporting laboratory and computer facilities, and a full staff. Eugene P. Orringer to WWM, November 23, 2004.

103. Berryhill, Medical progress at Chapel Hill, 1953.

104. SMEDAR, 1950–1951.

105. See chart on p. 9 of SMEDAR, 1960–1961.

106. SMEDAR, 1963–1964. In 2005–2006 UNC–CH received $593,390,527 for research, of

which $288,199,704 went to the medical school. For the fiscal year "grants marked a 2.4 percent increase from 2005's $579 million, more that doubling the amount UNC–CH collected as recently as 1997. This record funding also coincides with a cut in appropriations from the National Institutes of Health . . . that has historically accounted for slightly more than half of all research funding at UNC–CH." Stephanie Newton, Research funding sees spike, *Daily Tar Heel,* August 28, 2006.

107. Frank P. Graham, Inaugural Address as President at the University of North Carolina, November 11, 1931. NCC.

108. John B. Graham to WWM, February 12, 1999.

109. Richard M. Peters to FWD, May 1997.

110. Niven, Wesley Critz George, 1998, pp. 39 ff.

111. David Cecelski, Dr. James Slade: People that do right, *Raleigh News and Observer,* February 11, 2001.

112. Reynolds, Professional and hospital discrimination, 2004.

113. Robert R. Cadmus, quoted in Office of Medical Center Public Affairs, brochure, UNC Hospitals: 40 Years of Caring, September 2, 1992, p. 5. NCC.

114. Richard M. Peters to FWD, May 1997.

115. North Carolina Hospital and Medical Care Commission and Poe, *Hospital and Medical Care for All Our People,* 1947, p. 4.

116. Albert Maisel, So you can't get a doctor! *Collier's,* May 14, 1947, quoted in Thomas, I got these hands dirty saving a life, 1998, p. 33.

117. The suit in the 1930s by Thomas R. Hocutt, a graduate of North Carolina Central College, is recounted in Anderson, *Durham County,* 1990, 368–369. Gray, quoted in Thomas, I got these hands dirty saving a life, 1998, pp. 34–35.

118. Brown, A grudging acceptance, 2002.

119. Amy Stephens, Students remember racist past: the two first black students at UNC entered the School of Law in June 1951 and graduated in 1952, *Daily Tar Heel,* February 23, 1999.

120. Thomas, I got these hands dirty saving a life, 1998, pp. 34–45.

121. SMEDAR, 1950–1951.

122. WRB to Chancellor Robert House, December 2, 1953. Quoted in Thomas, I got these hands dirty saving a life, 1998, pp. 34–35.

123. Judson Van Wyk to Edward Curnen, February 5, 1954.

124. Walter Reece Berryhill to William Friday, July 13, 1955. UA. Quoted in Thomas, I got these hands dirty saving a life, 1998, p. 34.

125. Thomas, I got these hands dirty saving a life, 1998, p. 35.

126. David Cecelski, Dr. James Slade: People that do right, *Raleigh News and Observer,* February 11, 2001; Thomas, I got these hands dirty saving a life, 1998.

127. Brown, A grudging acceptance, 2002.

128. Since 1974 the UNC Schools of Medicine and Dentistry have offered an intensive "structured summer curriculum at the level of professional education to increase the ability of advanced pre-professional candidates, especially those who are disadvantaged, to compete successfully for admission to health professional schools." From 1974 to the early 2000s, "88% of the 1,886 students who have attended the MED summer program decided to apply to health profession schools. Ninety percent gained admission, with 80% matriculating into medical or dental school, and the remainder entering other health profession schools." UNC MED Web site, http://www.med.unc.edu/oed/med/ (accessed August 24, 2006). *Medical Alumni Bulletin,* Spring 2002:13.

129. Broom, What a milestone: The class of 1954, 2004.

130. BBM, p. 126.

131. SMEDAR, 1951–1952.

132. BBM, p. 127.

133. Berryhill, Medical progress at Chapel Hill, 1953.

134. *Bulletin of the School of Medicine,* April 1955;2(4):46.

135. BBM, p. 127.

136. Lewis Thorp to WWM, November 2, 1999.

137. BBM, pp. 119–120.

138. SMEDAR, 1951–1952, p. 10.

139. BBM, p. 127.

140. Walter Reece Berryhill, Final Report to the Medical Alumni of the UNC School of Medicine, WRBP., nd (most likely an address at the spring 1964 Medical Alumni Meeting in Chapel Hill).

141. BBM, p. 128.

142. WRB to Chancellor William Aycock, May 15, 1963. Berryhill personnel file. UA.

143. Chancellor William Aycock to WRB, June 21, 1963. Berryhill personnel file. UA.

144. Henry T. Clark to WRB, July 9, 1963. Berryhill personnel file. UA.

145. In 1990 the North Carolina Memorial Hospital and the other subsequent hospitals at the site were collectively designated as UNC Hospitals. In 1998 UNC Hospitals, the School of Medicine, UNC Physicians and Associates, and various affiliated practices and hospitals became the UNC Health Care System. The dean of the School of Medicine now (2006) serves also as CEO of the health system and vice chancellor. See Appendix M.

146. Berryhill, Final Report to the Medical Alumni of the UNC School of Medicine, nd (probably spring 1964), unpublished address. WRBP. See also: expanded version of his remarks in *Bulletin of the School of Medicine,* April 1964;11(4):13 ff.

147. SMEDAR, 1963–1964, pp. 1–3.

148. Charles Craven, Dean Berryhill visualized topflight medical center: Now it's a reality at UNC, *Raleigh News and Observer,* September 1, 1963.

CHAPTER 9: Community Medical Education and the Final Years

1. Strand, Physician assistants, 2002.

2. See the issue of the *North Carolina Medical Journal* devoted to the Office of Rural Health and the work of James D. Bernstein (1942–2005). It quoted Bernstein: "State government could not merely issue edicts or dangle money; it had to engage in meaningful partnerships, be prepared to make long-term investments in communities and nurture the leadership needed to deliver the desired improvements." DeFriese, Contemporary issues in rural healthcare, 2006.

3. Henderson, The President, 1915.

4. BBM, 1979, pp. 107–108. See also W. P. Richardson, A history of medical postgraduate education in North Carolina, in: Medicine in North Carolina, 1972, vol. II, 553–563. Richardson states that "this was the first program of this kind anywhere, and it attracted a great deal of favorable opinion nationally, providing a model by which other states with large numbers of rural and small town physicians set up programs of refresher courses." He credited Dr. W. S. Rankin, the state health officer, for initiating the program, but listed various others who helped made it possible. Rankin, in a presentation to a joint meeting of the state board of health and the state medical society, "pointed out that the amount of postgraduate work done by the average general practitioner was quite negligible, and that the reason was the matter of expense. The income of the general practitioner ranged from $1,000 to 1,800 a year, and a six weeks postgraduate course [usually at a northern medical school or hospital] would cost at least $400. On the other hand, a circuit course could be

sent to six locations for $2,000 which, assuming 60 physicians participated, would come to $33.33 each."

5. Berryhill, A proposed program, 1946.

6. North Carolina Hospital and Medical Care Commission and Poe, *Hospital and Medical Care for All Our People,* 1947, p. 71.

7. National Committee for the Medical School Survey, 1946. SHC.

8. See the Minority Report by Graham L. Davis and Victor Johnson, MD, of the Sanger Commission in the Official Report of the Medical Care Commission on the Expansion of the Medical School of the University of North Carolina, 1946.

9. Report of the Committee on Medical School Expansion, Doctor Whitaker, Chairman, p. 23, in Official Report of the Medical Care Commission on the Expansion of the Medical School of the University of North Carolina, 1946.

10. A. J. Warren, Some modern health care problems, address delivered at the 160th annual commencement at UNC–CH, June 7, 1954. SHC.

11. Berryhill, What about the road ahead?, 1955.

12. Virtually an absurdity, *Charlotte Observer,* July 20, 1946. JMSS in SHC.

13. G. Dixon, A rural doctor protests, *Charlotte Observer,* July 22, 1946. JMSS in SHC.

14. The health program, *Charlotte Observer,* July 23, 1946. JMSS in SHC.

15. C. Glenn Pickard, Jr., to authors, 2002.

16. Madison, Historical and contemporary meanings of "primary care," 2002, observes, "The proportion of American general practitioners [had] declined precipitously (from three quarters of all physicians just before World War II to one third by the mid-1960s)."

17. Kerr L. White recalled in a 1998 interview that in 1953–1954 "the Rockefeller Foundation, represented by John Grant, one of its most creative officers, had offered to put up a building for us [at UNC] and to finance a prepaid faculty group practice to demonstrate its feasibility for providing medical care, conducting research, and educating medical students [in primary care] . . . But this subversive plan was turned down by the medical faculty. It was really off-the-wall in those days." Later in the 1960s White told an Edinburgh physician, who held the first chair of general practice created anywhere, "General and Practice are now two dirty words in [US] academic circles. The medical school faculties don't want anything to do with preparing generalists. Specialization is the cry of the day." Kerr L. White, interview by Edward Berkowitz in Charlottesville, VA, March 12, 1998, http://www.med.virginia.edu/hs-library/historical/kerr-white/biography/kwinterv.html (accessed May 14, 2003).

18. Kerr L. White, interview by Edward Berkowitz in Charlottesville, VA, March 12, 1998, http://www.med.virginia.edu/hs-library/historical/kerr-white/biography/kwinterv.html, accessed May 14, 2003.

19. White, The ecology of medical care, 1961. See also: DeFriese, The visualization of primary care, 2002.

20. T. F. Williams, D. A. Martin, and R. R. Huntley to WRB, May 18, 1963. UA, Dean of School of Medicine files.

21. W. R. Berryhill, Whitehead Lecture, 1964, unpublished manuscript. SHC.

22. Citron, Dr. Berryhill's third career, 1984.

23. BBM, pp. 128–129.

24. WRB to Commonwealth Fund, March 1964. WRBUA.

25. Citron, Dr. Berryhill's third career, 1984.

26. Berryhill, Robert Alexander Ross, 1966.

27. NCB to WWM, April 19, 2002.

28. Dan A. Martin to Dean Isaac M. Taylor, April 21, 1965. UA.

29. A Policy Statement of the Faculty, School of Medicine, UNC–CH, Adopted January 10, 1966. UA.

30. William J. Cromartie to Isaac M. Taylor, Proposal Regarding the Establishment of a Division of Health and Medical Care Research in the School of Medicine of the University of North Carolina, June 22, 1965. UA.

31. W. J. Cromartie to I. M. Taylor, July 9, 1965. UA.

32. T. F. Williams to I. M. Taylor, July 29, 1965. UA.

33. I. M. Taylor to WRB, December 27, 1965. UA.

34. BBM, p. 140.

35. The 1946 Sanger Report recognized the necessity for off-site clinical instruction for the state's proposed four-year medical school: "Strong argument might be made for locating the medical school in a large metropolitan center if one existed in North Carolina . . . Therefore, it is better to take advantage of the University environment . . . In fact there is no possible medical location in the whole State which would not require sending students for short periods to other communities for supplemental instruction in order to secure maximal educational results." Sanger, Bishop, Davis, et al. *National Committee for the Medical School Survey,* 1946, p. 5.

36. C. Glenn Pickard, Jr., to WWM, 2002.

37. Robert R. Huntley to authors, 1997 and 2002.

38. C. Glenn Pickard, Jr., to the authors, 2001–2003.

39. Lawrence M. Cutchin to authors, 2002.

40. R. R. Huntley, interview by WWM and C. Glenn Pickard, Jr., January 31, 2002.

41. WRB to Isaac M. Taylor, March 15, 1966. UA.

42. Teaching Community Medicine in North Carolina: Report of a Conference held March 12, 1966, in the Private Dining Room of North Carolina Memorial Hospital, Chapel Hill, NC. UA.

43. WRB to Members, Advisory Committee, Division of Education and Research in Community Medical Care, May 17, 1966. UA. Minutes of the Advisory Committee to the Division of Education and Research in Community Medicine, June 24, 1966. UA.

44. C. Glenn Pickard, Jr., to authors, January 24, 2002. Community physicians' suggestion to build a community hospital in Chapel Hill had provoked much debate. Allowing practicing physicians to teach and have staff privileges at the North Carolina Memorial Hospital was an effort to head off the community hospital threat.

45. News notes from Duke University Medical Center: Department of Community Health Sciences. *North Carolina Medical Journal,* 1966; 27: 450.

46. WRB to I. M. Taylor, August 11, 1966. UA. It is likely that the date on Berryhill's letter is incorrect, since articles about the UNC program were in the August 11, 1966, issues of the *Durham Morning Herald* and the *Raleigh News and Observer.*

47. *Durham Morning Herald* and *Raleigh News and Observer,* August 11, 1966. NCC.

48. News notes from UNC School of Medicine: A new division of education and research in community medical care has been established. *North Carolina Medical Journal,* 1966; 27: 495–496.

49. Louis G. Welt to WRB, April 10, 1967. UA.

50. WRB to Louis Welt, April 18, 1967. UA.

51. C. Glenn Pickard, Jr., interview by Karen K. Thomas, September 12, 1997.

52. William B. Herring to WWM, 2002.

53. Wilson, The organizational structure, 1971.

54. C. Glenn Pickard, Jr., to WWM, January 24, 2002.

55. White, The ecology of medical care, 1997.

56. Summary of the Activities of the Division of Education and Research in Community Medical Care, December 8, 1970. UA.

57. Wilson, The organizational structure, 1971.

58. http://www.piedmonthealth.org/ (accessed March 21, 2006).

59. C. Glenn Pickard, Jr., to WWM, January 24, 2002.

60. Robert R. Huntley, interview by WWM and C. Glenn Pickard, Jr., January 31, 2002.

61. Louis Welt, quoted by Robert R. Huntley in interview by WWM and C. Glenn Pickard, Jr., January 31, 2002.

62. C. Glenn Pickard to WWM, 2001.

63. BBM, pp. 143–146.

64. Summary of the Activities of the Division of Education and Research in Community Medical Care, December 8, 1970. UA.

65. http://www.med.unc.edu/ahec/medair.htm (accessed March 21, 2006).

66. WRB to I. M. Taylor, October 20, 1966. UA.

67. Summary of the Activities of the Division of Education and Research in Community Medical Care, December 8, 1970. UA.

68. Glenn Wilson, The need for funds in fiscal 1971–72, April 14, 1971. UA.

69. BBM, pp. 153–154.

70. William J. Cromartie, Affiliation of Community Hospitals with the School of Medicine: Goals and Requirements, October 7, 1965. UA.

71. Berryhill, The university and the community, 1975.

72. Berryhill, The university and the community, 1975.

73. BBM, pp. 74–77.

74. WRB, SMEDAR, 1947.

75. William J. Cromartie to WWM, June 2002.

76. Herring, The history of medical education in Greensboro, 1991.

77. Robert R. Cadmus and Rachael E. Long, The potential for graduate medical education at the Moses H. Cone Hospital, 1966, unpublished report in Greensboro Historical Medical Library at the Moses H. Cone Memorial Hospital, Greensboro, NC.

78. Hospital Affiliates with UNC Medical School. *Moses Cone Hospital Review,* vol. 2; 1967:1.

79. Samuel Ravenel, introduction to Martha Sharpless, The history of pediatrics in Greensboro, in R. L. Phillips, ed. *The History of Medicine in Greensboro, North Carolina,* 1991:130–131.

80. William B. Herring to WWM, May 20, 2002, and January 13, 2007.

81. John H. Bradley, Jr., to WWM, November 4, 2001.

82. William B. Herring to WWM, May 20, 2002.

83. Lafferty, *The North Carolina Medical College,* 1946.

84. BBM, p. 33.

85. For a history of Charlotte Memorial Hospital and Carolinas Medical Center, see: Shinn, *A Great, Public Compassion,* 2002.

86. Citron, Dr. Berryhill's third career, 1984.

87. Citron, Dr. Berryhill's third career, 1984.

88. B. Galusha to WWM, personal communication, 2004.

89. B. Galusha to WWM, personal communication, 2004.

90. R. R. Huntley, interview by WWM and C. Glenn Pickard, Jr., January 31, 2002.

91. Report to the Advisory Committee of the Division, December 8, 1970. UA.

92. Glenn Wilson to I. M. Taylor, April 14, 1971. UA.

93. WRB to I. M. Taylor, August 28, 1969. UA.

94. I. M. Taylor to WRB, September 13, 1969. UA.

95. WRB personnel records. UA.

96. BBM, pp. 142–143.

97. Berryhill, The university and the community, 1975.

98. Glenn Wilson, quoted in Citron, Berryhill's third career, 1984.

99. Carnegie Commission on Higher Education. Higher Education and the Nation's Health, 1970. HSL. One physician has called the 1970 Carnegie Report the "second half of the Carnegie Report by Flexner in 1910." Larry Cutchin to WWM, June 6, 2002.

100. BBM, pp. 163–164.

101. BBM, p. 163.

102. B. Galusha to WWM, June 4, 2002.

103. L. M. Cutchin to WWM, June 6, 2002.

104. F. Pickard to WWM, February 11, 2003.

105. BBM, pp. 162, 164.

106. Bennett, *A Statewide Plan*, 1973.

107. AHEC, Berryhill honored by American College of Physicians, *Chapel Hill Newspaper*, February 13, 1977.

108. AHEC, Berryhill honored by American College of Physicians, *Chapel Hill Newspaper*, February 13, 1977.

109. On the occasion of Reece Berryhill's passing [editorial]. *Greensboro Daily News,* January 5, 1979.

110. C. Glenn Pickard, Jr., in an interview by Karen K. Thomas, September 12, 1997, commented on the ECU medical school fight, which he said "was one of the most bitter fights I've ever been in politically. I think it was really what killed Dr. Berryhill; I don't think he ever got over losing the East Carolina struggle . . . Some of the very people who had helped us build the [community medicine and AHEC] program in the east turned and were advocates for the East Carolina med school . . . These were very, very powerful people in positions of authority, and when he learned that they were supporting the East Carolina med school he was absolutely devastated . . . [One problem] was that the aspirations and agenda of the people who created East Carolina University [medical school] were the same as ours." Pickard said, "We didn't deny that eastern North Carolina needed a major regional medical center and that we could not supply that need [but] . . . that was our notion of what the eastern AHEC" should evolve into. He said we felt that "the undergraduate medical school was just going to be a drain on state resources that's not going to accomplish anything." But ECU President Leo Jenkins believed that "the way to build East Carolina University was to get a med school. He could have built the best history department, the best English department . . . [but he would have] never attracted the funding and/or the status that he got by building a med school . . . I don't deny that he understood the problems, and he was sincere in his effort to address them. But he also was an unbridled political opportunist who was extraordinarily skillful. And he just beat us to death" with issues such as the fact that most of the eastern politicians had had at least one relative turned down for admission to UNC–CH and that ECU was going to produce "real doctors," not nurse practitioners, for eastern North Carolina. For another view of the fight for the ECU Medical School, see: Pories, The Brody School of Medicine, 2006. One writer in this overview of the history of the ECU medical school describes the school's establishment as the story of "how a university, practicing physicians, and community leaders across a large, poor, and underserved region realized a vision to 'grow their own' doctors in spite of concerted opposition from an elitist academic establishment and a self-interested profession."

111. Tom Bacon, NC AHEC Program, to WWM, January 2007.

112. James Harper to WWM, April 2007.

113. Finland, *The Harvard Unit at Boston City Hospital,* 1982.

114. Dr. Berryhill dies here at 78, *Chapel Hill News,* January 2, 1979.

115. H. R. Roberts to FWD, July 30 1997.

116. BBM.

117. NCB to WWM, April 19, 2002.

118. Norma Connell Berryhill, "first lady" of UNC School of Medicine, dies at 103, 2005, UNC–CH News Services, July 8, 2005.

119. Bondurant, in McLendon, Blythe, and Denny, *Norma Berryhill Lectures,* 2000, pp. xi–xii.

120. McLendon, Blythe, and Denny, *Norma Berryhill Lectures,* 2000.

Epilogue: W. Reece Berryhill and North Carolina's Good Health Movement

1. Harold R. Roberts to FWD, July 30, 1997.

2. Ross, Walter Reece Berryhill, MD, 1955.

3. Sam Summerlin, Tar Heel of the Week: Walter Reece Berryhill, *Raleigh News and Observer,* February 26, 1950.

4. Noted medical educator dies, *Raleigh News and Observer,* January 2, 1979.

5. BBM, p. 162.

6. Manire, Carolina: A research university, p. 48.

7. See special "UNC Medical Center Edition," *Raleigh News and Observer,* April 19, 1953, p. 5, "Surveys." This quotes a recent US Public Health Service publication showing that North Carolina had added 4,017 hospital beds since the end of World War II, putting it behind only Texas (5,581 beds) and New York (4,551 beds) among the forty-eight states.

8. Quote and data from the UNC Roadmap Web site, www.med.unc.edu/roadmap/about.htm.

9. H. S. Earp III, Director's message, *Cancer Lines,* UNC Lineberger Comprehensive Cancer Center (Spring 2004), p. 1.

10. Henderson, The president, 1915.

11. Sanger, Bishop, Davis, et al., *National Committee,* 1946.

12. Carnegie Commission on Higher Education, *Higher Education and the Nation's Health,* 1970.

13. Osborn, "Bimodal" medical schools, 1996.

14. M. Ehlers, One busy country doctor, *Raleigh News and Observer,* December 11, 2003.

15. See: Francis Collins, *The Language of God,* 2006.

16. Handout for George F. Sheldon, The university, the school of medicine and the department of surgery in the 21st century, Norma Berryhill Lecture, 2000.

17. Research Triangle Park Web site, http://www.rtp.org/ (accessed April 23, 2007).

18. North Carolina Biotechnology Center Web site, http://www.ncbiotech.org/resource_center/accolades/index.html (accessed April 16, 2007).

19. BBM, p. 61.

20. North Carolina Hospital and Medical Care Commission and Poe, *Hospital and Medical Care for All Our People,* 1947.

Bibliography

Anderson JB, Historic Preservation Society of Durham. *Durham County.* Durham, NC: Duke University Press; 1990.

Ashby W. *Frank Porter Graham: A Southern Liberal.* Winston-Salem, NC: John F. Blair; 1980.

Association of American Medical Colleges. *Directory of American Medical Education.* Washington, DC: 2000–2001.

Ayers EL. *The Promise of the New South: Life after Reconstruction.* New York: Oxford University Press; 1992.

Ayers EL. The first occupation: what the Reconstruction period after the Civil War can teach us about Iraq. *New York Times Magazine.* May 29, 2005:20–21.

Beardsley EH. *A History of Neglect: Health Care for Southern Blacks and Mill Workers in the Twentieth-Century South.* Knoxville: University of Tennessee Press; 1987.

Beecher HK, Altschule MD. *Medicine at Harvard: The First Three Hundred Years.* Hanover, NH: University Press of New England; 1977.

Bennett IL. *A Statewide Plan for Medical Education in North Carolina: Report of the Panel of Medical Consultants to the Board of Governors of the University of North Carolina.* Raleigh, NC: Board of Governors of the University of North Carolina; September 1973.

Berryhill WR. Primary atypical pneumonia, etiology unknown. *North Carolina Medical Journal.* 1943;4:421–430.

Berryhill WR. A proposed program for more adequate medical care and hospitalization in North Carolina. *Southern Medical Journal.* 1946;39:421–426.

Berryhill WR. The location of a medical school: consideration in favor of locating a medical school on a university campus. *Proceedings of the Annual Congress on Medical Education and Licensure.* Chicago: Council on Medical Education and Hospitals of the American Medical Association;1950:1–12. See Appendix K.

Berryhill WR. Medical progress at Chapel Hill: A new and yet an old school. *Bulletin of the UNC School of Medicine.* October 1953; 1(1):6–9.

Berryhill WR. What about the road ahead? *Bulletin of the UNC School of Medicine.* April 1955;2:37–40.

Berryhill WR. Robert Alexander Ross. *North Carolina Medical Journal.* November 1966; 27(11):506–509.

Berryhill WR. The university and the community. *North Carolina Medical Journal.* 1975; 36(9):535–539.

Berryhill WR. W. Reece Berryhill: 1927–1929. In: Finland M, ed., *The Harvard Medical Unit at Boston City Hospital.* Vol. 2, Part 1. Boston: Distributed by the University Press of Virginia for the Countway Library of Medicine; 1982:55–61.

Berryhill WR, Blythe WB, Manning IH. *Medical Education at Chapel Hill: The First Hundred Years.* Chapel Hill, NC: Medical Alumni Office, University of North Carolina; 1979.

Blythe WB. Walter Reece Berryhill: physician, medical educator, and innovator. *North Carolina Medical Journal.* 1984;45(10):615–619.

Bonner TN. *Iconoclast: Abraham Flexner and a Life in Learning.* Baltimore: Johns Hopkins University Press; 2002.

Bowles MD, Dawson VP. *With One Voice: The Association of American Medical Colleges, 1876–2002.* Washington, DC: Association of American Medical Colleges; 2003.

Breeden JO. Disease as a factor in Southern distinctiveness. In: Savitt TL, Young JH, eds., *Disease and Distinctiveness in the American South.* Knoxville: University of Tennessee Press; 1988:1–28.

Brinkhous KM, Graham JB. Hemophilia in the female dog. *Science.* 1950;111:723–724.

Broom D. What a milestone: the class of 1954: the first four-year class in the School of Medicine's history gathers 50 years later. *UNC Medical Bulletin;* 2004.

Broughton JM, Corbitt DL. *Public Addresses, Letters and Papers of Joseph Melville Broughton: Governor of North Carolina, 1941–1945.* Raleigh: State of North Carolina Council of State; 1950.

Brown DE. A grudging acceptance. *Carolina Alumni Review.* 2002;91(3):20–29.

Calvin J. *Institutes of the Christian Religion.* Book 3, Section 7: Calvin Translation Society; 1845. Accessed April 24, 2007 at http://www.ccel.org/ccel/calvin/institutes.iv.iii.viii.html.

Campbell WE, High M. *Foundations for Excellence: 75 Years of Duke medicine.* Durham, NC: Duke University Medical Center Library; 2006

Carnegie Commission on Higher Education. *Higher Education and the Nation's Health: Policies for Medical and Dental Education.* New York: McGraw-Hill; 1970.

Carpenter CC. *The Story of Medicine at Wake Forest University.* Chapel Hill: University of North Carolina Press; 1970.

Cherry RG, Corbitt DL. *Public Addresses and Papers of Robert Gregg Cherry, Governor of North Carolina, 1945–1949.* Raleigh: Council of State, State of North Carolina; 1951.

Citron DS. Dr. Berryhill's third career, 1964–1978. *North Carolina Medical Journal.* 1984;45(10):625–628.

Clark HT. *After 71 Years: First Report of the Administrator of the Division of Health Affairs.* Chapel Hill: University of North Carolina; 1950.

Clark HT, Gray G, Cadmus RR, et al. The complete story of every department of the North Carolina Memorial Hospital. *Hospital Management.* 1953;76(4):33–131.

Cochran RJ. *Catalogue of Public Schools in Mecklenburg County, North Carolina, 1901–1907.* Charlotte, NC: Queen City Printing; 1907.

Collins FS. *The Language of God : A Scientist Presents Evidence for Belief.* New York: Free Press; 2006.

Covington HE. *Favored by Fortune: George W. Watts & the Hills of Durham.* Chapel Hill: University of North Carolina at Chapel Hill Library; 2004.

Davison WC. *The Duke University Medical Center: Reminiscences of W. C. Davison, Dean, 1927–1960.* Durham, NC: Duke University Medical Center; 1966.

DeFriese GH. The visualization of primary care: the White-Williams-Greenberg diagram. *North Carolina Medical Journal.* 2002;63(4):186–188.

DeFriese GH, et al. Contemporary issues in rural healthcare in honor of James D. Bernstein (1942–2005). *North Carolina Medical Journal.* 2006;67(1):22–89.

Denny Jr. FW. Growth and development of pediatrics in North Carolina and at the University of North Carolina School of Medicine. In: McLendon WW, Blythe WB, Denny FW, eds., *Norma Berryhill Lectures, 1985–1999, the School of Medicine, the University of North Carolina at Chapel Hill.* Chapel Hill: Medical Foundation of North Carolina; 2000:66–85.

Denny Jr. FW, ed. *From Infancy to Maturity: The History of the Department of Pediatrics, the University of North Carolina at Chapel Hill, 1952–1995*. Chapel Hill: Department of Pediatrics, University of North Carolina; 1996.

Dunlap SV. Dr. Berryhill, my boss: 1942–1964. *North Carolina Medical Journal*. 1984;45(10): 628–629.

Durden RF. *The Launching of Duke University, 1924–1949*. Durham, NC: Duke University Press; 1993.

Edel L. Interview of Leon Edel. In: Plimpton G, ed., *Writers at Work: The* Paris Review *Interviews, Eighth Series*. New York: Viking; 1988.

Editorial. *Journal of the American Medical Association*. December 28, 1918;71(26):2154.

Ehle J, Kuralt C. *Dr. Frank: Life with Frank Porter Graham*. Chapel Hill, NC: Franklin Street Books; 1993.

Felts JH. Abraham Flexner and medical education in North Carolina. *North Carolina Medical Journal*. 1995;56(11):534–540.

Few WP, Woody RH. *The Papers and Addresses of William Preston Few, Late President of Duke University*. Durham, NC: Duke University Press; 1951.

Finland M. *The Harvard Medical Unit at Boston City Hospital*. Vol. 2, Part 1. Boston: Distributed by the University Press of Virginia for Countway Library of Medicine; 1982.

Flexner A. *Medical Education in the United States and Canada: A Report to the Carnegie Foundation for the Advancement of Teaching*. New York: Carnegie Foundation; 1910.

Flexner A. *I Remember: The Autobiography of Abraham Flexner*. New York: Simon and Schuster; 1940.

Flexner S, Flexner JT. *William Henry Welch and the Heroic Age of American Medicine*. New York: Viking Press; 1941.

Garrison DS, Applegate WB. *Wake Forest University: one hundred years of medicine*. Winston-Salem, N.C.: Wake Forest University Health Sciences Press; 2002.

George R. Minot (1885–1950): inquiring physician. *Journal of the American Medical Association*. May 15, 1967;200(7):159–160.

Giduz R. *Who's Gonna Cover 'Em Up?: Chapel Hill Uncovered, 1950–1985*. Chapel Hill, NC: Citizen; 1958.

Gifford JF. *The Evolution of a Medical Center: A History of Medicine at Duke University to 1941*. Durham, NC: Duke University Press; 1972.

Gottschalk CW. Carolina's contributors to nephrology. In: McLendon WW, Blythe WB, Denny FW, eds., *Norma Berryhill Lectures, 1985–1999, the School of Medicine, the University of North Carolina at Chapel Hill*. Chapel Hill: Medical Foundation of North Carolina; 2000:131–147.

Gottschalk CW, Mylle M. Micropuncture study of the mammalian urinary concentrating mechanism: evidence for the countercurrent hypothesis. *American Journal of Physiology*. 1959:927–936.

Gottschalk CW, Mylle M. Micropuncture study of the mammalian urinary concentrating mechanism: evidence for the countercurrent hypothesis. Reprint in: *Journal of the American Society of Nephrology*. 1997;8(1):153–164.

Grady HW. The New South: address delivered at the banquet of the New England Club, New York, December 21, 1886. In: Alderman EA, Harris JC, eds., *Library of Southern Literature*. Vol. V. New Orleans: Martin & Hoyt; 1907:1964–1970.

Graham FP. A challenge to the medical schools and the medical profession [an address at the dedication of the UNC Medical Center, April 1953]. *Pediatrics*. January 1954;13: 92–102.

Graham FP. Inaugural address of President Frank P. Graham at the University of North Carolina, November 11, 1931. In: Ehle J, Kuralt C, eds., *Dr. Frank: Life with Frank Porter Graham*. Chapel Hill, NC: Franklin Street Books; 1995.

Graham JB. Walter Reece Berryhill: dean of medicine, 1941–1964. *North Carolina Medical Journal.* 1984;45(10):619–625.

Graham JB. *How It Was: Pathology at UNC, 1896–1973.* Chapel Hill: University of North Carolina; 1996.

Grant DL. *Alumni History of the University of North Carolina.* 2nd ed. Durham, NC: Christian & King; 1924.

Greensboro Chamber of Commerce. *Greensboro as the Site of the Medical School of the University of North Carolina.* Greensboro, NC; 1946.

Grisham JW. From morbid anatomy to pathogenomics: a century of pathology at UNC. In: McLendon WW, Blythe WB, Denny FW, eds., *The Norma Berryhill Lectures, 1985–1999, the School of Medicine, the University of North Carolina at Chapel Hill.* Chapel Hill: Medical Foundation of North Carolina; 2000:275–301.

Hachiya M, Wells W. *Hiroshima Diary: The Journal Of A Japanese Physician, August 6–September 30, 1945.* Chapel Hill: University of North Carolina Press; 1955.

Hachiya M, Wells W. *Hiroshima Diary: The Journal Of A Japanese Physician, August 6–September 30, 1945: Fifty Years Later.* Chapel Hill: University of North Carolina Press; 1995.

Hall JK. The University of North Carolina, the Old Medical School, Dr. Richard H. Whitehead, Dr. Charles S. Mangum. *North Carolina Medical Journal.* 1940;1(5):3–12.

Halperin EC. Frank Porter Graham, Isaac Hall Manning, and the Jewish quota at the University of North Carolina Medical School. *North Carolina Historical Review.* 1990;67(4):385–410.

Henderson A. The president. *University Magazine.* 1915;45(7):280–286.

Henderson A. *The Campus of the First State University.* Chapel Hill: University of North Carolina Press; 1949.

Hendricks CH, Cefalo RC, Easterling WW. *Obstetrics & Gynecology at the University of North Carolina at Chapel Hill: The First Half Century.* Chapel Hill: Department of Obstetrics and Gynecology, University of North Carolina at Chapel Hill; 2000.

Herring WB. The history of medical education in Greensboro. In: Phillips RL, ed., *The History of Medicine in Greensboro, North Carolina, during the 19th and 20th Centuries: A Series of Essays by Prominent Health Care Providers.* Vol. 1. Greensboro, NC: Printworks; 1991:71–94.

Historical Committee of 1976. *The History of Steele Creek Presbyterian Church, 1745–1978.* 3rd ed. Charlotte, NC: Craftsman; 1978.

House RB. *The Light That Shines: Chapel Hill, 1912–1916.* Chapel Hill: University of North Carolina Press; 1964.

Kagarise MJ, Thomas CGJ. *Legends and Legacies: A Look inside Four Decades of Surgery at the University of North Carolina at Chapel Hill, 1952–1993.* Chapel Hill: Department of Surgery, University of North Carolina at Chapel Hill; 1997.

Knudtzon K, Crandell C. *From Quonset Hut to Number One and Beyond: A History of the UNC School of Dentistry.* Chapel Hill: University of North Carolina Dental Alumni Association; 1982.

Kolata GB. *Flu: The Story of the Great Influenza Pandemic of 1918 and the Search for the Virus That Caused It.* New York: Farrar Straus & Giroux; 1999.

Korstad RR. *Dreaming of a Time: The School of Public Health, the University of North Carolina at Chapel Hill, 1939–1989.* Chapel Hill: School of Public Health, University of North Carolina at Chapel Hill; 1990.

Lafferty RH. *The North Carolina Medical College: Davidson and Charlotte, North Carolina.* Charlotte, NC: Privately published; 1946.

Langdell RD, Wagner RH, Brinkhous KM. Effect of antihemophilic factor on one-stage clotting tests: presumptive test for hemophilia and a simple one-stage antihemophilic assay procedure. *Journal of Laboratory and Clinical Medicine.* 1953;41:637–647.

Leuchtenburg WE. *Franklin D. Roosevelt and the New Deal, 1932–1940.* New York: Harper & Row; 1963.

Long D. *Medicine in North Carolina: Essays in the History of Medical Science and Medical Service, 1524–1960.* Raleigh, NC: North Carolina Medical Society; 1972.

Ludmerer KM. *Learning to Heal: The Development of American Medical Education.* Baltimore: Johns Hopkins University Press; 1996.

Ludmerer KM. *Time to Heal: American Medical Education from the Turn of the Century to the Era of Managed Care.* New York: Oxford University Press; 1999.

MacNider, W de B. *The Good Doctor and Other Selections from the Essays and Addresses of William de Berniere MacNider.* Chapel Hill: University of North Carolina Press; 1953.

Madison DL. Historical and contemporary meanings of "primary care." *North Carolina Medical Journal.* 2002;63(4):197–205.

Manire GP. Tribute to Isaac M. Taylor. *UNC School of Medicine and Medical Alumni Association Bulletin.* 1971;18:4.

Manire GP. Carolina: a research university. In: McLendon WW, Blythe WB, Denny FW, eds., *Norma Berryhill Lectures, 1985–1999, the School of Medicine, the University of North Carolina at Chapel Hill.* Chapel Hill, NC: Medical Foundation of North Carolina; 2000:40–59.

Manire GP. *The First Hundred Years, 1897–1979: History of the Department of Bacteriology and Immunology at Chapel Hill.* Chapel Hill, NC: Department of Microbiology and Immunology; 2002.

Mann R, ed. *Medical Education at Chapel Hill: Centennial Alumni Directory.* Chapel Hill: School of Medicine, University of North Carolina; 1979.

McCain PP, Vernon JW, Haywood HB, et al. To the governor of North Carolina from a committee of the medical profession [letter]; 1944. [See Appendix E.]

McDevitt NB. *A History of the Nathan A. Womack Surgical Society.* Chapel Hill: Nathan A. Womack Surgical Society; 1995.

McLendon WW. Edenborough Medical College: North Carolina's first chartered School of Medicine. *North Carolina Medical Journal.* 1958;19:433. Reprinted in Long, D. Medicine in North Carolina, Vol II. Raleigh, NC: North Carolina Medical Society; 1972: 351–363.

McLendon WW, Blythe WB, Denny FW, eds. *Norma Berryhill Lectures, 1985–1999, the School of Medicine, the University of North Carolina at Chapel Hill.* Chapel Hill: Medical Foundation of North Carolina; 2000.

Morris N, Maternal and child health. In Denny et al., *From Infancy to Maturity: The History of the Department of Pediatrics, the University of North Carolina at Chapel Hill, 1952–1995.* Chapel Hill: Department of Pediatrics, University of North Carolina; 1996. pp. 522–527.

News notes from UNC School of Medicine: a new Division of Education and Research in Community Medical Care has been established. *North Carolina Medical Journal.* 1966;27:495–496.

News notes from Duke University Medical Center: Department of Community Health Sciences. *North Carolina Medical Journal.* 1966;27:450.

Niven S. Wesley Critz George: scientist and segregationist. *North Carolina Literary Review.* 1998;7:39–41.

Noble A. *The School of Pharmacy of the University of North Carolina.* Chapel Hill: University of North Carolina Press; 1961.

North Carolina Hospital and Medical Care Commission, Poe C. *Hospital and Medical Care for All Our People: Reports of Chairman and Sub-Committees of the North Carolina Hospital and Medical Care Commission.* Raleigh, NC: 1947.

North Carolina Medical Care Commission. *The Official Report of the Medical Care Commission on the Expansion of the Medical School of the University of North Carolina to Governor R. Gregg Cherry and the Board of Trustees.* Raleigh, NC: 1946.

Orr OH. *Charles Brantley Aycock.* Chapel Hill: University of North Carolina Press; 1961.

Osborn EHS, O'Neal EH. "Bimodal" medical schools: excelling in research and primary care. *Academic Medicine.* 1996;71(9):941–949.

Osler W. *Aequanimitas: With Other Addresses to Medical Students, Nurses and Practitioners of Medicine.* 3rd ed. Philadelphia: Blakiston; 1932.

Osler W. *Osler's "A Way of Life" and Other Addresses, with Commentary and Annotations.* Ed. Hinohara S, Niki H. Durham: Duke University Press; 2001.

Parkins LE. *The Harvard Medical School and Its Clinical Opportunities.* Boston: Press of R. W. Hadley; 1916.

Peabody FW. The care of the patient. *Journal of the American Medical Association.* 1927;88(12):877–882.

Peabody FW. *Doctor and Patient: Papers on the Relationship of the Physician to Men and Institutions.* New York: Macmillan; 1930.

Peacock EE, Jr. Nathan Womack and the first Department of Surgery at the University of North Carolina. *North Carolina Medical Journal.* 1989;50(1):31–37.

Phillips RL. *The History of Medicine In Greensboro, North Carolina During The 19th And 20th Centuries: A Series Of Essays.* Greensboro, NC: The Printworks, 1991.

Pleasants JM, Burns AM. *Frank Porter Graham and the 1950 Senate Race in North Carolina.* Chapel Hill: University of North Carolina Press; 1990.

Poe C. *My First 80 Years.* Chapel Hill: University of North Carolina Press; 1963.

Pories WJ. The Brody School of Medicine. In: Ferrell J, Henry C, eds., *Promises Kept: East Carolina University, 1980–2007.* Greenville, NC: East Carolina University; 2006:246–298.

Powell WS. *Higher Education in North Carolina.* Raleigh, NC: State Department of Archives and History; 1964.

Powell WS. *North Carolina through Four Centuries.* Chapel Hill: University of North Carolina Press; 1989.

Powell WS. *The First State University: A Pictorial History of the University of North Carolina.* 3rd ed. Chapel Hill: University of North Carolina Press; 1992.

Ravenel S. Introduction of Martha K. Sharpless, MD. In: Phillips RL, ed., *The History of Medicine in Greensboro, North Carolina, during the 19th and 20th Centuries: A Series of Essays by Prominent Health Care Providers.* Vol. 1. Greensboro, NC: Printworks; 1991:130–131.

Reynolds PP. Professional and hospital discrimination and the U.S. Court of Appeals, Fourth Circuit, 1956–1967. *American Journal of Public Health.* 2004;94(5):710–720.

Reynolds PP, Liles J. *Watts Hospital of Durham, North Carolina, 1895–1976: Keeping the Doors Open.* Durham, NC: North Carolina School of Science and Mathematics; 1991.

Richardson WP. A history of medical postgraduate education in North Carolina. In: Long, D, ed. *Medicine in North Carolina: Essays in the History of Medical Science and Medical Service, 1524–1960.* Vol II. Raleigh: The North Carolina Medical Society; 1972:553–563.

Ross RA. Walter Reece Berryhill MD. *Bulletin of the UNC School of Medicine.* 1955;2(4): 25–26.

Royster HA and University of North Carolina Medical Department at Raleigh Alumni Association. *Historical Sketch of the University of North Carolina Medical Department at Raleigh with Biographical Notes of its Graduates.* Chapel Hill NC, The Alumni Association, 1941.

Sanger WT, Bishop EL, Davis GL, et al. *National Committee for the Medical School Survey.* Raleigh, NC: North Carolina Medical Care Commission; 1946. See Appendix I.

Saunders JM. Chapel Hill letter: hospital and health affairs "hill" dedicated. *UNC Alumni Review.* April 1953:170–172.

Saunders JM. New medical-public health building is opened. *UNC Alumni Review.* December, 1939.

Seaman WB. Ernest Harvey Wood, MD, 1914–1975. *Radiology.* 1975;116:494.

Shinn J. *A Great, Public Compassion: The Story of Charlotte Memorial Hospital and Carolinas Medical Center.* Charlotte, NC: University of North Carolina–Charlotte; 2002.

Sketches of Charlotte: North Carolina's Finest City. Promotional brochure. No. 4. Charlotte, NC: Wade H. Harris; 1902.

Snider WD. *Light on the Hill: A History of the University of North Carolina at Chapel Hill.* Chapel Hill: University of North Carolina Press; 1992.

Spies T, Berryhill WR. The calcification of experimental intraabdominal tuberculosis. *American Review of Tuberculosis.* 1932;26(3):275–281.

Strand J. Physician assistants. *North Carolina Medical Journal.* 2002;63(4):225–227.

Taubenberger JK, Morens DM. 1918 influenza: the mother of all pandemics. *Emerging Infectious Diseases.* 2006;12(1):15–22. http://www.ncbi.nlm.nih.gov/entrez/query.fcgi?cmd= Retrieve&db=PubMed&dopt=Citation&list_uids=16494711. 2006;12(1):15–22.

Thomas KK. "I got these hands dirty saving a life": oral histories of three African-American North Carolina physicians. *North Carolina Literary Review.* 1998;7:28–50.

Tuchman BW. Biography as a prism of history. In: Pachter M, ed., *Telling Lives: The Biographer's Art.* Washington: New Republic Books/National Portrait Gallery; 1979:133–147.

United States Office of Scientific Research and Development, Bush V. *Science, the Endless Frontier: A Report to the President.* Washington, DC: US Government Printing Office; 1945.

University of North Carolina Catalogue. Chapel Hill: University of North Carolina; 1923–1924; 1924–1925; 1938–1939; 1941–1942.

Venable FP. The university and the state: an address delivered by President Venable on University Day. *University Record.* 1900;6(11):9–15.

Whitaker PF, Hubbard FC. The history of the North Carolina Medical Care Commission. In: Long D, ed., *Medicine in North Carolina: Essays in the History of Medical Science and Medical Service, 1524–1960.* Vol. 1. Raleigh, NC: North Carolina Medical Society; 1972:330–349.

White KL. The ecology of medical care: origins and implications for population-based healthcare research. *HSR: Health Services Research.* 1997;32(1):11–21.

White KL, Williams TF, Greenberg B. The ecology of medical care. *New England Journal of Medicine.* 1961;265(18):885–892.

Wilkerson Jr. IO. History of the North Carolina Medical Care Commission. *North Carolina Medical Journal.* 1992;53(1):42–48.

Williams WC. *Beginning of the School of Medicine at East Carolina University, 1964–1977.* Greenville, NC: Brookcliff; 1998.

Wilson CR, Ferris WR. *Encyclopedia of Southern Culture.* Chapel Hill: University of North Carolina Press; 1989.

Wilson G. The organizational structure of a comprehensive medical care program in a university medical center. *UNC School of Medicine and Medical Alumni Association Bulletin.* 1971;18:6–8, 59.

Wilson LR. *The University of North Carolina, 1900–1930: The Making of a Modern University.* Chapel Hill: University of North Carolina Press; 1957.

Wilson LR. *Historical Sketches.* Durham, NC: Moore; 1976.

Wolfe T. *Look Homeward, Angel: A Story of the Buried Life.* New York: Charles Scribner's Sons; 1929.

Woodward CV. *Origins of the New South, 1877–1913.* Baton Rouge: Louisiana State University Press; 1951.

Wooten L, Broom D. *Jubilee: A 50-Year Illustrated Retrospective of the North Carolina Memorial Hospital and UNC School of Medicine.* Chapel Hill: Medical Foundation of North Carolina; 2002.

Yackety Yack. Chapel Hill: University of North Carolina; 1919–1942.

Index

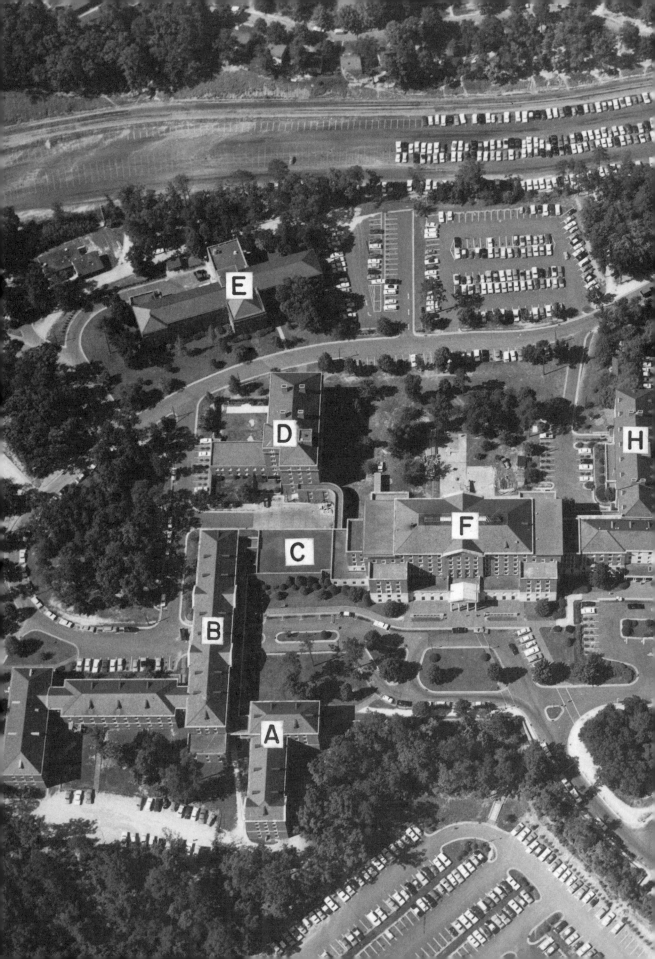